Manual of Neurologic Therapeutics:
With Essentials of Diagnosis

DR. B. A. SPILKER

MANUAL OF
NEUROLOGIC
THERAPEUTICS
WITH ESSENTIALS OF DIAGNOSIS

EDITED BY MARTIN A. SAMUELS, M.D.

Instructor in Neurology, Peter Bent Brigham Hospital, Harvard Medical School;
Junior Associate in Medicine (Neurology), Peter Bent Brigham Hospital, Boston;
and Chief, Neurology Section, Veterans Administration Hospital, West Roxbury,
Massachusetts

Little, Brown and Company   Boston

Cover: Untreated (left) and treated (right) communicating hydrocephalus originally described by R. D. Adams, C. M. Fisher, S. Hakim, et al. Symptomatic occult hydrocephalus with "normal" cerebrospinal-fluid pressure: A treatable syndrome. *N. Engl. J. Med.* 273:117, 1965.

This manual is dedicated to Raymond D. Adams, M.D., on the occasion of his retirement from the Bullard Professorship of Neuropathology, Harvard Medical School, and as Chief of the Neurology Service, Massachusetts General Hospital.

The contributing authors are among the last group of neurology residents fully trained by Dr. Adams. Throughout his 25-year tenure, Dr. Adams's extraordinary talents as a neuroscientist—and particularly as a neuropathologist—have been well known, placing him in the vanguard of the profession.

Those of us who have had the privilege of training under him know of another talent equally impressive but less generally known: his skill as a clinician. His incredible abilities, not only as a superb diagnostician but also as the classic bedside physician, have made him the role model for all of us concerned with the art of clinical medicine.

It seems appropriate, then, that a manual on the treatment of neurologic disease should be inspired by, and dedicated to, this premier neurologic therapist.

Contributing Authors

Telmo M. Aquino, M.D.
Consultant in Neurology,
Second Chair of Internal Medicine,
Hospital de Clinicas, Asunción, Paraguay

Raymond J. Fernandez, M.D.
Assistant Professor of Pediatrics and
Director, Pediatric Neurology Section,
University of South Florida College of Medicine,
Tampa, Florida

Robert D. Helme, M.B.B.S., Ph.D.
Senior Lecturer,
Department of Pathology and Immunology,
Monash University School of Medicine,
Victoria, Australia

Daniel B. Hier, M.D.
Instructor in Neurology,
Massachusetts General Hospital,
Harvard Medical School;
Clinical and Research Fellow in Neurology,
Massachusetts General Hospital,
Boston, Massachusetts

Richard C. Hinton, M.D.
Instructor in Neurology,
Massachusetts General Hospital,
Harvard Medical School;
Clinical and Research Fellow in Neurology,
Massachusetts General Hospital,
Boston, Massachusetts

Stephen M. Sagar, M.M.Sc., M.D.
Research Fellow, Department of Neurology,
Harvard Medical School;
Assistant in Neurology,
Children's Hospital Medical Center,
Boston, Massachusetts

Martin A. Samuels, M.D.
Instructor in Neurology,
Peter Bent Brigham Hospital,
Harvard Medical School;
Junior Associate in Medicine (Neurology),
Peter Bent Brigham Hospital, Boston;
and Chief, Neurology Section,
Veterans Administration Hospital,
West Roxbury, Massachusetts

Thomas M. Walshe, M.D.
Assistant Professor of Neurology,
Boston University School of Medicine, Boston;
Neurologist, Geriatric Research,
Education, and Clinical Center,
Bedford Veterans Administration Hospital,
Bedford, Massachusetts

Howard D. Weiss, M.D.
Assistant Professor of Neurology,
Johns Hopkins Medical School;
Attending Neurologist,
Sinai Hospital,
Baltimore, Maryland

Preface

Until very recently the neurologist's primary task was to categorize and organize the structure and pathologic alterations of the nervous system. In fact, neurology has long been known as a discipline with elegantly precise and specific diagnostic capabilities but little or no therapeutic potentiality. Further, many surgeons, pediatricians, and internists have traditionally thought of the neurologist as an impractical intellectual who spends countless hours painstakingly localizing lesions while ignoring pragmatic considerations of treatment. Perhaps this conception is largely attributable to the peculiar complexity of the nervous system and the consequent relative naivete of physicians in their understanding of its functions.

Many of the classic descriptions of disease states in other medical disciplines were completed in the last century; in neurology, these have only been described in the past generation, and only in the last ten years has neurology begun to be characterized by subcellular mechanistic concepts of disease. This maturity has meant that the neurologist is now as much involved in the therapeutic aspects of his specialty of medicine as any of his colleagues. Certain neurologic diseases, such as epilepsy, have been treatable for relatively long periods of time, but understanding of the subcellular mechanisms of other diseases has led to newer, more effective forms of therapy.

An example of this is the enlarged understanding we now have of the biochemical alterations in Parkinson's disease, and the resultant therapeutic implications. Now, much as the endocrinologist treats diabetes with insulin and the cardiologist treats congestive heart failure with digitalis, the neurologist treats Parkinson's disease with L-dopa. In all these situations, the underlying condition is not cured; rather, an attempt is made to alter the pathophysiologic processes by utilizing a scientific understanding of the function of the diseased system.

This manual embodies a practical, logical approach to the treatment of neurologic problems, based on accurate diagnosis, that should prove useful to both clinician and student. No attempt is made to reiterate the details of the neurologic examination; it is assumed that the reader is competent to examine the patient—although particularly important or difficult differential diagnostic points are mentioned when appropriate. In this regard, it should be emphasized that this manual is only a guide to diagnosis and therapy, and each patient must be treated individually. The manual is organized to best meet the needs of the clinician facing therapeutic problems. Thus, the first seven chapters are concerned with symptoms, such as dizziness and headache, while the last ten consider common diseases, such as stroke and neoplasms.

I thank the many colleagues and friends whose criticism and comments were useful in the preparation of this book, in particular Drs. G. Robert DeLong, C. Miller Fisher, George Kleinman, James B. Lehrich, Steven W. Parker, Henry C. Powell, E. P. Richardson, Jr., Maria Salam, Bagwan T. Shahani, Peter Weller, James G. Wepsic, and Robert R. Young. In addition, I am indebted to Sara Nugent and Helen Hyland for their assistance in the preparation of the many manuscripts, and to Diana Odell Potter, formerly of Little, Brown and Company, for her editorial skills. Jane Sandiford, formerly of Little, Brown and Co., and Kathleen O'Brien and Carmen Thomas of Little, Brown provided invaluable assistance in the final preparation of this material. Deep appreciation goes to Lin Richter, Editor in Chief of the Medical Division, Little, Brown and Company for her support throughout this effort. I further thank Jon Paul Davidson, also formerly of Little, Brown, for his valuable encouragement and help early in the course of this project. Much support and encouragement was derived from my new colleagues in the Peter Bent Brigham Hospital Neurology Section, The Longwood Avenue Neurology Program, and the West Roxbury Veterans Administration Hospital. A great deal of inspiration came from the birth of my daughter Marilyn, and my deepest thanks go to my wife, Linda, who provided constant encouragement, editorial skill, and infinite patience.

M.A.S.

Contents

PART I
NEUROLOGIC SYMPTOMS

Telmo M. Aquino

Coma and Alterations
in Consciousness

I. **GENERAL PRINCIPLES.** When confronted with a patient with impaired consciousness the clinician proceeds in an orderly, systematic manner. He gathers information at the same time as he is performing specific therapeutic maneuvers aimed at maintaining vital functions and avoiding further neurologic damage. The patient should never be left on a stretcher unattended while the history is obtained.

Impairment of consciousness may derive from a variety of causes. The first priority is to define and treat, as expeditiously as possible, those causes that are potentially reversible (see sec **V**).

II. **PATHOPHYSIOLOGY. Consciousness,** which commonly connotes the state of awareness of self and environment, in clinical neurologic practice is considered to be the behavioral state of arousal and responsiveness to various stimuli.

Consciousness involves the sum of all cerebral cortical functions including memory, language, intelligence, and particularly **arousal.** The mechanism responsible for arousal is located in the upper brainstem, largely in the midbrain, and is called the *ascending reticular activating system* (ARAS). It receives collaterals from the main sensory pathways and projects to the cortex via thalamic relay nuclei. The ARAS acts as an "off-on" switch that keeps the hemispheres awake.

Consciousness may be impaired by three major mechanisms:

A. **Supratentorial lesions,** by virtue of occupying space, displace the hemisphere downward, secondarily distorting and compressing the brainstem ARAS. Examples are brain tumors, abscesses, and hematomas. They frequently begin with unilateral hemispheric lateralizing or **focal signs** (e.g., hemiparesis, hemisensory loss, dysphasia, hemianopia).

B. **Infratentorial lesions** affect the brainstem directly. Examples are pontine infarction and cerebellar masses compressing the brainstem. Physical signs and symptoms may be bilateral, and frequently there are cranial nerve palsies, dysconjugate eye movements, or pupillary abnormalities.

C. **Metabolic processes** affect both brainstem and hemispheres to a variable extent. Examples are uremia, diabetic ketoacidosis, hypoglycemia, hypoxia, hepatic encephalopathy, and drug effects. They are generally characterized by symmetric motor abnormalities and preservation of pupillary reaction (unless the patient is using glutethimide or atropine) and extraocular movements (unless the patient is taking barbiturates).

III. **DIAGNOSIS**

A. **History.** Frequently the patient is brought to the emergency ward unresponsive, and no information at all is available. Whenever possible, family, friends, ambulance personnel, and physicians who have previously treated the patient are contacted. **Important features** of the history are trauma, previous illnesses, medications, addiction to drugs or alcohol, and psychiatric disorders.

B. **General physical examination** should pay special attention to:

1. **Vital signs:** patency of the airway, and circulatory and ventilatory status.

2. **Skin:** signs of trauma, stigmata of liver disease, needle marks, infective or embolic phenomena.

3. **Head:** Battle's sign (indicates mastoid fracture), raccoon's eyes (orbital fracture), localized tenderness or crepitus, hemorrhage of ear or nostrils (basilar skull fracture).

4. **Neck** (*Do not manipulate if there is suspicion of cervical spine fracture*): stiffness may be indicative of infection or subarachnoid bleeding.

5. **Chest, abdomen, heart,** and **extremities** are examined, and **rectal** and **pelvic** examinations are done, in the usual manner. A **stool guaiac** also is done.

6. **Breath:** may exhibit fetor hepaticus ("liver breath"), the fruity smell of ketoacidosis, the smell of liquor, or the uriniferous smell of uremia.

C. **A neurologic examination** is performed in all patients and recorded. With the goal of defining the presence, location, and nature of the process causing impaired consciousness, special emphasis is placed on the following:

1. **Observation of the patient**

   a. Observe if the patient **lies in a natural, comfortable position,** as though in natural sleep. If so, unconsciousness is probably not very deep. Yawning and swallowing have the same significance.

   b. **Jaw and lid tone** are also indications of the severity of unconsciousness. Open lids and hanging jaw indicate severe unresponsiveness.

2. **Level of alertness.** Consciousness comprises a continuum from full alertness to total unresponsiveness. It is useful in clinical practice to subdivide consciousness into stages of progressive unresponsiveness. Because there is much confusion surrounding these terms, it is good practice to describe in detail on the record the responses of the patient to various stimuli.

   a. **Drowsiness** is also termed *lethargy, somnolence,* or *obtundation.* This state is characterized by ready arousal, ability to respond verbally, and fending-off movements induced by painful stimuli in the absence of hemiparesis or aphasia.

   b. **Stupor** is characterized by incomplete arousal to painful stimuli. Response to verbal commands is inconsistent and vague. No verbal response or moaning is elicited. The motor responses are still of the purposeful, fending-off type.

   c. **Light coma** is characterized by primitive and disorganized motor responses to painful stimuli. There is no response to attempts at arousal.

   d. **Deep coma** is characterized by absence of response to even the most painful stimuli.

   e. When there is a question of **psychogenic unresponsiveness,** try to obtain a forced conscious response by, for example, letting the patient's hand fall toward the face. Avoid applying noxious stimuli to eyes, testicles, breasts, or other sensitive areas.

3. **Respiration.** The respiratory pattern is helpful in localizing and, in certain instances, determining the nature of the process.

   a. **Cheyne-Stokes respiration** is characterized by periods of hyperventilation tapering off gradually to apnea of variable duration; respirations then resume and gradually build up again to hyperventilation. It indicates bilateral deep hemispheric and basal ganglionic dysfunction. The upper brainstem also may be involved. (**Note** Cheyne-Stokes respiration may also be observed in nonneurologic conditions, such as congestive heart failure.)

   b. **Central neurogenic hyperventilation** (CNHV) refers to continued rapid and regular respirations at a rate of about 25/min. It has no segmental localizing significance. Regularity rather than rate is an unfavorable prognostic sign, since increasing regularity correlates with increasing depth of coma.

Hypoxemia should be excluded (two Po_2 determinations over 70 mm Hg in 24 hours is considered adequate for this purpose) before it is concluded that hyperventilation is of neurologic origin.

c. **Apneustic breathing** consists of a prolonged inspiratory phase followed by apnea in expiration, at a rate of about one and one-half cycles/min. It may be followed by **cluster breathing,** which consists of closely grouped respirations followed by apnea. Either pattern implies lower pontine damage.

d. **Ataxic breathing** and **gasping breathing** imply damage to the medullary respiratory centers. In ataxic breathing respirations are chaotic. Gasping breathing is characterized by gasps followed by apnea of variable duration. Both are agonal events and usually precede respiratory arrest.

e. **Depressed breathing** consists of shallow, slow, and ineffective breathing caused by medullary depression, usually produced by drugs.

f. **Coma with hyperventilation** is seen frequently in metabolic disorders.

   (1) **Metabolic acidosis** (e.g., diabetic ketoacidosis, uremia, ingestion of organic acids, lactic acidosis).

   (2) **Respiratory alkalosis** (e.g., hepatic encephalopathy, salicylate poisoning)

4. **Position of the head and eyes.** The normal cerebral hemisphere tends to move both head and eyes conjugately toward the opposite side. In hemispheric lesions, the healthy hemisphere becomes unopposed and, as a result, the head and eyes look toward the lesion and away from the hemiparesis. The reverse occurs in pontine lesions, in which the eyes deviate toward the hemiparesis and away from the lesion.

5. **Visual fields and funduscopy**

   a. In patients who are not completely unresponsive, visual fields should be tested with threatening movements, which should evoke a blink. Asymmetry of the blink response indicates hemianopia (in the absence of blindness or optic nerve damage). Air movement into the eyes can produce a false positive response.

   b. Funduscopy may reveal papilledema suggestive of increased intracranial pressure. A **subhyaloid hemorrhage**—a rounded, well-defined clot on the surface of the retina—is commonly associated with ruptured aneurysms.

6. **Pupils.** Note size, roundness, and equality in reaction to light, tested both binocularly and consensually.

   a. **Midposition (3–5 mm) nonreactive pupils** are evidence of midbrain damage.

   b. **Reactive pupils** indicate midbrain intactness. In the presence of unresponsiveness and absent extraocular movements and corneal reflexes, reactive pupils are suggestive of metabolic abnormality (e.g., hypoglycemia) or drug ingestion (e.g., barbiturate).

   c. **A unilaterally dilated and unreactive pupil** in a comatose patient is a sign of third-nerve compression due to temporal lobe herniation. Other components of third-nerve dysfunction (e.g., drooping of the eyelid and abduction of the eye as the result of unopposed action of the lateral rectus muscle) may be concomitant with or follow pupillary dilatation. Less frequently, midbrain damage caused by compression or direct damage is expressed by a dilated nonreactive pupil.

d. **Small but reactive pupils.** These signify pontine damage, as in infarction or hemorrhage. Opiates and pilocarpine also produce pinpoint reactive pupils. A magnifying glass may be helpful in the examination.

e. **Dilatation** of the pupils in response to a painful stimulus in the neck (the normal ciliospinal reflex) indicates lower brainstem integrity.

7. **Extraocular movements** (EOMs). If the patient is responsive enough to follow commands, saccadic and pursuit eye movements should be tested. A large number of ocular and gaze palsies may be present. In addition, spontaneous abnormal displacements of the eyes may be observed. **The most useful tests** are:

a. **Doll's head maneuver** (DHM), or **oculocephalic reflex.** (*Do not perform this maneuver when there is a question of cervical spine injury.*) DHM is performed by turning the patient's head with quick lateral and vertical displacements. **The reflex is normal or preserved** if the eyes move in the orbits in the direction opposite to the rotating head, maintaining their position in relation to the environment. **Abnormal response** (no movement of the eyes in the orbits, or asymmetry of movement) is suggestive of a destructive lesion at the pontine-midbrain level. Barbiturate poisoning also may abolish the reflex.

b. **Ice water calorics,** or the **oculovestibular reflex,** are reflex eye movements in response to irrigation of the tympanic membrane with cold water.

(1) **Position the head** 30 degrees with respect to the horizontal. Make certain that the canal is not occluded with cerumen, and that the tympanic membrane is intact. **Instill** between 10 and 30 ml of ice water into the canal and observe the eyes.

(2) The **normal response in a conscious patient** consists of tonic deviation of the eyes toward the stimulated side, followed by a quick corrective nystagmus toward the opposite side. **In an unconscious patient** only the slow component is present, provided that the brainstem is intact.

(3) **Absence of eye deviation** is evidence of structural pontine-midbrain damage. As with the doll's head maneuver, ice water calorics may be abolished by barbiturates and some other drugs.

8. **Motor responses** may be spontaneous, induced, or reflexive.

a. **Spontaneous**

(1) **Seizures** may be focal, in which case they have some localizing value. Generalized seizures do not help in localizing the lesion. Multifocal seizures are suggestive of a metabolic process.

(2) **Myoclonic jerks** also point to metabolic encephalopathies (e.g., hypoxia, hepatic failure, uremia). **Asterixis** has the same significance.

(3) **Absence of movements** in one side of the body, or asymmetry of movements, is suggestive of hemiparesis.

b. **Induced movements** (e.g., fending-off or other complex, purposeful movements, such as scratching the nose in response to tickling of the nostril) require integrity of the corresponding corticospinal tract. Poorly organized, incomplete movements, especially when unilateral, are suggestive of corticospinal tract dysfunction or damage.

c. **Reflex movements** are always elicited by a stimulus and have a certain time relationship between stimulus and response.

(1) **Decorticate movements** consist of flexion and adduction of the arms

and extension of the legs. The lesion is deep hemispheric or just above the midbrain.

(2) Decerebrate movements consist of extension, adduction, and internal rotation of the arms and extension of the legs. The lesion is in the upper brainstem between the red nucleus and the vestibular nuclei.

9. Sensory system. In drowsy or obtunded patients, the response to pain may be asymmetric, evidencing a hemisensory defect in the absence of paralysis. Facial and corneal sensation should be tested, since they also may be asymmetric.

IV. "PSEUDOCOMA" STATES

A. Psychogenic unresponsiveness. The patient appears unresponsive but is physiologically awake. The neurologic examination is otherwise normal, there is active opposition to attempts at eye-opening by the examiner, and with ice water calorics there will be a slow and a quick component. The EEG is normal.

B. The "locked-in" syndrome. In this situation a destructive process (usually basilar artery occlusion with brainstem infarction) interrupts the descending corticobulbar and corticospinal tracts, sparing only the fibers controlling blinking and vertical eye movements. The patient is able to communicate by means of blinks but is otherwise completely paralyzed.

V. ETIOLOGY.
Causes of impaired consciousness are multiple and, of these, many are not primarily neurologic. This is the reason why a detailed history derived from all available sources, thorough physical and neurologic examinations, and extensive laboratory screening is often needed. **Causes of impaired consciousness** can be categorized as follows:

A. Coma due to primary brain injury or disease is usually associated with a demonstrable structural lesion.

1. Trauma

  a. Concussion

  b. Contusion

  c. Laceration or traumatic intracerebral hemorrhage

  d. Subdural hematoma

  e. Epidural hematoma

2. Vascular disease

  a. Intracerebral hemorrhage

  (1) Hypertensive (putaminal, thalamic, pontine, cerebellar, or lobar)

  (2) Ruptured aneurysm with intraparenchymatous hematoma

  (3) Arteriovenous malformation

  (4) Miscellaneous (e.g., bleeding disorders, intratumoral hemorrhages)

  b. Subarachnoid hemorrhage

  (1) Ruptured aneurysm

  (2) Arteriovenous malformation

  (3) Secondary to trauma (e.g., contusion, laceration)

  c. Infarct

  (1) Thrombosis of intracranial and extracranial vessels

  (2) Embolism

(3) Vasculitis

(4) Malaria

d. Infections

(1) Meningitis

(2) Encephalitis

(3) Abscess

e. Neoplasms

(1) Primary intracranial

(2) Metastatic

(3) Nonmetastatic complications of malignancy (e.g., progressive multifocal leukoencephalopathy)

f.   Seizures (status epilepticus)

B. Coma due to systemic diseases (affecting the brain secondarily)

1. Metabolic encephalopathies

a. Hypoglycemia

b. Diabetic ketoacidosis

c. Hyperglycemic nonketotic hyperosmolar states

d. Uremia

e. Hepatic encephalopathy

f. Hyponatremia

g. Myxedema

h. Hypercalcemia and hypocalcemia

2. Hypoxic encephalopathies

a. Severe congestive heart failure

b. Chronic obstructive pulmonary disease with decompensation

c. Severe anemia

d. Hypertensive encephalopathy

3. Toxic

a. Heavy metals

b. Carbon monoxide

c. Drugs (e.g., opiates, barbiturates)

d. Alcohol

4. Physical

a. Heat stroke

b. Hypothermia

5. Deficiency states (Wernicke's encephalopathy)

VI. LABORATORY SCREENING

A. Routine. CBC, urinalysis, electrolytes, BUN, creatinine, blood sugar, Ca, PO_4, liver function studies, enzymes, osmolality, ECG, and chest x-ray.

B. Toxic screen should be obtained, when clinically indicated, in blood, urine, and gastric aspirate, including screening for opiates, barbiturates, antidepressants, and alcohol.

C. Special studies

 1. Skull x-rays

 2. Brain scan

 3. EEG

 4. CT scan (see sec **VI.C.6**)

 5. Angiography

 6. Lumbar puncture should be done if there is suspicion of intracranial infection (e.g., meningitis or encephalitis). Keep in mind the possibility of temporal lobe or cerebellar herniation in cases of increased intracranial pressure.

   The advent of CT scanning has made it possible to diagnose intracranial hemorrhage without resorting to lumbar puncture in the majority of cases. When the hemorrhage is small enough to escape undetected by CT scanning, lumbar puncture is safe and will determine whether angiography is needed.

VII. MANAGEMENT

A. Immediate therapeutic measures in all comatose patients are initiated promptly to forestall further neurologic damage.

 1. **Establish a good airway.** Intubation and artificial ventilation may be necessary.

 2. **Insert a large-bore IV catheter.**

 3. **Draw blood** for routine studies and toxic screen if indicated (see sec **VI**).

 4. In possible **Wernicke's encephalopathy,** give thiamine 100 mg IV to prevent acute deficiency due to the administration of dextrose.

 5. Give 50 ml of **dextrose 50%** in water IV.

 6. If there is some evidence that coma results from **opiate overdose,** give **naloxone,** 0.4 mg IV every 5–10 minutes, until consciousness returns. In patients with opiate addiction this might provoke an acute withdrawal state requiring narcotic therapy. The duration of action of naloxone is shorter than that of methadone, so repeated doses may be necessary.

B. Management of the specific processes (e.g., trauma, infections, tumor) is covered in the corresponding chapters.

C. Nursing care of the comatose patient is a crucial point in management. Fastidious nursing care is essential to prevent the multiple complications of the unresponsive state.

 1. **Circulation.** Give **fluids** in order to maintain blood pressure at levels to insure adequate cerebral, myocardial, and renal perfusion. In the initial stages at least, **cardiac monitoring** is useful.

 2. **Ventilation. Adequate oxygenation** and **prevention of infection, aspiration,** and **hypercapnia** are the goals.

  a. Remove dentures.

  b. Insert and tape a short oropharyngeal airway of adequate size to prevent the tongue from obstructing air flow.

  c. Prevent aspiration by suction of secretions.

   (1) Suction the nasopharynx and mouth frequently.

   (2) Place the patient in the lateral decubitus position, with the neck

slightly extended and the face turned toward the mattress. If there are no contraindications (e.g., raised intracranial pressure), the Trendelenburg position is helpful for drainage of tracheobronchial secretions.

  d. If ventilation is unsatisfactory and/or secretions are uncontrollable, insert a cuffed endotracheal tube. If intubation is necessary for longer than three days, consider tracheostomy.

  e. Insert a nasogastric tube and evacuate gastric contents to improve ventilation and prevent aspiration.

  f. Obtain arterial blood gases as often as necessary to make sure ventilation is adequate.

3. Skin. Turn the patient every 1–2 hours. Keep sheets tightly drawn. Pad bony prominences to prevent formation of sores.

4. Nutrition should be provided by IV solutions initially. Later, when the situation is stable, tube feedings are started. Vitamin supplements are used.

5. Bowel care. Diarrhea may result from tube feedings, antacids given concomitantly with steroids, and fecal impaction. Frequent rectal examinations for impaction are necessary.

6. Bladder care

  a. A condom catheter may be used in male patients. Penile maceration should be avoided.

  b. If an indwelling catheter becomes necessary, a three-way catheter should be used, with continuous irrigation with acetic acid 0.25% solution. This acidifies the urine and prevents stone formation.

  c. Clamp the catheter intermittently to maintain bladder tone. Release every 3–4 hours.

7. Eyes. Avoid corneal injury by taping the eyelids closed or using methylcellulose eye drops, two drops in each eye BID or TID.

8. Restlessness and agitation. In the recovery phase of many metabolic processes and drug intoxications, agitation and restlessness may occur. *Avoid unnecessary sedation.* If heavy sedation becomes necessary due to excessive severity or duration of agitation, chlordiazepoxide (Librium), 25 mg IM every 4–6 hours, may be indicated. A phenothiazine such as chlorpromazine (Thorazine), 25–50 mg IM every 4–6 hours, also may be used.

D. Management of cerebral edema and increased intracranial pressure. A number of processes (e.g., trauma, hemorrhage, large infarcts, tumors) may result in cerebral edema and a consequent rise in intracranial pressure. When the capacity of the brain to accommodate the increased intracranial volume is surpassed, cerebral tissue herniates through certain weak points.

  In many instances neurologic deterioration is caused by edema and is potentially reversible. Treatment of cerebral edema may be lifesaving until definitive therapy aimed at correcting the specific pathologic process can be carried out. **If the process is left unchecked,** local circulatory disturbances cause secondary brainstem hemorrhages, irreversible brain damage, and death.

1. Avoid hypotonic IV solutions. Restrict fluids and monitor blood pressure, serum osmolality, and urine output.

2. Hyperventilation produces hypocapnia and respiratory alkalosis decreasing cerebral blood flow and effectively reducing intracranial pressure. Its effects are immediate. The Pco_2 should be lowered to between 25 and 35 mm Hg.

3. Mannitol 20% may be given at a dose of 1.0 gm/kg IV over 10–30 minutes, according to the severity of the situation. The usual dose for a normal adult is 250 ml of the 20% solution or 50 gm of mannitol. The dose may be repeated every 12 hours. The effect is immediate and lasts several hours. An indwelling bladder catheter is necessary. Monitor vital signs, electrolytes, BUN, and osmolality frequently.

   4. Steroids. Give dexamethasone (Decadron) 10 mg by rapid intravenous infusion and follow with 4–6 mg IV or IM every 6 hours. The effect begins in 4–6 hours and peaks at 24 hours.

E. Seizures should be vigorously treated. See Chapter 6 for details.

SELECTED READING

Fisher, C. M.   The neurological evaluation of the comatose patient. *Acta Neurol. Scand.* *45* [Suppl. 36] 1:56, 1969.

Hinterbuchner, L. P.   Evaluation of the unconscious patient. *Med. Clin. North Am.* 57:1363, 1973.

Luzecky, M.   Neurologic Emergencies: Coma, In E. C. Boedeker and J. H. Dauber (Eds.), *Manual of Medical Therapeutics,* 21st ed. Boston: Little, Brown, 1974. P. 393.

Plum, F., and Posner, J. B.   *Diagnosis of Stupor and Coma,* 2nd ed. Philadelphia: Davis, 1972.

Posner, J. B.   The comatose patient. *J.A.M.A.* 233:1313, 1972.

Posner, J. B.   Delirium and Exogenous Metabolic Brain Disease, in P. B. Beeson and W. McDermott (Eds.), *Textbook of Medicine,* 14th ed. Philadelphia: Saunders, 1975. Pp. 544–552.

2

Headache

Headache is one of the complaints most frequently faced by internists and neurologists in their office practices. Most people accept an occasional headache as part of their lives. Patients come to physicians because of **chronic or recurrent headaches,** which have persisted unabated or occurred repeatedly over months or years, or **acute severe headaches,** unrelated to previous headaches and characterized by a violent onset or relentless progression. Most chronic recurrent headaches are of vascular or psychogenic origin, while acute severe headaches carry a more ominous prognosis and may reflect serious underlying disease.

I. EVALUATION OF THE PATIENT WITH HEADACHE

A. History. A careful history provides both the data necessary for correct diagnosis and the therapeutic rapport necessary for successful treatment of most headaches. **Special inquiry** should be made into the quality of the head pain, its frequency, its duration, its location, and any associated symptoms (Table 2-1). The family headache history and the patient's psychosocial history also are essential to the evaluation.

B. Physical examination. Each patient with a complaint of headache should undergo careful neurologic and general physical examination. Occasionally the examination will yield clues as to the etiology of the headache (see Table 2-2), but generally it will serve to reassure both patient and physician that nothing serious is causing the pain.

C. Ancillary tests. Any headache patient in whom **neurologic examination discloses an abnormality** should undergo further studies. When the **neurologic examination is normal,** no further studies are indicated **except** when:

1. An element of the history suggests a specific diagnosis (e.g., epilepsy or brain tumor).

2. The headaches have developed a new quality, are more severe, or have become intractable to treatment.

3. The headaches are atypical (e.g., trigeminal neuralgia in a patient under age 30).

II. MIGRAINE HEADACHE

A. Description. Migraine is a recurrent, throbbing headache of vascular origin. Although the headache is usually unilateral, opposite sides of the head may be affected during different attacks.

1. In **classic migraine** a visual aura precedes the throbbing headache by 10 to 20 minutes. Commonly this prodrome consists of scintillating and migrating scotomata or waviness and blurriness of vision. The prodrome is followed by a unilateral throbbing headache that intensifies over 1–6 hours. The headache usually abates in 6–24 hours but occasionally lasts longer. Vomiting, nausea, photophobia, irritability, and malaise are common.

   Most patients experience the first migraine headache between the ages of 10 and 30 years, although about 25% will recall childhood vomiting attacks or motion sickness. About 60 to 75% of patients are women.

2. **Migraine variants**

   a. In **common migraine** the characteristic throbbing headache occurs without the visual prodrome of classic migraine. Common migraine usually has a slightly longer course than classic migraine.

Table 2-1. Important Features of the Pain in the Evaluation of Chronic Recurrent Headaches

Headache	Quality	Location	Duration	Frequency	Associated Symptoms
Common migraine	Throbbing	Unilateral head	6–48 hr	Sporadic (often several times monthly)	Nausea, vomiting, malaise, photophobia
Classic migraine	Throbbing	Unilateral head	3–12 hr	Sporadic (often several times monthly)	Visual prodrome, vomiting, nausea, malaise, photophobia
Cluster	Boring, sharp	Unilateral head (especially orbit)	15–120 min	Closely bunched clusters with long remissions	Ipsilateral tearing, facial flushing, nasal stuffiness, Horner's syndrome
Psychogenic	Dull, pressure	Diffuse, bilateral	Often unremitting	May be constant	Depression, anxiety
Trigeminal neuralgia	Lancinating	Fifth nerve distribution	Brief (15–60 sec)	Many times daily	Identifiable trigger zone
Atypical facial pain	Dull	Unilateral or bilateral face	Often unremitting	May be constant	Often depression, occasionally psychosis

Table 2-2. Important Physical Findings in the Evaluation of Headache

Physical Finding	Possible Etiology
Optic atrophy, papilledema	Mass lesion, hydrocephalus, benign intracranial hypertension
Focal neurologic abnormality (hemiparesis, aphasia)	Mass lesion
Stiff neck	Subarachnoid hemorrhage, meningitis, cervical arthritis
Retinal hemorrhages	Ruptured aneurysm, malignant hypertension
Cranial bruit	Arteriovenous malformation
Thickened, tender temporal arteries	Temporal arteritis
Trigger point for pain	Trigeminal neuralgia

      b. In cases of **migraine associée,** the headache is accompanied by a transient neurologic deficit. Examples of migraine associée are ophthalmoplegic migraine, hemiplegic migraine, and migraine with aphasia. Usually the neurologic deficit precedes the headache, but it may follow it or even occur in the absence of headache (*migraine dissociée*).

      c. Rarely these neurologic deficits persist, suggesting that cerebral infarction has occurred **(complicated migraine).** In these patients potent vasoconstrictors (e.g., ergotamine) should be used with caution or not at all, because of the danger of exacerbating cerebral infarction.

      d. "Lower-half" headaches are unilateral facial pains affecting the nose, palate, cheek, and ear. These pains, believed to represent attacks of atypical migraine, may be associated with nausea and vomiting. Lower-half headaches also may respond to treatment with ergotamine.

B. Mechanism of migraine. Current hypotheses as to the etiology of migraine stress the role of vasoconstriction and vasodilatation. The prodromal phase of classic migraine is believed to be produced by vasoconstriction and cerebral ischemia, and decreases in cerebral blood flow during this prodromal phase have been documented. Vasodilatation follows upon vasoconstriction, and headache is produced by the pulsatile flow of blood through dilated arteries. Because concomitant increases in cerebral blood flow occur during the headache phase of migraine, therapy with vasoconstrictors (e.g., oxygen, epinephrine, ergotamine) may prevent development of this painful vasodilatation phase (see sec **II.C.2**).

C. Treatment of migraine

   1. General measures

      a. In many patients **inciting factors** can be identified and partially controlled. Some patients report an increase in the frequency and severity of their migraine attacks in relation to smoking, drinking, lack of sleep, stress, fatigue, or the ingestion of certain foods, especially chocolate and tyramine-containing cheeses.

      b. Anxiety and **depression** should be treated with appropriate psychotherapy and medication.

      c. In about one-third of women with migraine who are taking **oral contraceptives,** the incidence of headaches is increased. It is worth a trial period off oral contraceptives in these women. On the other hand, another one-third of women with migraine who start on oral contraceptives experience improvement in their headaches. We do not consider the control of migraine to be an indication for the use of oral contraceptives; in fact, there is preliminary evidence that the combination of oral contraceptives and migraine may be particularly conducive to the development of stroke. (However, there does not appear to be an increased incidence of stroke in most patients with migraine.)

d. **Cerebral arteriography** is usually contraindicated during an attack of migraine, since vasospasm and cerebral infarction have been reported to occur as rare complications during acute attacks. The incidence of migraine in patients with either saccular aneurysms or arteriovenous malformations is not much higher than in the general population, so migraine alone is not an indication for neuroradiologic procedures. However, when migraine is accompanied by permanent neurologic deficits, seizures, or a history suggestive of subarachnoid hemorrhage, cerebral arteriography is warranted.

2. **Abortive therapy** should be initiated as early as possible. The patient with classic migraine can begin therapy at the onset of the prodrome, while the patient with common migraine must await the onset of headache. Some authorities recommend awaiting the onset of headache in either case, since some migrainous prodromes will not be followed by headache.

   Once the headache has been well established for a period of hours (sometimes the patient will arise from sleep with a migraine headache); there is little to be gained from abortive therapy measures. Both **ergotamine** and **isometheptene** have proved superior to placebo in aborting migraine attacks. Placebo alone ameliorates the course of about a third of migraine attacks.

   a. **Ergotamine.** Ergotamine may be administered alone or in combination with antiemetics, analgesics, or sedatives. Many preparations contain caffeine (Cafergot, Wigraine) which also is capable of producing cerebral vasoconstriction and is known to potentiate the action of ergotamine. When the oral route is unsatisfactory because of nausea or vomiting, ergotamine may be administered rectally, sublingually, or by inhalation (Table 2-3). We do not routinely use ergotamine parenterally, since its potent vasoconstrictive properties occasionally precipitate angina.

      Ergotamine preparations are contraindicated in the presence of peripheral artery or coronary artery disease, hepatic or renal disease, hypertension, or pregnancy (Table 2-4). Side effects of ergotamine include nausea, vomiting, and cramps. Rare cases of ergotism with mental changes and gangrene have been reported even at therapeutic dosages.

      The usual dosage is 1 mg at onset followed by 1 mg every half-hour, to a maximum of 5 mg/attack or 10 mg/week. (See Table 2-3.)

   b. **Isometheptene.** Isometheptene either alone (Octin) or in combination (Midrin) is somewhat less effective than ergotamine but has fewer contraindications and adverse reactions (see Table 2-4). The usual dosage is two capsules at onset followed by one capsule each hour, to a maximum of five per attack, or until the headache is relieved (see Table 2-3).

3. **Preventive therapy** should be considered only in patients with frequent or disabling attacks of migraine (Table 2-5).

   a. **Ergotamine (Gynergen).** Ergotamine at a dosage of 1 mg BID will sometimes abolish recurrent attacks of migraine. No more than 10 mg should be given weekly. Rarely, prolonged usage of ergotamine leads to ischemic complications. **Bellergal** (ergotamine 0.3 mg/belladonna 0.1 mg/phenobarbital 20 mg combination) at a dose of two to four tablets daily is of benefit to some patients.

   b. **Methysergide (Sansert).** About three-quarters of patients respond favorably to methysergide (4–8 mg daily in divided doses). Although this drug has been implicated as a rare cause of retroperitoneal, cardiac valvular,

Table 2-3. Drugs Useful in the Abortive Therapy of Migraine Headaches

Drug	Dosage
Ergotamine 1 mg (Gynergen) tablets	1 tablet PO immediately, repeat every ½ hr to maximum of 5 mg/attack or 10 mg/week.
Ergotamine 1 mg/caffeine 100 mg (Cafergot) tablets	1 or 2 tablets PO immediately, repeat to maximum of 5/attack or 10/week.
Ergotamine 1 mg/belladonna 0.1 mg/caffeine 100 mg/phenacetin 130 mg (Wigraine) tablets	1 tablet PO immediately, repeat every ½ hr to maximum of 5/attack or 10/week.
Ergotamine 2 mg sublingual (Ergomar)	1 tablet sublingually, repeat in ½ hr if necessary to maximum of 3 tablets/day.
Ergotamine/caffeine (Cafergot) suppositories	1 suppository immediately, repeat in 1 hr if necessary.
Ergotamine/caffeine/ phenacetin/belladonna (Wigraine) suppositories	1 suppository immediately, repeat in 1 hr if necessary.
Ergotamine inhaler (Medihaler-Ergotamine)	1 inhalation immediately, repeat in 5 min if necessary, to maximum of 6 inhalations/day.
Isometheptene 130 mg (Octin)	1 tablet immediately, then 1 every hr to maximum of 5/day or 10/week.
Isometheptene 65 mg/ acetaminophen 325 mg/ dichloralphenazone 100 mg (Midrin) capsules	2 capsules immediately, then 1 every hr to maximum of 5/day as needed or 10/week.

and pulmonary fibrosis; in most cases the fibrosis is reversible if the drug is discontinued. Methysergide should be prescribed with utmost caution, however, and its usage is contraindicated during pregnancy or in the presence of cardiac valvular, collagen vascular, coronary artery, peripheral vascular, pulmonary, or fibrotic disease. No patient should be continued on the drug for longer than 6 months at a time, and patients should be monitored for the appearance of azotemia, dyspnea, or cardiac murmurs. A 1-month "vacation" from the drug every 6 months of use is usually adequate to avoid serious complications.

   c. **Propranolol (Inderal),** 40–160 mg daily in divided doses, has been used with some success to prevent migraine headaches. Its mechanism of action is uncertain but may be related to the prevention of β-adrenergic–mediated vasodilatation. Propranolol should not be used in patients with asthma or congestive heart failure. If the patient is already under treatment for hypertension, it is sometimes useful to substitute propranolol for one of the antihypertensive drugs. Excessive drowsiness and depression occur in some patients.

   d. **Amitriptyline (Elavil),** 50–75 mg in divided doses or at bedtime, has been shown to provide effective migraine prophylaxis for some patients. Its action against migraine appears to be independent of its antidepressive action. Nervousness, tremor, and anticholinergic side effects can be troublesome in certain patients.

   e. **Cyproheptadine (Periactin),** 8–16 mg daily in divided doses, is an antihistamine that, like methysergide, has antiserotonin properties; fibrotic complications have not been reported. However, this drug lacks the effectiveness of methysergide. Drowsiness, especially at higher dosages, is bothersome to some patients.

Table 2-4. Adverse Reactions and Contraindications for Drugs Used in Treatment of Headache

Drug	Indications*	Adverse Reactions	Contraindications†
Ergotamine preparations (Cafergot, Wigraine, Gynergen, Ergomar)	Migraine	Nausea, vomiting, angina, numbness and tingling, cramps	Renal and hepatic failure, coronary artery and peripheral vascular disease, pregnancy, hypertension
Methysergide (Sansert)	Migraine, cluster	Retroperitoneal, valvular, and pulmonary fibrosis; vasoconstriction; nausea; vomiting; drowsiness; neutropenia	Pregnancy; fibrotic and collagen diseases; renal, valvular, pulmonary, and hepatic disease; hypertension; coronary artery and peripheral vascular disease
Isometheptene preparations (Midrin, Octin)	Migraine	Dizziness	Glaucoma; severe cardiac, renal, or hepatic disease
Tricyclic antidepressants (Elavil, Tofranil)	Psychogenic, migraine*	Dry mouth, tremor, urinary retention, glaucoma, arrhythmias, agitation	Coronary artery disease, MAO inhibitors
Propranolol (Inderal)	Migraine, cluster*	Bronchospasm, heart failure, bradycardia, hypotension, drowsiness, depression	Heart failure, asthma, bradycardia, MAO inhibitors
Cyproheptadine (Periactin)	Cluster, migraine*	Drowsiness, dry mouth	MAO inhibitors, glaucoma
Carbamazepine (Tegretol)	Trigeminal neuralgia	Bone marrow depression, hepatic dysfunction, ataxia, drowsiness, nausea, vomiting	MAO inhibitors, bone marrow depression, hepatic disease
Phenytoin (Dilantin)	Trigeminal neuralgia, migraine*	Gingivitis, rash, ataxia, macrocytic anemia	

*Usage is not routine.
† All drugs cited are contraindicated in the presence of allergy or hypersensitivity.

Table 2-5. Drugs Useful in the Preventive Therapy of Migraine

Drug	Dosage
Methysergide (Sansert)	4–8 mg daily, in divided doses (Do not continue drug for longer than 6 months at a time)
Ergotamine (Gynergen)	1 mg BID, not to exceed 10 mg weekly (2 days/week must be skipped)
Ergotamine/belladonna/ phenobarbital (Bellergal)	2–4 tablets daily
Propranolol (Inderal)	10–40 mg QID
Cyproheptadine (Periactin)	2–4 mg QID
Amitriptyline (Elavil)	50–75 mg daily, in divided doses
Phenytoin (Dilantin)	200–400 mg daily

   f. Phenytoin (Dilantin). Some patients with migraine benefit from phenytoin (200–400 mg daily). Certain of these patients probably have
   headaches as seizure equivalents. The existence of "migrainous epilepsy"
   as a distinct entity is controversial, and this drug should not be considered
   as a standard treatment for migraine. However, at a dose of 5 mg/kg/day,
   phenytoin seems to be of benefit in children with migraine.

4. Symptomatic therapy

   a. Many patients obtain adequate relief of **occasional migraine headaches**
   with aspirin or acetaminophen. Some patients get better relief when a
   small amount of barbiturate is added (Fiorinal, Minotal). Propoxyphene
   (Darvon) may be useful when aspirin is poorly tolerated.

   b. Severe headaches should be treated with codeine, 30–60 mg, or morphine, 4–8 mg, every 3–4 hr.
      Nausea and vomiting may be produced by the headache itself, by
   ergotamine, or by narcotics. Vomiting can be controlled with promethazine (Phenergan) 25–50 mg, or prochlorperazine (Compazine) 5–10
   mg. Allowing the patient to sleep by administering a hypnotic, such as
   flurazepam (Dalmane) 15–60 mg, is generally an effective way of ending
   the migraine.

   c. In cases of **severe, prolonged,** or **unremitting migraine** (status mi-
   grainosus) a short course of prednisone (40–60 mg daily) may be of benefit.

III. CLUSTER HEADACHE

   A. Description. Cluster headache (histamine cephalalgia, Horton's headache) is a
   periodic, paroxysmal headache disorder. Excruciating unilateral head pain (often
   localized to the orbit) occurs in brief episodes (15 minutes to 2 hours) without
   prodrome. The headaches are distributed into clusters, occurring daily for 3
   weeks to 3 months, then remitting entirely for months or years. The pain is sharp
   and piercing and unaccompanied by either nausea or vomiting.
      Headaches are most common late at night or early in the morning. This is one of
   the few headaches that awaken patients from their sleep. Some patients experience facial flushing, Horner's syndrome, nasal stuffiness, or eye tearing ipsilateral to the headache. Men are affected five times as frequently as women, and
   most patients have their first attack between the ages of 20 and 40. Exacerbation
   of the headaches due to alcohol consumption is common. The mechanism underlying cluster headache is not well understood but is believed to be vascular.

   B. Treatment

      1. Ergotamine. The lack of aura and the short duration of cluster headaches
      make abortive therapy of these headaches difficult. Occasionally a patient

can successfully end a cluster headache by promptly taking an ergotamine preparation (e.g., Cafergot, Ergomar). Other patients may improve with ergotamine (Gynergen) 1 mg BID.

2. **Methysergide (Sansert).** About 50–80% of patients are substantially improved on methysergide (4–8 mg daily in divided doses). Caution must be exercised in the use of this drug (see Table 2-4), but a bout of cluster headaches is self-limited, and it is rare to continue the drug for longer than 3 months.

3. **Cyproheptadine** (Periactin). If methysergide is contraindicated, poorly tolerated, or ineffective, cyproheptadine (8–16 mg daily in divided doses) is sometimes of benefit.

4. **Propranolol** (Inderal). Uncontrolled studies have indicated that propranolol (40–160 mg daily in divided doses) is effective in certain patients.

5. **Prednisone.** Some authors recommend a short course of prednisone (20–40 mg daily, followed by a gradual tapering) for refractory cases of cluster headaches.

6. **Histamine desensitization** is of historical interest but rarely indicated.

7. **Narcotics.** Symptomatic relief of cluster headaches may require narcotic agents (e.g., codeine 30–60 mg every 3–4 hr).

IV. PSYCHOGENIC HEADACHES

A. **Description.** The term *psychogenic headache* encompasses several entities including **tension headache, muscle contraction headache,** and the headaches of **anxiety** and **depression.** The individual with sporadic headaches that are relieved by aspirin or acetaminophen, or with occasional neck and scalp muscle tightness that is relieved by massage, rarely consults a physician. In contrast, most patients with psychogenic headaches who seek medical attention have had daily or unremitting headaches for months or years that are not relieved by simple analgesics or even narcotics (unlike the headaches of intracranial masses).

   In our experience the great majority of these **patients are depressed;** signs of depression, including tearfulness, hopelessness, insomnia, anorexia, and an inability to enjoy life, are often prominent. These patients describe ill-defined, diffuse aching or pressure sensations. The **pain** may be occipital, temporal, or frontal in distribution, but it is almost invariably bilateral. Unilateral throbbing pain characteristic of migraine is uncommon.

B. **Treatment**

   1. **General measures**

      a. Initiation of **therapeutic rapport** between physician and patient is very often the first step to improvement. Some patients respond positively to the physician's forceful reassurance that nothing is physically wrong inside their brains or heads, which dispels fears of brain tumor or other intracranial disease.

      b. An assessment should be made as to whether **anxiety** or **depression** is present. Some patients accept the suggestion that their headaches are related to depression and encourage a therapeutic program directed against it, while other patients can be foreseen to be uncomfortable with this diagnosis, even though indicated. For the latter, emphasis is better left on treating the headache. Depression and anxiety can sometimes be controlled by examination and modification of the life events contributing to these emotions. When the depression is severe, refractory to treatment, or complicated by threats of suicide, the patient should be referred to a psychiatrist.

2. **Tricyclic antidepressants.** Aspirin or acetaminophen may be of value for some patients with psychogenic headaches, but when depression is prominent the use of analgesics is usually futile, and sedating tranquilizers may deepen the depression. Several controlled studies have shown tricyclic antidepressants to be superior to analgesics or minor tranquilizers in the treatment of these headaches. **Imipramine** or **amitriptyline** may be started as a single bedtime dose of 25 to 50 mg and gradually increased to 150 mg over 2 weeks (see also Chap. 9). Treatment should be continued for at least 4 weeks before being judged ineffective. Both these drugs have mild sedating properties, so administration at bedtime helps to correct the sleep disturbance of these depressed patients.

3. **Benzodiazepines.** In the smaller group of patients in whom muscle contraction and anxiety predominate, treatment with **diazepam** (Valium) 5–30 mg daily, **chlordiazepoxide** (Librium) 10–75 mg daily, or **oxazepam** (Serax) 30–90 mg daily, in conjunction with aspirin or acetaminophen, is useful.

4. **Relaxation techniques.** The value of hypnosis, biofeedback, meditation, and other relaxation techniques in the treatment of psychogenic headaches has not been established.

V. TRIGEMINAL NEURALGIA

A. Description. Trigeminal neuralgia (tic douloureux) is characterized by brief, lancinating paroxysms of pain, lasting for seconds or minutes, in the distribution of the fifth cranial nerve. The third and second divisions of the trigeminal nerve are affected more frequently than the first, and **trigger points** often can be found on the face. Attacks occur spontaneously or during toothbrushing, shaving, chewing, yawning, or swallowing.

Onset in over 90% of patients with trigeminal neuralgia occurs after age 40, with women affected somewhat more frequently than men. In most cases no etiology for trigeminal neuralgia can be found. When it is associated with **hypesthesia** in the distribution of the fifth cranial nerve, with **other cranial nerve palsies,** or with **onset before the age of 40,** so-called symptomatic trigeminal neuralgia should be suspected. Further investigation may reveal multiple sclerosis (in as many as 3% of patients with trigeminal neuralgia, in some series) or a posterior fossa tumor.

B. Treatment

1. **Phenytoin** (Dilantin). Many patients get relief from **phenytoin** alone, 200–400 mg daily.

2. **Carbamazepine** (Tegretol). About 80% of patients with trigeminal neuralgia respond to initial treatment with **carbamazepine** (400–1200 mg daily); in fact, response to carbamazepine is helpful in differentiating trigeminal neuralgia from certain cases of atypical facial pain (see sec **VI.A.**). Both phenytoin and carbamazepine can produce troublesome ataxia (especially when used concurrently). Rare complications of carbamazepine are leukopenia, thrombocytopenia, and liver function abnormalities, so its use requires monthly monitoring of white blood cell count, platelet count, and liver function. After initial improvement, many patients develop **recurrent pain** despite adequate blood levels of one or both of these drugs.

3. **Surgery.** Patients who relapse during drug treatment or fail to tolerate the drugs should be referred for possible surgical management. The current procedure of choice is **electrocoagulation of the gasserian ganglion** by percutaneous insertion of a radio frequency electrode. This procedure can be performed under local anesthesia in conjunction with short-acting narcotics and barbiturates. Use of the radio frequency electrode permits selective destruction of the pain-related nerve fibers with relative sparing of the

tactile-related fibers, minimizing the potential for complications such as corneal abrasion and analgesia algera. This technique also makes an intracranial approach to the trigeminal nerve unnecessary. Over 90% of patients experience relief, and recurrences are uncommon.

VI. ATYPICAL FACIAL PAIN

A. Description. Atypical facial pain must be carefully distinguished from trigeminal neuralgia. Commonly it is seen in young or middle-aged patients as a unilateral boring or aching facial pain that lacks both the paroxysmal quality and the well-defined anatomic distribution characteristic of trigeminal neuralgia. The etiology of atypical facial pain is unknown.

B. Treatment. Patients are unimproved by either phenytoin or carbamazepine. Surgical procedures on the trigeminal nerve are not indicated, since they do not relieve the pain and may produce analgesia algera. For depressed patients, imipramine or amitriptyline should be tried. When the pain has a delusional quality, a major tranquilizer may be of benefit. Many cases prove frustratingly difficult to treat.

VII. TEMPORAL ARTERITIS (giant cell arteritis)

A. Description. Temporal arteritis, a systemic illness of elderly patients, is characterized by inflammatory infiltrates of lymphocytes and giant cells in cranial arteries. It presents variously as **temporal headache, visual loss,** or generalized **malaise.** *When* **visual loss** *is present, it should be considered a medical emergency.* It is estimated that only about one-half the patients complain of headache or have tender temporal arteries, although nearly all patients have some systemic symptoms including low-grade fever, weight loss, anorexia, or weakness. The erythrocyte sedimentation rate (ESR) is elevated in all patients, usually to between 60 and 120 mm/hr. Onset before age 50 is distinctly uncommon. Visual loss occurs in 10 to 40% of untreated patients. The diagnosis should be confirmed by temporal artery biopsy, since this procedure can be performed easily under local anesthesia even in debilitated patients. Rarely the biopsy will be normal in the presence of active arteritis because of patchy involvement of the temporal artery.

The relationship of temporal arteritis to **polymyalgia rheumatica** is controversial. There appears to be considerable overlap between the two illnesses, and some patients with polymyalgia rheumatica exhibit giant cell arteritis on temporal artery biopsy.

B. Treatment

1. High-dose **corticosteroids** should be initiated immediately to avoid visual loss. When the diagnosis is suspected, initiation of therapy should not await the pathology report of the temporal artery biopsy. **Prednisone** (45 mg daily) will abolish systemic symptoms and normalize the ESR within 4 weeks in most patients. The dose can then be gradually reduced to 5–10 mg daily over a period of several months.

2. **A rise in ESR** or a **recrudescence of systemic symptoms** sometimes necessitates a temporary increase in corticosteroid dosage.

3. Temporal arteritis is **self-limited,** and corticosteroids can usually be discontinued within 6 months to 2 years.

4. Patients must be observed for **complications** of high-dose corticosteroid therapy including psychosis, osteoporosis, vertebral body collapse, and gastrointestinal hemorrhage.

VIII. POSTCONCUSSION SYNDROME

A. Description. Following cerebral concussion, patients may complain of decreased concentration, vague headaches, dizziness, fatigue, and photophobia. The forcefulness of these complaints does not correlate with either the severity of the concussion or any objective finding, except that the complaint of **dizziness** is sometimes correlated with the finding of **nystagmus.** The postconcussion syndrome usually remits spontaneously, but occasionally it runs a protracted course over years (especially if litigation is pending). The **etiology** of this syndrome is largely psychogenic; fear that cerebral damage has been suffered plays a role in some cases.

B. **Treatment. Anxiety** should be allayed with repeated assurances that nothing is amiss. Benzodiazepine tranquilizers may be added if necessary. **Depressive symptoms** may require short-term psychotherapy or a brief course of tricyclic antidepressants. The management of **dizziness** is discussed in Chapter 4. Some cerebral concussion patients describe **headaches** that are vascular in nature, which respond to migraine headache therapy. When litigation is pending, all forms of therapy may prove futile.

IX. BENIGN INTRACRANIAL HYPERTENSION (pseudotumor cerebri)

A. **Description.** Benign intracranial hypertension is a syndrome of increased intracranial pressure without evidence of mass lesion or hydrocephalus. **Headache** and **papilledema** are uniformly present. About 90% of the patients are both obese and female. Occurrence after age 45 is rare. The **etiology** of most cases is unknown, although occasionally vitamin A intoxication, tetracycline use, corticosteroid use or withdrawal, or dural sinus thrombosis have been implicated. About 5% of the patients experience a **decrease in visual acuity** associated with the papilledema; this loss may be permanent if increased intracranial pressure persists unrelieved. **Localizing neurologic signs** do not occur, although unilateral or bilateral sixth nerve palsies may occasionally produce diplopia.

B. **Diagnosis**

1. **Headache** and **papilledema** should always prompt a thorough investigation for mass lesions or hydrocephalus.

2. The **CT scan** delineates most supratentorial lesions as well as many infratentorial lesions capable of producing papilledema. The ventricles are either diminished in size (slitlike) or normal in configuration. Enlarged ventricles cast great doubt on the diagnosis and suggest hydrocephalus. When CT scanning is unavailable, **technetium brain scanning** and an **EEG** should be performed.

3. When these preliminary tests are **normal,** and localizing signs are absent, **lumbar puncture** can be safely performed in the presence of papilledema. The diagnosis of benign intracranial hypertension is confirmed by the finding of normal CSF under increased pressure (usually 250 to 500 mm H_2O). Any abnormality of the CSF (cytology, protein, sugar) should prompt further investigation.

4. When the EEG, technetium brain scan, or CT scan is **abnormal,** it may be necessary to proceed to arteriography or ventriculography before lumbar puncture.

C. **Treatment**

1. About one-third of these patients have spontaneous remission after the first lumbar puncture. Most other cases can be successfully managed by repeated lumbar punctures, daily at first, then every third day, weekly, or even monthly as needed. Sufficient CSF (up to about 30 ml) should be removed at each lumbar puncture to reduce the CSF pressure to less than 180 mm H_2O.

2. Patients **who do not respond** to repeated lumbar punctures may be tried on **prednisone** (40–60 mg daily) or **dexamethasone** (6–12 mg daily). Response to corticosteroids generally occurs within 1 week. In refractory cases, especially when visual loss is occurring, **neurosurgical consultation** should be

obtained. Subtemporal decompression may be considered when cortico-steroids, oral glycerol (15–60 mg, 4 to 6 times daily), acetazolamide (250 mg TID), and repeated lumbar punctures fail to control intracranial pressure, and visual loss is progressing.

3. **Visual acuity** should be measured daily until the intracranial pressure is controlled.

X. OTHER HEADACHE SYNDROMES

A. Headache in association with **fever** and **stiff neck** (with or without mental changes) can be due to **encephalitis** or **meningitis** (see Chap. 8).

B. The **violent onset** of headache (with or without loss of consciousness) followed by stiff neck suggests **subarachnoid hemorrhage** (see Chap. 10). The headache is often described in dramatic terms, such as "the worst headache of my life" or "a headache like something snapped in my head." **Photophobia** and **malaise** may be present. **Funduscopy** may reveal preretinal (subhyaloid) hemorrhages. The headache of ruptured saccular aneurysm is generally more severe than that of leaking arteriovenous malformations. A **dull unremitting headache** that persists for days following a subarachnoid hemorrhage is sometimes due to the increased intracranial pressure of **communicating hydrocephalus** (see Chap. 3). The headache may be relieved by lumbar puncture. Occasionally a shunting procedure is necessary to control the hydrocephalus.

C. Headache occurs with a variety of **intracranial mass lesions** such as subdural hematoma (Chap. 12), brain tumor (Chap. 11), and brain abscess (Chap. 8). The headache of **brain tumors** is usually paroxysmal at first (often worst early in the morning upon arising). Later the headaches become unremitting and may be complicated by vomiting. The initial side of the headache may reflect the side of the tumor, but this is not a highly reliable sign. Headache is the first symptom of about 80% of posterior fossa tumors and 30% of supratentorial tumors.

D. The headache of **increased intracranial pressure** (Chap. 11) may be intensified by coughing, sneezing, or bending over. **Cough headache** also exists as a benign entity without known intracranial pathology.

E. **Occipital headache** associated with pain on movement of the neck may be due to **cervical arthritis.** Arthritic changes can be confirmed by plain x-ray examinations of the cervical spine. A trial of aspirin in combination with diazepam (Valium), 5–30 mg daily, gives relief to some patients. Cervical collars and cervical traction are occasionally of benefit.

1. **In refractory cases,** phenylbutazone (Butazolidin), 400 mg in divided doses daily, or indomethacin (Indocin), 100 mg in divided doses daily, may be tried, but their usage may be complicated by adverse hematologic and gastrointestinal reactions.

2. When signs of **radiculopathy** or **myelopathy** are present, cervical myelography may reveal spinal cord or nerve root compression by a spondylitic bar or herniated disc. An electromyogram (EMG) may also confirm radiculopathy. Surgical management is indicated in most such cases.

F. The headache that occurs **after lumbar puncture** is exacerbated by standing and relieved by lying down. These headaches appear to be due to persistent leakage of cerebrospinal fluid from the subarachnoid space; most can be prevented by use of a small-bore needle (20 or 22-gauge). Post–lumbar puncture headaches usually can be managed by a combination of bedrest, analgesics, and hydration. When conservative measures fail, an epidural patch with autologous blood usually gives relief.

G. Tumors of the **foramen magnum** produce an occipital headache that worsens on recumbency and is relieved by standing.

H. Nasal stuffiness or discharge associated with pain on percussion over the sinuses suggests that the headache may be due to **acute sinusitis.**

I. Headache in association with a red painful eye can be produced by **acute closed-angle glaucoma.** Open-angle glaucoma (which is more common) does not produce headache.

J. There is no correlation between headache and moderate elevations of blood pressure. An occasional patient with **hypertension** has relief of early morning headaches with control of blood pressure, but hypertension should not be considered a common cause of headache.

SELECTED READING

General
Dalessio, D. J.   *Wolff's Headache and Other Head Pain* (3rd ed.). New York: Oxford, 1972.
Diamond, S., and Dalessio, D. J.   *The Practicing Physician's Approach to Headache.* New York: Medcom, 1973.
Friedman, A. P.   Headache, in A. B. Baker and L. H. Baker (Eds.), *Clinical Neurology.* New York: Harper & Row, 1971. Chap. 13.
Lance, J. W.   *The Mechanism and Management of Headache.* London: Butterworth, 1969.
Vinken, P. J., Bruyn, G. W. (Eds.)   *Headaches and Cranial Neuralgias.* Handbook of Clinical Neurology, Vol. 5. Amsterdam: North-Holland Publishing Co., 1968.

Migraine and Cluster Headaches
Couch, J. R., Ziegler, D. K., and Hassanein, R.   Amitriptyline in the prophylaxis of migraine. *Neurology* 26:121, 1976.
Diamond, S., and Medina, J. L.   Isometheptene—a non-ergot drug in the treatment of migraine. *Headache* 15:211, 1975.
Graham, J. R.   Methysergide for prevention of headache. *N. Engl. J. Med.* 270:67, 1964.
Graham, J. R., Suby, H. I., LeCompte, P. R., and Sadowsky, N. L.   Fibrotic disorders associated with methysergide therapy for headache. *N. Engl. J. Med.* 274:359, 1966.
Kalendorsky, L., and Austin, J. H.   "Complicated migraine." Its association with increased platelet aggregability and abnormal plasma coagulation factors. *Headache* 15:18, 1975.
Leviton, A., Malvea, B., and Graham, J. R.   Vascular diseases, mortality, and migraine in the parents of migraine patients. *Neurology* 24:669, 1974.
Weber, R. B., and Reinmuth, O. M.   The treatment of migraine with propranolol. *Neurology* 21:404, 1971.

Psychogenic Headache
Budzynski, T. H., Soyra, I. M., Adler, C. S., and Mullaney, D. J.   EMG biofeedback and tension headache: a controlled outcome study. *Psychosom. Med.* 35:484, 1973.
Lance, J. W., and Curran, D. A.   Treatment of chronic tension headache. *Lancet* 1:1236, 1964.
Okasha, A., Ghaleb, H. A., and Sadek, A.   A double-blind trial for the clinical management of psychogenic headaches. *Br. J. Psychol.* 122:181, 1973.

Trigeminal Neuralgia and Atypical Facial Pain
Delaney, J. F.   Atypical facial pain as a defense against psychosis. *Am. J. Psychol.* 133:10, 1976.
Gardner, W. J.   Trigeminal neuralgia. *Clin. Neurosurg.* 15:1, 1968.
Killian, J. M., and Fromm, G. H.   Carbamazepine in the treatment of neuralgia. *Arch. Neurol.* 19:129, 1968.
Sweet, W. H., and Wepsic, J. G.   Controlled thermocoagulation of the trigeminal ganglion and rootlets for differential destruction of pain fibers. Part 1: trigeminal neuralgia. *J. Neurosurg.* 39:143.

Temporal Arteritis
Fauchald, P., Rygvold, O., and Oystese, B.   Temporal arteritis and polymyalgia rheumatica, clinical and biopsy findings. *Ann. Intern. Med.* 77:845, 1972.

Hunder, G. G., Sheps, S. G., Allen, G. L., Yoyce, J. W.   Daily and alternate-day cortico-steroid regimens in treatment of giant cell arteritis, comparison in a prospective study. *Ann. Intern. Med.* 82:613, 1975.

Benign Intracranial Hypertension

Greer, M.   Management of benign intracranial hypertension (pseudotumor cerebri). *Clin. Neurosurg.* 15:11, 1968.

Weisberg, L.   Benign intracranial hypertension. *Medicine* (Baltimore) 54:197, 1975.

Other Headache Syndromes

Gormley, J. B.   Treatment of postspinal headache. *Anesthesiology* 21:565, 1960.

Lidvall, H. F., Linderoth, B., and Norlin, V.   Causes of the postconcussional syndrome. *Acta Neurol. Scand.* [Suppl] 56:3, 1974.

Weiss, N. S.   Relationship of high blood pressure to headache, epistaxis, and selected other symptoms. *N. Engl. J. Med.* 287:631, 1972.

3 Raymond J. Fernandez and Martin A. Samuels

Intellectual Dysfunction:
Mental Retardation and Dementia

Intelligence refers to the ability to comprehend ideas and their relationships and to reason about them. This obviously extremely complex function consists, in neurologic terms, of multiple capacities including those for general knowledge, memory, acquisition of new knowledge, attention, comprehension, judgment, abstract thinking, verbalization, understanding of mathematic concepts, orientation, perception, and association.

Mental retardation is defined as static subnormal development of intelligence. *Dementia* describes progressive deterioration, or loss, of intellectual functions that had previously developed; the term generally excludes confusion, delirium, obtundation, and other abnormalities in level of consciousness. Psychiatric illnesses in particular are excluded from the category of dementia (see sec **III**). Further, isolated abnormalities of one cortical function (e.g., isolated aphasias, pure memory loss) are not generally considered dementias despite their ability to produce impairment of intellect.

I. **MEASUREMENT OF INTELLIGENCE.** Attempts to quantify intelligence and developmental level have been made using many psychological testing methods, the most common of which are:

A. The **Wechsler Adult Intelligence Scale** (WAIS) provides a verbal, nonverbal, and overall intelligence quotient (IQ) and is appropriate for people over the age of 16.

B. The **Weschler Intelligence Scale for Children** (WISC) is designed for children between 6 and 16 years old and also yields a verbal, nonverbal (performance), and full-scale IQ. A discrepancy between verbal IQ and performance IQ often provides a clue to perceptual handicaps.

C. The **Denver Developmental Screening Test** tests four areas of behavior: gross motor, fine motor, language, and personal-social and provides a measure of developmental delay in infancy and preschool years.

D. The **Stanford-Binet** test is appropriate for children between 2 and 8 years old and yields a mental age (MA) and an IQ. It is heavily weighted toward verbal performance and thus may underestimate the intelligence of children with specific communication disorders or perhaps from environments that have not stimulated their verbal capacity.

E. **Limitations on testing.** These tests are variously successful, but all suffer from poor reproducibility, especially in young subjects, and fail to correct successfully for the known effects on intelligence test scores of cultural and educational background, interest, motivation, and effort. Furthermore, certain psychiatric disorders—particularly depression and schizophrenia—may lower IQ. Whether this occurs because of actual lowering of intelligence or because of an artifact of the testing as a result of impaired motivation in these conditions is unknown.

Despite these drawbacks, psychological testing is presently the only scientific method of estimating intelligence and can be useful in evaluating and following patients with intellectual dysfunction—as long as the limitations of the tests are clearly understood.

II. **EVALUATION OF THE PATIENT WITH INTELLECTUAL DYSFUNCTION**

A. **History.** A careful history of the **onset and course of the intellectual dysfunction** is obtained.

1. In **children,** one must attempt to discern whether the problem is one of mental retardation or of dementia, since the further evaluation of the patient depends heavily on this distinction.

2. Exact descriptions of the abnormal behavior may help in ascertaining the **cortical distribution** of the dysfunction (i.e., frontal, parietal, temporal, or occipital).

3. The **course of the illness** deserves special consideration, particularly whether it occurred in steps or gradually, the former suggesting strokes and the latter a degenerative process.

4. History of possible **intracranial hemorrhage** strongly suggests **occult hydrocephalus.**

5. **A general medical history** is taken, with particular importance placed on:

   a. Prior gastric surgery (predisposing the patient to vitamin B_{12} deficiency).

   b. Thyroid disease.

   c. Use of drugs or ingestion of toxins, such as bromide-containing drugs.

   d. **Family history** of other neurologic or psychiatric illness.

6. In children, a careful history of the **pregnancy and delivery** is important.

B. **Physical examination**

1. The **general physical examination** is aimed at excluding any medical illness that may underlie the intellectual dysfunction, such as:

   a. Uremia

   b. Liver failure

   c. Anemia

   d. Hypertension

   e. Malignancy

2. In **children,** the condition underlying the intellectual dysfunction may be obvious on physical examination (e.g., Down's syndrome).

3. The **mental status examination** helps to define the extent and precise type of dysfunction. Functions to be tested include:

   a. Attention

   b. Orientation

   c. Alertness

   d. Speech

   e. Comprehension

   f. Memory

   g. Naming

   h. Repetition

   i. Reading

   j. Writing

   k. Calculations

   l. Right-left discrimination

   m. Praxis

   n. Developmental level in children

   4. The **neurologic examination** excludes signs of focal brain disease, such as:
      a. Hemiparesis
      b. Primary modality sensory loss
      c. Hemianopia
      d. Cranial nerve abnormalities
   5. In **children,** particular attention is paid to head size and rate of head growth.
   6. In infants under 18 months of age, transillumination of the skull is routinely done in order to detect a fluid-filled structure such as a subdural effusion, porencephalic cyst, or massive hydrocephalus.

C. **Laboratory tests** (see Table 3-1)

III. **CONDITIONS WITH INTELLECTUAL DYSFUNCTION AS A MAJOR MANIFESTATION**

   A. **Degenerative diseases**

      1. **Alzheimer's disease** and **Pick's disease** (presenile dementia and senile dementia)

         a. **Description.** Alzheimer's disease is the most common cause of dementia. The older concept of presenile (before age 65) and senile (after age 65) dementias now has little clinical relevance, since the **pathology** (i.e., decreasing number of cortical neurons with accumulation of lipofuscin in neurons and the presence of neurofibrillary degeneration of neurons; senile plaques; deepening cortical sulci; and increasing ventricular size with progressive decrease in brain weight) and the **clinical course** of Alzheimer's disease are known to be the same in all age groups.

            (1) **Symptoms and signs of dysfunction.** Since the cortical degeneration is widespread, one might expect nearly every part of the cerebral cortex to show dysfunction. In practice, most patients begin to have difficulty in parietal and temporal lobe function, with memory loss and spatial disorientation. As the disease progresses, signs of frontal lobe dysfunction appear, with loss of social inhibitions and concomitant incontinence and abulia (loss of spontaneity). Aphasia and apraxia may occur at any point in the course of the disease. However, this sequence of events is not always seen, and some patients will have extensive frontal lobe difficulty long before temporal and parietal lobe functions are disturbed.

            In a rare variant of Alzheimer's disease **(Pick's lobar atrophy),** only frontal and temporal pole degeneration is seen. In both Alzheimer's and Pick's diseases *it is exceedingly rare to see signs of pyramidal tract dysfunction* (i.e., hemiparesis, hyperreflexia, or Babinski signs) or *loss of primary sensory modalities.* Such findings should raise suspicion that a space-occupying lesion or areas of encephalomalacia account for the dementia.

            (2) **Patient behavior and prognosis.** Patients with Alzheimer's disease, particularly when there is severe frontal lobe degeneration, can be extremely difficult to manage. Such patients are commonly incontinent of urine and feces, may wander away from home and be unable to find their way back, may be agitated and confused intermittently (particularly at night), and may use embarrassingly inappropriate language and actions. Early in the course of the illness depression may be a major problem.

            The disease is progressive, inevitably terminating in complete incapacity and death. The course is extremely variable, but most patients die within 4 to 10 years of the time of diagnosis.

b. **Treatment.** There is no specific therapy aimed at reversing or arresting the underlying pathologic changes. However, several maneuvers are often useful palliatively.

   (1) **Abulia and apathy**

    (a) Methylphenidate (Ritalin) 10–60 mg PO daily, divided into 2 or 3 doses

    (b) Dextroamphetamine sulfate (Dexedrine) 10–60 mg PO daily, divided into 2 or 3 doses

   (2) **Depression**

    (a) Imipramine (Tofranil) 75–300 mg PO, once a day at bedtime

    (b) Amitriptyline (Elavil) 75–300 mg PO, once a day at bedtime

   (3) **Agitation and confusion**

    (a) Avoid periods of decreased sensory stimulation by keeping the lights on in the patient's room at night, if nighttime confusion and agitation ("sundowning") is a problem.

    (b) Haloperidol (Haldol) 1–6 mg PO daily, divided into 2 or 3 doses

    (c) Chlorpromazine (Thorazine) 30–75 mg PO daily, divided into 3 doses or at bedtime

2. **Progressive supranuclear palsy** (Steele-Richardson-Olszewski syndrome)

   a. **Description.** Progressive supranuclear palsy is a rare degenerative disease in which there is neurofibrillary and granular degeneration of neurons, chiefly in the nuclear structures of the reticular formation of the midbrain, pretectal regions, substantia nigra, globus pallidus, subthalamic nuclei, and dentate nuclei of the cerebellum. These lesions account for the **clinical picture** of progressive hypertonia, supranuclear ocular palsies (particularly conjugate downward gaze), and disturbances of wakefulness. There is a dementia similar to that seen in Alzheimer's or Pick's disease.

   b. **Treatment.** There is no specific treatment for the dementia, although the movement disorder may respond favorably to L-dopa or amantadine (see Chap. 15). Palliative measures as outlined in sec **III.A.1.b** may be useful.

3. **Parkinson's disease**

   a. **Description**

   (1) The triad of **tremor, rigidity,** and **akinesia** that characterizes Parkinson's disease is discussed in detail in Chapter 15.

   (2) It is the impression of most neurologists that there is an **increased incidence of dementia** in parkinsonian patients. This is difficult to prove for two reasons:

    (a) These patients are often extremely **difficult to test,** since their movement disorder may be so severe that it interferes with their ability to respond appropriately in the test situation.

    (b) **Alzheimer's disease is common** in the age group affected by Parkinson's disease, so undoubtedly some of the dementia seen in parkinsonian patients is due only to the coexistence of these two relatively common conditions.

   (3) It is generally agreed, however, that Parkinson's disease itself may occasionally be a dementing illness, with symptoms similar to those of classic Alzheimer's disease.

There is an interesting disease complex seen in the Marianas Islands, known as **Parkinson's dementia complex,** in which dementia is regularly seen with Parkinson's disease. Many patients with this disease go on to develop a motor neuron disease that is clinically indistinguishable from amyotrophic lateral sclerosis. The pathology of both conditions is characterized by prominent neurofibrillary and granulovacuolar neuronal degeneration, suggesting that these syndromes may be linked by a common pathophysiology.

    b. Treatment. The treatment for the movement disorder of Parkinson's disease is covered in Chapter 15. There is **no specific therapy for the dementia,** and it is unlikely to respond to standard antiparkinsonian drug therapy. Palliative measures as noted in sec **III.A.1.b** may be useful.

B. Multiple strokes

    1. Description. The syndrome of multiple strokes is a rare cause of dementia. The precise **clinical picture** depends on the locations of the infarctions or hemorrhages.

        a. When multiple lacunar infarctions have occurred in the basal ganglia, internal capsule, and pons, a **lacunar state** may develop that is characterized by rigidity, hyperreflexia, pseudobulbar palsy, and dementia. The **dementia** in this condition is primarily a frontal lobe type, with prominent abulia, apathy, and loss of social inhibitions. The reason for the development of this particular type of dementia is unknown.

        b. Dementia due to multiple strokes may often be **distinguished from Alzheimer's disease** on the basis of its history, which may show a stepwise development of symptoms rather than the insidious, smoothly progressing course of a degenerative disease.

        c. The presence of **hypertension** in a patient with a progressive dementing illness with signs of bilateral pyramidal tract disease, including pseudobulbar palsy, may **suggest the lacunar state,** though bilateral cerebral infarctions or hemorrhages could present a similar clinical picture. CT scanning will often reveal cerebral infarctions or hemorrhages but is much less likely to show small lacunar infarctions either supratentorially or infratentorially. These must be suspected on clinical grounds alone.

    2. Treatment. There is no specific treatment for the dementia of multiple strokes once it has developed, but it may be possible to **influence the development** or progression of this illness by treating the risk factors for stroke, particularly hypertension and sources for emboli (see Chap. 10). Palliative treatment as outlined in sec **III.A.1.b** may be useful.

C. Chronic hydrocephalus

    1. Terminology. Chronic hydrocephalus may produce dementia or mental retardation. (The syndrome of acute hydrocephalus is a neurologic emergency and does not present as a dementia [see Chap. 11].) The **terminology** of chronic hydrocephalus is summarized as follows:

        a. Nonobstructive *(ex vacuo)*

            (1) Alzheimer's disease

            (2) Pick's disease

            (3) Multiple cerebral infarctions

        b. Obstructive

            (1) Communicating (normal pressure, low pressure, tension)

                (a) Postsubarachnoid hemorrhage

(b) Postmeningitis

(c) Idiopathic

(2) Noncommunicating (internal)

(a) Aqueductal stenosis

(b) Masses compressing the fourth ventricle (e.g., cerebellar tumors)

(c) Malformations at the foramen magnum (e.g., Arnold-Chiari malformation and Dandy-Walker malformation)

2. **Description. Nonobstructive** or *ex vacuo* hydrocephalus is due to degeneration or destruction of cerebral cortex with secondary increase in ventricular size. **Obstructive hydrocephalus** is divided clinically according to the site of CSF blockage: if the blockage is within the ventricular system, the term *noncommunicating hydrocephalus* applies, while if the blockage is outside of the ventricular system, then the term *communicating hydrocephalus* is appropriate. It should be emphasized that in cases of obstructive hydrocephalus that present as dementia the blockage is never complete, since a total block of CSF flow would result in acute hydrocephalus, massively increased intracranial pressure, and death within a few hours (see Chap. 11).

   a. In **children** a common site of obstruction is within the ventricular system (noncommunicating hydrocephalus), due either to aqueductal stenosis or to incomplete development of the foramina of Magendie and Luschka. This type of abnormality, often only one manifestation of a generalized maldevelopment of the nervous system, is associated with such abnormalities as microgyria, macrogyria, porencephaly, agenesis of the corpus callosum, fusion of the cerebral hemispheres, agenesis of the cerebellar vermis, spina bifida, meningocele, encephalocele, syringomyelia, hydromyelia, and the Arnold-Chiari malformation. Children may also develop communicating hydrocephalus due to adhesions in the subarachnoid space at the base of the brain. These adhesions may be produced by perinatal subarachnoid or intraventricular hemorrhages.

   b. In adults chronic hydrocephalus is usually communicating, with the block at the base of the brain in the subarachnoid space. Rarely, noncommunicating hydrocephalus due to aqueductal stenosis is seen in adults.

3. **Diagnosis.** The diagnosis of hydrocephalus is suspected in **children** whose head circumference enlarges too rapidly and in **adults** who have a frontal lobe type of dementia (prominent abulia, incontinence, and gait disturbance with the intellectual deterioration) of unclear etiology. A history of intracranial hemorrhage or meningitis further raises the suspicion of chronic hydrocephalus. *A CT scan will reliably and safely reveal the presence of hydrocephalus.* Although the pattern of ventricular enlargement on CT scan gives clues to the site of blockage, either an air study (pneumoencephalogram or ventriculogram) or a CSF flow study (with either radioiodinated serum albumin [RISA] or radioactive Indium) is usually required to determine the exact site of the obstruction.

4. **Treatment**

   a. **Surgery**

      (1) Rationale. Theoretically, chronic hydrocephalus may be relieved by the **shunting of CSF** around the blockage. This will lower the pressure in the ventricular system proximal to the block and thereby prevent further damage to brain tissue. However, *shunting must be done before excessive irreversible loss of brain tissue has already taken place.* This can easily be done in **children** before the sutures and fontanelles have closed, since the diagnosis of hydrocephalus can be made early in the course of the illness. Once the sutures and fontanelles have closed irreversibly, head measurements are of no value in the diagnosis of hydrocephalus.

(2) When to shunt. It is not known how long a period can elapse prior to shunting before irreversible damage has occurred, but it appears that *the likelihood of a good result from shunting is inversely proportional to the length of time from the onset of symptoms to the time of diagnosis.* No specific time limit can be set beyond which surgery can be said to be of no benefit, but most studies in adults have shown much better results in patients who have had symptoms for less than 6 months. However, it should be emphasized that many patients with longer-term illness have improved with shunting.

In **children** the width of the cortical mantle does not necessarily correlate with the ultimate intellectual outcome, so all should be evaluated for shunting. However, in some early mild cases in children (usually a communicating hydrocephalus with a known etiology, such as ruptured aneurysm or postmeningitis) the patient may be carefully observed, with frequent serial head measurements and CT scans, in hopes that the process will arrest spontaneously, thereby avoiding a shunting procedure.

(3) Cortical atrophy. Since Alzheimer's disease is so much more common a cause of dementia in adults than in children, with an adult patient one should always be sure to rule out cerebral atrophy (hydrocephalus *ex vacuo*) as either the sole or partial cause of the dementia, because this aspect of the hydrocephalus will not respond to shunting procedures since there is no obstruction to CSF flow. Certain neuroradiologic criteria have been developed to differentiate *ex vacuo* from obstructive hydrocephalus.

(a) The **callosal angle** (the angle between the lateral ventricles as seen on PEG) is usually more obtuse (> 105 degrees) in *ex vacuo* hydrocephalus and more acute (< 105 degrees) in obstructive hydrocephalus.

(b) The **depth of the cerebral fissures and sulci** (particularly the sylvian fissure) as seen on either CT scan or PEG also adds weight to an estimate of the degree of cerebral atrophy.

When there is a significant degree of cerebral atrophy, even if there is a component of obstructive hydrocephalus, shunting procedures are unlikely to show good results.

(4) Indications for shunting. Patients who should have shunting procedures include:

(a) **Children** in whom the diagnosis of chronic progressive hydrocephalus has been made and in whom the likelihood of spontaneous arrest has been ruled out.

(b) **Adults** who have a relatively recent onset of dementia and who show a purely obstructive hydrocephalus by CT scan, PEG, and/or CSF flow studies.

(5) Procedures available. Many shunting operations are available but the two most commonly employed are ventriculoatrial (V-A) shunts and ventriculoperitoneal (V-P) shunts.

(6) Complications of shunting. Even in the ideal case, with good initial response to shunting, one must remain vigilant for complications of the shunt, including:

(a) Infection.

(b) Mechanical malfunction.

(c) Movement of the cannula, and consequent inadequate draining of the ventricles.

(d) Emboli and endocarditis (with V-A shunts).

(e) Ascites, peritonitis, and ruptured viscus (with V-P shunts).

If the shunt becomes infected, it must be removed and the infection treated as outlined in Chapter 8. Periodically, the reservoir of the shunt should be manually pumped to ensure its mechanical functioning. Any deterioration in mental functioning is an indication for reevaluation of ventricular size, preferably by CT scanning.

b. **Medical treatment.** Medical treatment of chronic obstructive hydrocephalus is relatively ineffective and should be used only when surgery is not possible. Occasionally in children in whom the diagnosis of mild hydrocephalus has been made, medical therapy may be used pending a decision about surgery. The rationale for medical management of chronic obstructive hydrocephalus is based on the observation that acetazolamide (Diamox) may decrease the rate of cerebrospinal fluid production by the choroid plexus. The dose of acetazolamide is 10–25 mg/kg/day PO, divided into three doses in children, and 250 mg divided into three doses in adults.

D. **Spongioform encephalopathies**

1. These rare diseases, which include kuru, and Creutzfeldt-Jakob Disease, are characterized by diffuse cerebral, basal ganglion, and spinal cord neuronal degeneration; glial proliferation; and spongy appearance of the cortex. They are characterized by a rapidly progressive, subacute dementia similar to Alzheimer's disease but usually accompanied by striking myoclonus and sometimes by cerebellar signs, rigidity, and weakness (see also Chap. 8).

2. **Treatment.** There is no specific therapy for the disease itself. Palliative measures as noted in sec **III.A.1.b** are sometimes useful. In addition, the myoclonus may respond to the use of one of the benzodiazepine derivatives such as:

   a. Clonazepam (Clonopin) 1.5–2.0 mg PO daily, divided into 3 doses

   b. Diazepam (Valium) 15–30 mg PO daily, divided into 3 doses

E. **Viral encephalitides** (see also Chap. 8)

1. **Description.** Many of the viral encephalitides may result in dementia due to destruction of cerebral cortex. Any of these diseases may be incriminated: arbovirus infections (eastern, western, Venezuelan, and California equine encephalitides), herpes simplex encephalitis, and subacute sclerosing panencephalitis. The critical factor in the development of dementia is presumably the amount of brain destroyed by the infection. However, the encephalitis itself may be inapparent, only presenting with the late onset of dementia. This is particularly true of herpes simplex encephalitis. In some patients only memory loss is seen, but in many others there is widespread higher cortical dysfunction.

2. **Treatment.** There is no effective treatment for the viral encephalitides except for the symptomatic treatment of cerebral edema and seizures. If dementia develops, the palliative maneuvers noted in sec **III.A.1.b** may be beneficial.

F. **Neurosyphilis** (see also Chap. 8)

1. **Description.** In the late stages of neurosyphilis in adults one may see the syndrome of *dementia paralytica,* or *general paresis of the insane.* The mental changes take many forms including frank psychosis, memory deficit, impairment of judgment, excessive lability of mood, and others. Usually pa-

tients who have congenital paretic syphilis have been known to be defective physically and mentally from birth. Between the ages of 6 and 21 years, often the affected child begins to function less well in school and has associated irritability and inattention. Psychometric tests show a decrease in IQ. Neurologic examination may or may not be abnormal but often shows pupillary abnormalities, choreiform movements, incoordination, spasticity, optic atrophy, or deafness.

2. **Treatment.** The treatment of neurosyphilis with penicillin is outlined in Chapter 8. The dementia often does not respond well to treatment, although the further progression of dementia is arrested in most treated patients. About one-third of adult patients have complete remission of symptoms and another 25% show a partial improvement. The degree of improvement depends on the stage of the disease when it is treated. Children with congenital syphilis have an even poorer prognosis for recovery of normal function than adults.

G. **Posttraumatic encephalopathies**

1. **Description.** Some patients who suffer head trauma fail to recover their full premorbid mental capacities. This is more common in patients who lose consciousness, particularly as a result of massive head trauma, than in trivial head injuries, but it may be seen in either situation. Older patients are more likely than younger ones to develop this posttraumatic dementia.

   If the patient appears to recover completely from the head trauma and subsequently begins to show a dementing illness, one must suspect development of either a communicating hydrocephalus, precipitated by blood in the subarachnoid space, or chronic subdural hematoma. Both of these conditions may require neurosurgical treatment. If the patient never fully regains normal mentation, various components of the so-called posttraumatic or postconcussion syndrome also may be seen, including headache, dizziness, insomnia, irritability, inability to concentrate, and personality changes. It is not known whether these symptoms are directly related to brain damage or are psychological in origin. Many of these symptoms resemble those of depression, and their resolution is often delayed when litigation is pending.

2. **Treatment**

   a. Of insomnia, irritability, restlessness, personality change, loss of ability to concentrate.

      (1) Imipramine (Tofranil) 75–150 mg PO daily

      (2) Amitriptyline (Elavil) 75–150 mg PO daily

   b. Of **headache:**

      (1) Aspirin 600 mg PO every 4 hours or as needed for pain.

      (2) Tricyclic antidepressants as in sec **III.G.2.a** above may also be useful if aspirin is not effective.

   c. **Dementia.** No specific therapy is available aside from those measures listed above. Reassurance is important since most patients show steady improvement, even though recovery may take several years. In a minority of patients (usually elderly patients who have survived massive head trauma) severe permanent intellectual dysfunction may require institutionalization and treatment as outlined in sec **III.A.1.b.**

H. **Congenital and early-acquired disorders**

1. **Definitions and classification.** Mental retardation may be defined as general intellectual capacity that is significantly below average, with associated deficits in adaptive behavior originating during the developmental period.

Individuals may, then, be classified according to their intellectual capacity as mildly, moderately, severely, or profoundly retarded.

a. The **mildly retarded (educable)** have IQ scores that range from 55 to 70. This group constitutes approximately 75% of the retarded population. They may never attain more than third- or fourth-grade educational skills, but as adults they should be able to function in the community with some degree of supervision.

b. The **moderately retarded (trainable)** have IQs between 45 and 55. Most are capable of learning self-care skills but will never attain significant academic achievement. Individuals within this group may live at home and attend sheltered workshops, but many are committed to residential care. They comprise approximately 20% of the retarded population.

c. The **severely retarded** (IQ 25–45) and **profoundly retarded** (IQ less than 25) are totally dependent, the majority being committed to residential care. Many are bedridden and never achieve any degree of socialization. This group comprises only approximately 5% of the retarded population. Behavior modification techniques are sometimes useful in teaching these individuals basic self-care skills and in controlling self-abusive behavior.

d. In the **overall assessment** of the individual with mental deficiency, the above classification is of limited value, but some generalizations may be made. Mildly retarded people are more common among socioeconomically disadvantaged groups and often have parents who are mentally dull. Multifactorial (polygenic and environmental) factors are thought to be involved, and it is usually not possible to establish a specific diagnosis. In contrast, individuals who are more severely retarded are more uniformly distributed among socioeconomic groups, and it is more often possible to make a specific diagnosis or to document structural CNS abnormalities.

2. Evaluation and treatment of the mentally retarded patient. Clinical classification is difficult, but one useful scheme is based on the time at which the illness is determined.

a. Prenatally determined

(1) Chromosomal abnormalities

(2) Hereditary syndromes with multiple anomalies but without identifiable chromosomal abnormalities

(3) Multifactorial inheritance (polygenic and environmental factors)

(4) Major malformations of uncertain etiology

(5) Metabolic and degenerative disorders

(a) Amino acid abnormalities

(b) Lysosomal storage diseases

(6) Congenital infections

(7) Maternal and environmental factors

b. Perinatally determined

(1) Birth injuries

(a) Hypoxic-ischemic-hemorrhagic insults

(b) Mechanical trauma

(2) Infections

(3) Toxic-metabolic abnormalities

(4) Cerebral palsy

c. Postnatally determined

(1) Infections

(2) Trauma

(3) Hypoxic-ischemic insults

(4) Toxic-metabolic disorders

(5) Neoplastic conditions

An appropriately detailed history and physical examination usually allow one to place the patient within a general category, and at times a specific diagnosis may be made. **Nonprogressive** intellectual (and motor) retardation must be distinguished from **progressive** deterioration, since the differential diagnosis and prognosis vary widely. If further diagnostic evaluation is necessary, as is often the case, it should be carried out as indicated by the history and physical examination. Routine biochemical, radiologic, and neurophysiologic studies for the initial evaluation of all retarded individuals are summarized in Table 3-1.

Table 3-1. Laboratory Testing in Dementia and Mental Retardation

Routine	If Specifically Indicated
Dementia	*Dementia*
Complete blood count (CBC)	Toxic screen of urine and/or blood
Erythrocyte sedimentation rate (ESR)	Pneumoencephalography
Serum electrolytes (Na, K, Cl, CO_2)	CSF flow study
Blood urea nitrogen (BUN) or serum creatinine	Arteriography
Serum calcium and phosphate	Skull x-rays
Liver function tests	Technetium brain scan (if CT scan is not available)
Serum vitamin B_{12}	Thyroid stimulating hormone (TSH) if T_4 is low-normal
Serum thyroxine (T_4)	
Serologic test for syphilis (STS)	
Computed tomography of the brain (CT scan)	
Retardation	*Retardation*
CBC	Serum titers for *Toxoplasma gondii,* rubella, cytomegalovirus, and herpesvirus (ToRCH titers)
Urine for amino acid screening	Berry spot test for mucopolysaccharidoses
Serum electrolytes	Toxic screen of urine and/or blood
BUN or serum creatinine	Specific enzyme studies
Liver function tests	Karyotyping
T_4	TSH
Skull x-rays	Nerve conduction velocities
STS	Nerve, muscle, and skin biopsies
CSF examination for cell count and protein	CSF flow study
CT scan	Arteriography
	Pneumoencephalography
	Technetium brain scan
	Brain biopsy

3. Causes of mental retardation

  a. **Chromosomal abnormalities.** Identifiable chromosomal abnormalities may often be diagnosed on clinical grounds alone and include trisomies 13, 18, and 21; Klinefelter's syndrome; and other less common disorders. Chromosome studies are indicated if these disorders are suspected and also in patients with mental retardation and associated multiple anomalies, abnormal dermatoglyphics with additional malformations, or an abnormal buccal smear. Chromosome studies are not routinely indicated in patients with mental retardation in the absence of associated physical anomalies.

  b. **Multiple anomalies.** Hereditary syndromes with multiple anomalies but without identifiable chromosomal abnormalities are varied, and individual description is beyond the scope of this text. These disorders may be classified according to associated defects; several atlases are available that may aid in establishing a diagnosis (see under Holmes and under Smith in the Selected Reading section).

  c. **Multifactorially determined conditions.** Conditions caused by multifactorial inheritances are found in a large percentage of mildly retarded persons and are heavily represented within socially disadvantaged groups. The inheritance of multiple genes from both parents who are often mentally dull is compounded by substandard environmental factors that further impair learning. Common isolated major malformations with severe mental retardation attributed to multifactorial inheritance include meningomyelocele, encephalocele, and anencephaly.

  d. **Isolated malformations.** Other isolated major malformations of diverse etiologies include primary and secondary microcephaly and various anomalies associated with hydrocephalus. Radiographic studies including skull x-rays, CT scanning, and pneumoencephalography or ventriculography may be indicated to define the exact nature and extent of the anomaly.

  e. **Amino acid disorders.** Amino acid disorders and related conditions (organic acid and urea cycle disorders) are a complex group of diseases that are difficult to distinguish from each other and from other degenerative diseases of the nervous system. After a variable period of normal development (at times extremely short, as in maple syrup urine disease) signs of diffuse involvement of the nervous system may become manifest, including delay or deterioration in intellectual or motor development, lethargy at times proceeding to coma, seizures, ataxia, and alterations of muscle tone. Several disorders may be associated with fairly consistent physical features and unusual odors, such as light pigmentation and eczema in phenylketonuria and the characteristic smell of the urine in maple syrup urine disease. Early diagnosis is essential since several of these disorders are treatable by exclusion or addition of dietary substances (Table 3-2). Blood and urine amino acid and organic acid analysis are essential for the diagnosis.

  f. **Lysosomal storage diseases.** The lysosomal storage disorders are a group of genetic diseases in which storage of certain metabolites occurs within lysosomes due to a specific enzyme deficiency. Table 3-3 lists lysosomal storage diseases with known enzyme deficiencies and the major accumulating metabolites. Disorders that primarily involve gray matter (such as the ganglioside storage diseases) result in dementia and seizures early in their course. As a rule, ataxia and spasticity appear early in the course of primary white matter degenerative disease, with seizures and dementia appearing later.

Table 3-2. Inborn Errors of Metabolism Associated with Mental Retardation that May Be Vitamin-responsive or Treated by Special Diets

Disorder	Diet	Vitamin Supplement*
Hyperammonemia	Restrict protein	. . . .
Argininemia	Restrict protein	. . . .
Argininosuccinic aciduria	Restrict protein	. . . .
Branched chain ketonuria (MSUD)	Restrict branched chain amino acids	Thiamine (rarely)
Citrullinemia	Restrict protein	. . . .
B-methyl crotonic aciduria	Restrict leucine	Biotin
Galactosemia	Eliminate galactose	. . . .
Hartnup disease†	. . . .	Niacin
Histidinemia†	Restrict histidine	. . . .
Homocystinuria	Low methionine, high cystine	Pyridoxine, B_{12} (rarely)
Isovaleric acidemia	Restrict leucine	. . . .
Methylmalonic aciduria	Restrict protein	B_{12}
Phenylketonuria	Restrict phenylalanine	. . . .
Propionic acidemia	Restrict protein	Biotin
Hypervalinemia	Restrict valine	. . . .
Xanthurenic aciduria†	. . . .	Pyridoxine

Source: Moser, H. W.   Biochemical Aspects of Mental Retardation. In D. B. Tower (Ed.), *The Nervous System*, Volume 2: *The Clinical Neuroscience*. New York: Raven Press, 1975. P. 371.
* The vitamin supplements usually must be given in amounts much larger than the normal requirement; almost all these disorders have vitamin-responsive and -unresponsive variants. The degree to which dietary constituents must be controlled, and the clinical effectiveness of dietary control, vary a great deal.
† For these disorders, it is not certain whether there is an increased incidence of mental retardation.

g. **Congenital infections.** Patients with mental retardation due to the recognizable congenital infections (e.g., herpesvirus, rubella, *Toxoplasma*, cytomegalovirus) usually have additional abnormalities including intrauterine growth retardation, neonatal jaundice, petechiae, hepatosplenomegaly, microcephaly or hydrocephalus, and intracranial calcifications. Patients with the congenital rubella syndrome frequently have cataracts and congenital heart lesions. Valuable laboratory studies during the neonatal period include attempted viral isolation in urine and total and specific IgM antibody determinations if available (if not, serial IgG titers must be obtained to differentiate passive transfer from active antibody production by the infant).

h. **Prenatal insults.** Prenatal maternal and environmental factors associated with mental retardation include chronic placental insufficiency, toxemia, diabetes, malnutrition, alcoholism, ingestion of certain drugs, and exposure to radiation.

Table 3-3. Lysosomal Storage Diseases

Disease	Enzyme Deficiency	Major Accumulating Metabolites
Glycogenosis		
Type 2 Pompe's disease	α-Glucosidase	Glycogen
Sphingolipidoses		
GM$_1$-gangliosidosis:	GM$_1$-ganglioside	GM$_1$-ganglioside,
Type 1—infantile, generalized	β-galactosidase	galactose-containing oligosaccharides
Type 2—juvenile		
GM$_2$-gangliosidosis:		
Tay-Sachs disease,	Hexosaminidase A	GM$_2$-ganglioside
Sandhoff-Jatzkewitz disease	Hexosaminidases A and B	GM$_2$-ganglioside, globoside
Sulfatidoses:		
Metachromatic leukodystrophy	Aryl sulfatase A	Sulfatide
Multiple sulfatase deficiency	Aryl sulfatases A, B, C; steroid sulfatase; iduronate sulfatase, heparan N-sulfatase.	Sulfatide, steroid sulfate, heparan sulfate, dermatan sulfate
Krabbe's disease	Galactocerebroside β-galactosidase	Galactocerebroside
Fabry's disease	α-Galactosidase	Ceramide trihexoside
Gaucher's disease:		
Infantile form	Total β-glucosidase	Glucocerebroside
Adult form	Membrane-bound β-glucosidase	Glucocerebroside
Niemann-Pick disease	Sphingomyelinase	Sphingomyelin
Farber's disease	Ceramidase	Ceramide
Mucopolysaccharidoses		
Hurler-Scheie syndrome	α-Iduronidase	Dermatan sulfate, heparan sulfate
Hunter's syndrome	Iduronate-sulfatase	Dermatan sulfate, heparan sulfate
Sanfilippo's syndrome:		
Type A	Heparan N-sulfatase-N-	Heparan sulfate
Type B	acetylglucose aminidase	Heparan sulfate
Morquio's syndrome	N-Acetylhexosamine-6-sulfate sulfatase	Keratan sulfate, chondroitin-6-sulfate
Maroteaux-Lamy syndrome	Aryl sulfatase B	Dermatan sulfate
β-Glucuronidase deficiency	β-Glucuronidase	Dermatan sulfate, heparan sulfate
Mucolipidoses		
I-cell disease & pseudo-Hurler polydystrophy	Cellular deficiency of many lysosomal enzymes; increased levels of same enzymes extracellularly	Mucopolysaccharide, glycolipid
Types 1 and 4	Unknown	Unknown

Table 3-3. (*Continued*)

Disease	Enzyme Deficiency	Major Accumulating Metabolites
Other Diseases of Complex Carbohydrates		
Fucosidosis	α-Fucosidase	Fucose-containing sphingolipids and glycoprotein fragments
Mannosidosis	Mannosidase	Mannose-containing oligosaccharides
Aspartylglycosaminuria	Aspartylglycosamine amide hydrolase	Aspartyl-2-deoxy-2-acetamidoglycosylamine
Other Lysosomal Storage Diseases		
Wolman's disease	Acid lipase	Cholesterol esters, triglycerides
Acid phosphatase deficiency	Lysosomal acid phosphatase	Phosphate esters

Source: Kolodny, E. H.   Lysosomal storage diseases. *N. Engl. J. Med. 294*: 1217, 1976.

    i. Perinatal insults to the developing brain may occur during labor, delivery, or the first several days of life. These may include hypoxic-ischemic injuries (often accompanied by intraventricular (periventricular) and/or subarachnoid hemorrhages, trauma, and infections) and toxic-metabolic disturbances. All perinatal injuries, with the possible exception of mechanical trauma, are more commonly seen in premature infants.

        (1) Periventricular hemorrhage, with intraventricular and subarachnoid extension, is essentially a disease of the premature infant. The majority of these infants die, but with the advent of CT scanning a significant number of patients with documented hemorrhages are known to survive. Hydrocephalus and chronic intellectual and motor disabilities are common complications.

        (2) Subarachnoid hemorrhage is also associated with hypoxic insults, and while more common in premature infants, occurs with significant frequency in full-term neonates as well. The immediate and long-term outcome is not bleak, as it is with intraventricular hemorrhage.

        (3) Acute subdural hemorrhage is uncommon in newborns but does occur in full-term infants, often following traumatic instrument deliveries. Subdural tap is indicated if this disorder is suspected.

        (4) Other important causes of permanent neurologic disability with onset during the perinatal period include meningitis, symptomatic hypoglycemia, and kernicterus.

    j. Postnatal factors in mental retardation include head trauma, CNS infections, hypoxic-ischemic insults, CNS neoplasms, and toxic-metabolic disturbances.

    k. Cerebral palsy. Chronic, nonprogressive motor disability, often associated with seizures and mental retardation, is commonly referred to as cerebral palsy and may be due to any of the above-mentioned perinatally determined factors, most often hypoxic-ischemic insults. This group of disorders may be classified by their neurologic signs into **spastic, choreoathetotic, ataxic,** and **mixed** varieties. Motor findings may evolve and not become manifest until the second year of life, making differentiation from a progressive neurologic disorder extremely difficult.

I. Demyelinating diseases

1. **Description.** Demyelinating diseases, of which the most common is **multiple sclerosis,** are discussed in detail in Chapter 13. When the disease becomes advanced, multiple lesions in the subcortical white matter may produce personality change, inappropriate emotional reactions, and intellectual deterioration. It is exceedingly rare, however, for multiple sclerosis to present as a dementia with no other associated abnormalities.

   Progressive multifocal leukoencephalopathy (PML) and **adrenal leukodystrophy** (Schilder's disease) are relatively rare demyelinating diseases, both of which may include dementia as a prominent feature. PML is usually associated with an underlying malignancy, most often lymphoma.

2. **Treatment** is outlined in Chapter 13. A dramatic reversal of the dementia in advanced demyelinating disease is unusual.

J. Intracranial space-occupying lesions

1. **Description.** Masses within the cranial cavity may produce dementia by directly destroying or compressing the brain, by producing increased intracranial pressure, or by producing hydrocephalus. Intracranial masses are found in some cases of dementia. Any mass within the cranial cavity may produce dementia, but the most common masses are primary brain tumors, brain abscesses, and chronic subdural hematomas. The specific clinical picture of each of these conditions is covered elsewhere in this book, but all should be diagnosable using the combination of history, physical examination, and CT scan.

2. **Treatment** varies according to the underlying condition but, in general, improvement of the dementia depends on surgical removal of the mass.

IV. SYSTEMIC DISEASES WITH CEREBRAL PATHOLOGY

A. Nutritional

1. Pellagra

a. **Description.** Pellagra is caused by nicotinamide (niacin) deficiency, although, as in most B-vitamin deficiency states, it is usually accompanied by signs of other B-vitamin deficiency diseases. It is seen in association with chronic alcoholism, dietary peculiarities, hyperthyroidism, pregnancy, and the stress of injury or surgical procedures. In the advanced state it is characterized by the classic "three Ds"—dermatitis, diarrhea, and dementia. Its earliest symptoms are often referable to the nervous system and include irritability, insomnia, weakness, memory loss, and paresthesias. Some patients may show a true dementia, but most show a confusional state. Irreversible intellectual deterioration may occur in untreated patients.

b. **Treatment.** Nicotinamide (Niacin) 500 mg PO daily for 7–10 days; then 50–100 mg PO daily until symptoms have ameliorated. The minimum daily requirement to prevent disease is 5–10 mg, depending on the patient's age.

2. Wernicke-Korsakoff disease

a. **Description.** Thiamine (vitamin B_1) deficiency, usually caused by chronic alcoholism but also occasionally by starvation states, may produce two syndromes that are often seen together.

      (1) Wernicke's encephalopathy is an acute, life-threatening disease, covered in detail in Chapter 14.

      (2) Korsakoff's psychosis may be caused by many disorders including ruptured anterior communicating artery aneurysm, encephalitis, posterior cerebral artery strokes, and head trauma, but is often the result of chronic or recurrent thiamine deficiency in alcoholics. It is characterized by poor memory, confusion, disorientation, and tendency to confabulate.

   b. Treatment. The Wernicke-Korsakoff syndrome is treated with thiamine (see Chap. 14 for details). However, once severe Korsakoff's psychosis is well established, a dramatic response to thiamine therapy is not expected.

3. Vitamin B_{12} deficiency

   a. Description. The neurologic implications of vitamin B_{12} deficiency are complex and are covered in more detail in Chapter 14. Vitamin B_{12} deficiency may produce a frontal lobe type of dementia for unknown reasons, even before it produces any hematologic or spinal cord abnormalities. For this reason, all patients being evaluated for dementia should have a serum vitamin B_{12} determination as part of the initial laboratory work.

   b. Treatment. Vitamin B_{12} 1000 mg IM daily for 5 days; then 1000 mg IM monthly.

B. Chronic metabolic insults

  1. Description. The major syndromes of chronic metabolic insults that may lead to intellectual dysfunction include hypoglycemia, hypoxia, uremia, and hepatic failure. The acute neurologic syndromes associated with these abnormalities are described in Chapter 14. The degree of chronic intellectual loss is related to the degree of cerebral damage induced by the metabolic insult. Once metabolic derangement has been corrected, the patient may be left with a permanent intellectual deficit.

   a. Hypoglycemia and hypoxemia. A history of repeated episodes of transient neurologic deficits, often with seizures, suggests recurrent attacks of hypoglycemia or hypoxemia. The former is most often seen in insulin-dependent diabetics or occasionally in patients on oral hypoglycemic agents, while the latter may be due to a number of conditions including ischemic anoxia (e.g., cardiac arrest), anoxemic anoxia (e.g., pulmonary insufficiency, carbon monoxide poisoning), or cytotoxic anoxia (e.g., cyanide poisoning). In the chronic state hypoxemic and hypoglycemic encephalopathy are difficult to distinguish from one another, since both consist of varying degrees of focal neurologic deficits (e.g., hemipareses, aphasias, apraxias, hemianopsias) and dementia.

   b. Uremia and hepatic failure. The neurologic impairments in uremia and liver failure are similar, consisting of various mixtures of confusion, irritability, convulsions, tremor, asterixis, myoclonus, and peripheral neuropathy.

  2. Treatment. There is no effective treatment for the dementia of any of these metabolic abnormalities once it is established. The acute confusional state may be treated by administering the appropriate agent (i.e., glucose, O_2) or treating the underlying condition (i.e., renal failure, hepatic failure) as outlined in Chapter 14. The aim is to prevent recurrent or prolonged periods of metabolic insult and thus prevent the development or progression of intellectual dysfunction.

C. Endocrine

  1. Hypothyroidism

   a. Description. Hypothyroidism may occur at any age and may be either primary (thyroid failure) or secondary (anterior pituitary failure). Primary hypothyroidism dating from birth is known as *cretinism*. Secondary hypothroidism may occur at any age due to thyroid stimulating hormone (TSH) deficiency as a result of anterior pituitary failure.

(1) Cretinism may be evident at birth, but more commonly it becomes obvious in the first several months of life. The infant shows the characteristic facies (broad, flat nose with widely spaced eyes, coarse features, thick lips, protruding tongue); a hoarse cry, and an umbilical hernia. Early diagnosis is vital, since the degree of intellectual impairment is related to the age at which therapy is initiated. Cretinism is an important treatable, although rare, cause of mental retardation and should be considered in every evaluation of a mentally retarded child, even if the physical stigmata mentioned previously are absent.

(2) Adult hypothyroidism. In the older child and adult, hypothyroidism is manifested by puffy eyelids; alopecia of the outer third of the eyebrows; dry, rough skin; brittle, dry hair; induration and doughiness of the subcutaneous tissues; slurred speech and hoarse voice; constipation; anemia; increased sensitivity to cold; cerebellar ataxia; muscle weakness and slowed deep tendon reflexes; and intellectual dysfunction. This intellectual impairment may represent any one of a wide range of syndromes including hallucinations, disorientation, agitation and confusion ("myxedema madness"), and true dementia (memory loss, incontinence, and lowered IQ).

Myxedema coma is a medical emergency not appropriately covered in this discussion. However, milder forms of hypothyroidism may present as a dementia, so every patient initially evaluated for intellectual dysfunction should have a serum thyroxine measurement. A serum TSH level is often useful when the thyroxine is in the low borderline range, since it is usually elevated in primary hypothyroidism. Furthermore, a very low TSH in the presence of a clearly low thyroxine suggests secondary hypothyroidism. Such patients should be referred to an endocrinologist for further evaluation of anterior pituitary function and treatment.

b. Treatment of primary hypothyroidism

(1) Cretinism

(a) Sodium L-thyroxine (Synthroid) 0.025 mg/day, increased at weekly or biweekly intervals to 0.3–0.4 mg/day, **or**

(b) Thyroid (USP) 15 mg PO daily, gradually increased at weekly or biweekly intervals to about 90–180 mg/day.

(2) Adult hypothyroidism

(a) Sodium L-thyroxine (Synthroid) 0.025 mg/day increasing at weekly intervals to 0.1–0.2 mg/day, **or**

(b) Thyroid (USP) 15 mg PO daily, gradually increased at weekly or biweekly intervals until the euthyroid state is achieved (usually about 90–180 mg/day).

c. Treatment of secondary and tertiary hypothyroidism depends on detailed endocrine evaluation of pituitary and hypothalamic function, which is beyond the scope of this manual.

D. Toxic

1. Heavy metal poisoning. Several varieties of chronic heavy metal poisoning may present with dementia, including poisoning by lead (Pb), mercury (Hg), arsenic (As), manganese (Mn), and thallium (Th). The diagnosis and treatment of these conditions are covered in Chapter 14.

2. Drug intoxications

a. Alcohol

(1) **Frontal lobe degeneration** may rarely occur with chronic use of alcohol. The dementia produced is indistinguishable from that of the Alzheimer-Pick degenerative diseases described in this chapter. There is no specific therapy, although discontinuance of the use of alcohol may prevent progression of the disease.

(2) **Marchiafava-Bignami disease** is a rare complication of alcohol abuse characterized pathologically by degeneration of the corpus callosum. The disease is indistinguishable clinically from the Alzheimer-Pick–type dementia. There is no specific therapy, but discontinuation of alcohol usage is recommended to prevent further progression of the process.

b. Medications.
Many drugs are capable of producing mental deterioration suggestive of dementia. Most, however, produce a **toxic confusional state** easily distinguished from true dementia by such signs and symptoms as hallucinations, tachycardia, changes in blood pressure, diaphoresis, dysarthria, and nystagmus. Any patient with apparent dementia in whom drug usage is suspected should have toxic screening of the urine and/or blood, depending on the agents suspected. Treatment of the common drug intoxications is covered in Chapter 14.

V. PSYCHIATRIC DISEASES.
A number of psychiatric illnesses may result in intellectual dysfunction caused by either interference with motivation or actual impairment of intellect, or both.

A. Depression
may simulate dementia in many respects, including inability to carry out tests of intellectual function. A therapeutic trial of antidepressant medication is of little value diagnostically, since many patients with Alzheimer's disease may be depressed early in the course of the illness. A slight response to antidepressant therapy does not exclude the diagnosis of a degenerative dementing disease. On the other hand, a patient with an apparent dementia who actually is suffering only from depression may benefit greatly from the therapy and has a much better prognosis than the patient with a degenerative disease. It is often difficult clinically to distinguish depression from dementia, but some guidelines are valuable.

1. Depressed patients usually have insight that they are functioning poorly, unlike most demented patients.

2. "Frontal lobe signs" and apraxias are often seen in dementias but rarely in primary depression.

3. Careful testing reveals no memory impairment in primary depression, in contrast to dementia.

4. Incontinence is more common in dementia, although it may be seen in very severe depression as well.

B. Schizophrenia
was originally called *dementia praecox* by Kraepelin and it can, in fact, result in a dementing illness similar in many respects to Alzheimer's disease. The age of the patient is of considerable value in making this distinction, but Alzheimer's disease certainly occurs rarely in younger patients in the age group at risk for schizophrenia. Apraxias and aphasias, common components of Alzheimer's disease, are not seen in schizophrenia, but when these are absent the distinction may be more difficult than it initially seems. The course of the illness should help to make the distinction; the schizophrenia will wax and wane over many years, with only very slow deterioration of intellect, whereas Alzheimer's disease progresses inexorably, with development of unmistakable features within a few years.

SELECTED READING

Dementia

Barnett, R. E.   Dementia in adults. *Med. Clin. North. Am.* 56:1405, 1972.

Feldman, R. G., Chandler, K. A., Jerry, L. L., et al.   Familial Alzheimer's disease. *Neurology* 13:811, 1963.

Heston, L. L., Lowther, D. L. W., and Leventhal, C. M.   Alzheimer's disease. *Arch. Neurol.* 15:225, 1966.

Marsden, C. D., and Harrison, M. J. G.   Outcome of investigation of patients with presenile dementia. *Br. Med. J.* 2:249, 1972.

Pearce, J., and Miller, E.   *Clinical Aspects of Dementia.* London: Baillière, Tindall, 1973.

Pollack, M., and Hornabrook, R. W.   The prevalence, natural history and dementia of Parkinson's disease. *Brain* 89:429, 1966.

Saunders, V.   Neurologic manifestations of myxedema. *N. Engl. J. Med.* 266:547, 1962.

Steele, J. C., Richardson, J. C., and Olszewski, J.   Progressive supranuclear palsy. *Arch. Neurol.* 10:333, 1964.

Strachan, R. W., and Henderson, J. G.   Psychiatric syndromes due to avitaminosis B_{12} with normal blood and marrow. *Q. J. Med.* 34:303, 1965.

Terry, R. J.   Dementia: a brief and selective review. *Arch. Neurol.* 33:1, 1976.

Wells, C. E. (Ed.)   *Dementia.* 2nd Edition. Philadelphia: F. A. Davis, 1977.

Mental Retardation

De Myer, W.   Congenital Anomalies of the Central Nervous System, in D. B. Tower (Ed.), *The Nervous System.* New York: Raven Press, 1975. Pp. 347–357.

Holmes, L. B.   *Mental Retardation: An Atlas of Diseases with Associated Physical Abnormalities.* New York: Macmillan, 1972.

Kolodny, E. H.   Lysosomal storage diseases. *N. Engl. J. Med.* 294:1217, 1976.

Moser, H. W.   Biochemical Aspects of Mental Retardation, in D. B. Tower (Ed.), *The Nervous System.* New York: Raven Press, 1975. Pp. 369–379.

Salam, M. Z., and Adams, R. D.   Research in the Clinical Expressions and Pathologic Basis of Mental Retardation, in D. B. Tower (Ed.), *The Nervous System.* New York: Raven Press, 1975. Pp. 359–367.

Smith, D. W.   *Recognizable Patterns of Human Malformations: Genetic, Embryologic and Clinical Aspects.* Philadelphia: Saunders, 1970.

Warkany, J.   *Congenital Malformations.* Chicago: Year Book, 1971.

4
Dizziness

Howard D. Weiss

"Dizziness" is one of the most common complaints that people bring to their physicians. The dizziness itself is not life-threatening, but it can be extremely disabling, and sometimes it heralds the onset of potentially serious disease. Because a variety of disorders in the realms of otolaryngology, neurology, psychiatry, cardiology, ophthalmology, and hematology may lead to the complaint of dizziness, a systematic approach is necessary to reach the correct diagnosis and institute appropriate therapy. This chapter will first review the general evaluation of the dizzy patient and then discuss treatment of the individual disorders that cause dizziness. (See Figs. 4-1 and 4-2.)

I. **DEFINITIONS.** *Dizziness* is an ambiguous term that patients use to describe several entirely different subjective states. Therefore, it is imperative to obtain an accurate description of the patient's subjective experience using words more descriptive than *dizzy*. The complaint of dizziness generally can be divided into the following four categories; initial classification of a patient with dizziness in one of these categories is an important first step in arriving at the correct diagnosis.

A. **Vertigo** is defined as an illusion or sensation of rotation or movement of the patient or of his surroundings. The vertiginous movement may be described as spinning, whirling, tilting, or swaying. The presence of vertigo implies a disturbance at some point along the peripheral or central nervous system pathways of the vestibular apparatus. The examining physician should be aware, however, that some patients use the word *vertigo* synonymously with the generic term *dizzy*.

B. **Syncope** is a sense of impending loss of consciousness or fainting. Syncope is generally a manifestation of transient circulatory insufficiency to the brain, such as might occur in orthostatic hypotension, hypersensitive carotid sinus syndrome, cardiac disease (e.g., bradycardia, ectopic tachycardias), or vasodepressor attacks. Thus, the implications of syncope are entirely different from those of vertigo and require both medical and cardiologic evaluation. (See Chap. 6 for more details.)

C. **Dysequilibrium,** or loss of balance without concomitant peculiar head sensations, occurs in some neurologic disorders. By depriving patients of adequate sensory information, **combined deficits** in proprioception, tactile sensation, vision, and/or vestibular function can produce a subjective feeling of dysequilibrium. Also, many patients with ataxia due to **cerebellar dysfunction** will describe their dysequilibrium as dizziness.

D. **Ill-defined or psychogenic dizziness.** Patients suffering from various **psychiatric disorders**—including hysterical neurosis, anxiety neurosis, and depression—often complain of dizziness. In these patients the complaint is usually of an ill-defined lightheadedness, faintness, or fear of falling that is distinct from vertigo (sense of motion), dysequilibrium (loss of balance), or syncope (faint). In many such instances the symptoms of dizziness are precipitated by acute episodes of hyperventilation (*hyperventilation syndrome*).

II. **CLINICAL EVALUATION OF PATIENTS WITH VERTIGO.** Patients with vertigo must be carefully evaluated to distinguish between peripheral disorders and central disorders of the vestibular system. The standard neuro-otologic testing procedures are as follows.

A. **Dizziness simulation battery.** It is often helpful to put the patient through a series of maneuvers that can trigger the various types of dizziness. This "dizziness

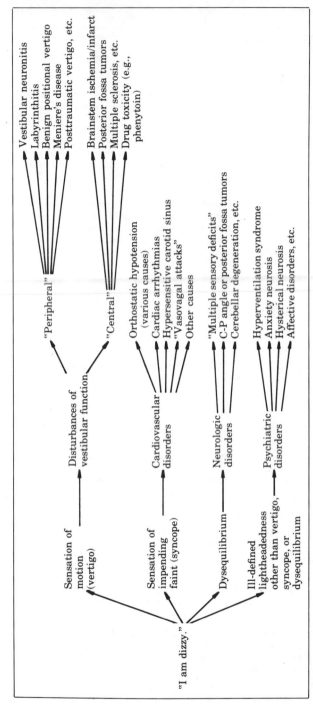

Fig. 4-1. Clinical spectrum of dizziness.

48

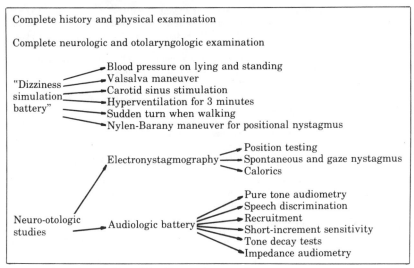

Fig. 4-2. Clinical evaluation of the dizzy patient.

simulation battery" helps the patient identify the sensation most closely resembling his own complaint. Six standard maneuvers are performed.

1. **Blood pressure** lying and standing (immediately and after 3 minutes).

2. A **Valsalva maneuver** (forced expiration for 15 seconds).

3. **Carotid sinus stimulation** (with ECG monitoring and appropriate cardiotonic drugs readily accessible).

4. Vigorous **hyperventilation** for 3 minutes.

5. **Sudden turns** when walking.

6. The **Nylen-Barany test** for positional vertigo (see sec **II.C**).

After each maneuver in the dizziness simulation battery the patient is asked if the sensation of dizziness (if any is elicited) matched his own complaint. In cases of hyperventilation syndrome, orthostatic hypotension, positional vertigo, and related disorders, these tests may exactly reproduce the patient's symptom and thereby yield important diagnostic information.

B. **Spontaneous nystagmus.** The vestibular and oculomotor systems are closely interrelated. Therefore, the spontaneous occurrence or the induction of nystagmus is a useful indicator of vestibular function or malfunction in patients with vertigo. Most **acute peripheral vestibular disorders** produce unidirectional nystagmus, with the slow phase beating toward the affected ear and the rapid phase beating away from the affected ear. The nystagmus increases in intensity as the eyes are deviated in the direction of the rapid component (i.e., toward the normal ear). Patients with **acute vestibular disorders** experience vertigo as a sensation that the *environment* is spinning in the direction of the fast component of the nystagmus, or that their *bodies* are spinning in the direction of the slow component. They tend to past-point and veer in the direction of the slow phase of their nystagmus (i.e., toward the diseased ear). When these patterns for nystagmus, vertigo, and past-pointing are not as described, the disorder *must* be located in the **central nervous system.**

For example, multidirectional nystagmus is more commonly seen in connection with drug intoxications or brainstem–posterior fossa disorders. Nystagmus that is present only on ocular fixation and absent when the eyes are closed is also typical of central nervous system disorders. Ocular fixation tends to abolish nystagmus of peripheral origin. Vertical nystagmus (particularly when persistent) is almost pathognomonic of brainstem or midline cerebellar disorders. **Hearing loss** and/or **tinnitus** frequently accompanies vestibular disorders due to coinvolvement of auditory apparatus; auditory symptoms are less common in central nervous system disorders.

C. **Positional vertigo and nystagmus.** Patients with vertigo often find that their problem is related to specific head positions or to the movement from one position to another. This phenomenon, called *positional vertigo,* can occur in disorders of the labyrinth or of the central nervous system; the Nylen-Barany test may be useful in making this important distinction. The test is performed by moving the patient from the sitting position to a lying position with the head extended 45 degrees backward. This maneuver is repeated with the head extended and turned to the right and then to the left. The patient is observed for the development of vertigo and nystagmus. The latency, duration, direction, and fatigability of the nystagmus reveal important diagnostic information (Table 4-1).

1. In positional vertigo due to **vestibular disorders:**

   a. There is a latent period of several seconds before the vertigo and nystagmus appear.

   b. The nystagmus is transient.

   c. Nystagmus decreases on repetition of the maneuver.

2. In positional nystagmus due to **brainstem and cerebellar abnormalities** (demyelination, brainstem ischemia, and posterior fossa tumors):

   a. The onset of nystagmus is immediate on assuming the provocative posture.

   b. The duration is prolonged.

   c. The response does not fatigue.

Table 4-1. Nylen-Barany Maneuver for Positional Nystagmus

Sign	Peripheral (Vestibular) Disorder	Brainstem–Posterior Fossa Disorder
Latent period before onset of positional nystagmus	2–20 sec	None
Duration of nystagmus	<1 min	>1 min
Fatigability	Nystagmus disappears with repetition of maneuver	Nonfatiguing
Direction of nystagmus in one head position	One direction	May change direction in a given head position
Intensity of vertigo	Severe	Slight or none
Head position	A single critical head position elicits vertigo	More than 1 position
Clinical examples	Benign positional vertigo	Acoustic neuroma, vertebro-basilar ischemia, multiple sclerosis

D. Caloric stimulation. Normal physiologic stimuli always affect both vestibular organs at the same time. Caloric stimulation is the most convenient clinical method of investigating the function of each labyrinth separately. The test is performed with the patient recumbent with his head flexed 30 degrees. In this position, with the horizontal semicircular canal perpendicular to the ground, the tympanic membrane in each ear is individually irrigated with cool water (30°C or ice water) and then with warm water (40°C).

Cool water induces a flow of endolymph that "turns off" the neural impulses from the horizontal canal on that side. This normally results in nausea and vertigo accompanied by horizontal nystagmus, with the slow component toward the side of cool-water stimulation and the fast component toward the contralateral side. These manifestations of cold-water irrigation are identical to the effects of a **vestibular destructive lesion** (e.g., vestibular neuronitis and labyrinthitis). **Warm water** causes the opposite effects, with the slow component of nystagmus away from, and the rapid component toward, the irrigated side.

The direction, duration, and amplitude of the nystagmus should be carefully observed. A reduced response in one ear implies a disorder in the vestibular labyrinths, vestibular nerve, or the vestibular nuclei on that side. The test should not be performed unless the tympanic membranes are intact.

E. Electronystagmography. The retina is electronegative to the cornea; thus, eye movements cause changing electric fields and currents. A technique known as electronystagmography (ENG) involves placing skin electrodes around the eye that can detect these changes and provide a means for objectively recording eye movements. The ENG provides quantitative data regarding direction, velocity, and duration of the eye movements in nystagmus. ENG is routinely used to record spontaneous nystagmus, positional nystagmus, and caloric-induced nystagmus, and it can also record nystagmus when the eyes are closed. Since ocular fixation often tends to suppress nystagmus, ENG recording with the eyes closed provides additional useful information that is not available on routine clinical examination.

F. Audiologic evaluation

   1. Pure tone audiometry. Because of the topographic-anatomic proximity of the vestibular and cochlear systems, audiologic testing often provides useful diagnostic information in patients with vertigo. Pure tone audiometry measures the listener's threshold of hearing as a function of the frequency and intensity of a sound stimulus. The threshold by air conduction is compared to that by bone conduction.

      a. If both air conduction and bone conduction are impaired to a similar degree (i.e., there is no "air-bone gap"), it strongly suggests that the disorder is *sensorineural* in nature, and the site of the lesion can be located somewhere central to the middle ear (i.e., cochlea or eighth nerve).

      b. Impaired air conduction with normal bone conduction implies a *conductive* hearing loss (e.g., otosclerosis).

      c. Mixed conductive and sensorineural hearing loss patterns also may be seen.

      c. Unfortunately, the pure tone audiogram usually does not distinguish sensorineural hearing loss of cochlear origin from that which is retrocochlear (eighth nerve) in origin. Since this distinction is a major focus of the audiologic evaluation of patients with vertigo, further audiometric testing is necessary (Table 4-2).

   2. Speech discrimination testing. There is often a markedly reduced ability to understand words (impaired *speech discrimination*) in ears affected by **retrocochlear lesions.** Cochlear lesions usually do not markedly reduce speech discrimination if the words are presented with suprathreshold intensity.

Speech discrimination testing consists of presenting monosyllabic words at suprathreshold intensity levels to one ear. The percentage of words that the listener repeats correctly is recorded. A useful rule of thumb has been that if the discrimination score (in percent) plus the speech reception threshold (in decibels) is less than 100, an eighth nerve lesion (e.g., acoustic schwannoma) should be suspected. If the sum is greater than 100, the lesion is probably cochlear.

3. **Recruitment.** In some cases loud sounds may seem to have the same intensity in the abnormal ear as in the normal ear. This phenomenon is referred to as *recruitment*. Recruitment commonly occurs with **cochlear** hearing deficits but usually not with retrocochlear lesions. The **alternate binaural loudness balance** (ABLB) test is a standard method for measuring recruitment and thus is useful in distinguishing cochlear from retrocochlear disorders.

4. **The short increment sensitivity index (SISI) test** was also devised to differentiate between cochlear and retrocochlear involvement on the basis of how the ear reacts to very small changes in sound intensity. Patients with **cochlear** deficits have an enhanced ability to perceive small increases in sound intensity and therefore will detect a high percentage (70–100%) of brief (200-msec) 1-decibel bursts of sound superimposed on a steady test tone. Patients with retrocochlear lesions (e.g., acoustic schwannoma) often detect fewer than 20% of these bursts. SISI scores in the 20–70% range are equivocal and of little localizing value.

5. **Tone decay.** When normal or cochlea-damaged ears are subjected to a long, steady tone, there is only a slight decrease in audibility of the sound (*tone decay*). **Retrocochlear** lesions (e.g., acoustic schwannoma) are sometimes associated with rapid and severe tone decay. Tone decay tests therefore form another useful part of the audiologic test battery (see Table 4-2).

Important: the combination of audiologic tests shows greater validity in predicting the site of a lesion than any single test does.

III. DIAGNOSIS AND TREATMENT OF DISEASES CAUSING VERTIGO

A. Vestibular neuronitis

1. **Description.** Vestibular neuronitis is characterized by a sudden and severe attack of vertigo, with nausea and vomiting. Spontaneous nystagmus occurs, with the rapid phase toward the normal ear, and there is reduced caloric excitability in the diseased ear. Positional nystagmus is present in one-third of cases. Tinnitus or a sensation of fullness in the ear occurs in about 40% of cases, but hearing remains unimpaired. Audiologic tests are normal. Except

Table 4-2. Audiologic Evaluation of Cochlear and Retrocochlear Disorders

	Cochlear Lesions	Retrocochlear (Eighth nerve) Lesions
Pure tone audiometry	Sensorineural hearing loss	Sensorineural hearing loss
Speech discrimination	Good	Poor
Recruitment	Yes	No
Short increment sensitivity index	Yes (70–100%)	No (<20%)
Tone decay	No	Yes
Clinical examples	Meniere's disease	Acoustic schwannoma

for some mild unsteadiness or lateral pulsion, there are no neurologic signs (e.g., diplopia, dysarthria, sensory loss, weakness) to suggest brainstem disease. The disorder mainly affects adults between the ages of 20 and 60 years. The vertigo resolves spontaneously over several days to weeks, but the patient may remain unsteady for several months. The disability from vestibular neuronitis lasts an average of four weeks. Follow-up studies reveal that about 60% of patients are not troubled by further attacks of vertigo, while the remainder have multiple episodes. The cause of vestibular neuronitis remains unknown. Many suspect a viral etiology, but this has not been proved. Careful neurologic and neuro-otologic examination, as outlined, indicates a "peripheral" disorder in patients with vestibular neuronitis and rules out the more ominous "central" disorders.

2. Treatment

a. Drugs. Since vestibular neuronitis is a **self-limited illness** of unknown cause, treatment is directed at suppressing the symptoms (Table 4-3).

The drugs listed in Table 4-3 are of approximately equal effectiveness in suppressing vertigo due to vestibular neuronitis, motion sickness, or other vestibular disorders. When **vomiting** is a severe problem, the antivertigo drugs can be administered via suppository or parenterally.

(1) Antihistamines

(a) Mechanism of action. Suppression of vertigo is not a general property of all antihistamines, and does not seem to correlate with their peripheral potency as histamine antagonists. The activity of those antihistamines that do counteract vertigo **(dimenhydrinate, diphenhydramine, meclizine, and cyclizine)** seems specific and not simply a matter of suppression of the brainstem vomiting center —many commonly used antiemetics are of little value in relieving patients with vertigo.

The drugs that can suppress vertigo are all effective in **antagonizing the effect of acetylcholine** in the central nervous system. In fact, the anticholinergic agent scopolamine was one of the first drugs found to be effective in preventing the vertigo and nausea of motion sickness. This central anticholinergic property may be the underlying biochemical mechanism of antivertigo activity, but this is unproved.

(b) Side effects. The major side effect of these agents is **sedation.** The ability to induce somnolence is somewhat more pronounced during therapy with dimenhydrinate or diphenhydramine. In severely vertiginous patients, sedation may be a desirable side effect. However, for patients who do not desire as much sedation, meclizine or cyclizine may be preferable.

Anticholinergic side effects, such as dry mouth or blurred vision, occasionally occur with these drugs. The relatively long half-life of meclizine enables the patient to take medication only once or twice a day as compared to three or more times per day with the other drugs.

(2) Belladonna alkaloids. For treatment of severe acute episodes of vertigo, some neurologists recommend the use of **scopolamine** 0.6 mg (PO or SQ) every 6 hours in addition to one of the other drugs listed in Table 4-3. The side effects (parasympathetic blockade) and contraindications for scopolamine therapy are similar to those for other belladonna alkaloids. **Scopolamine hydrobromide,** *not* scopolamine methylbromide, should be used, since the latter drug is a quaternary salt derivative that lacks central nervous system anticholinergic activity.

Table 4-3. Drugs Useful in the Symptomatic Treatment of Vertigo

Generic Name	Trade Name	Duration of Activity	Usual Oral Adult Dose	Relative Levels of Sedation	Other Modes of Administration
Buclizine	Bucladin-S	6–12 hr	50 mg B.I.D.	+	. . . .
Cyclizine	Marezine	4–6 hr	50 mg q6h	+	Rectal, IM
Dimenhydrinate	Dramamine	4–6 hr	50 mg q6h	++	Rectal, IM, IV
Diphenhydramine	Benadryl	4–6 hr	50 mg q6h	++	IM, IV
Diphenidol	Vontrol	4–6 hr	25–50 mg q6h	+	Rectal, IM, IV
Meclizine	Bonine, Antivert	12–24 hr	25–50 mg every morning	+	. . . .
Promethazine	Phenergan	4–6 hr	25 mg q6h	++	Rectal, IM, IV
Scopolamine	Aluscop, Bar-Don, Eldonal	4 hr	0.6 mg (1–2 tabs) q6h	+	SC, IV

(3) **Phenothiazines** comprise a large group of drugs with **antiemetic effects.** Not all antiemetics are effective antimotion sickness or anti-vertigo agents—for example, chlorpromazine (Thorazine) and pro-chlorperazine (Compazine) are highly effective against chemically induced nausea but are relatively ineffective against motion sickness. However, one widely used phenothiazine derivative, **promethazine** (Phenergan), also has significant antihistaminic properties. Promethazine has been the most effective phenothiazine for treating vertigo and motion sickness, ranking with the other antihistamines listed in Table 4-3. **Drowsiness** is the major limiting **side effect** in the use of promethazine; it is much less likely to induce acute dystonias or other extrapyramidal reactions than the other phenothiazines are.

b. **Other measures.** There are some simple maneuvers **the patient can perform** to lessen the sensation of vertigo.

(1) **Visual fixation** tends to inhibit nystagmus and diminish the subjective feeling of vertigo in patients with peripheral vestibular disorders, such as vestibular neuronitis. Fixing one's gaze on a nearby object, such as a picture or outstretched finger, may be preferred by the patient to lying down with his eyes closed.

(2) Since intellectual activity or mental concentration may facilitate vertigo, the discomfort is best minimized by **mental relaxation** coupled with intense visual fixation.

(3) **When vertigo is not relieved.** Many patients with acute peripheral vestibular disorders will not have dramatic symptomatic improvement as the result of any of the medications or maneuvers described. The patient feels acutely ill and may become extremely fearful of future attacks. Many physicians recommend **mild tranquilizers,** e.g., diazepam (Valium) or chlordiazepoxide (Librium) for these patients. However, an important aspect of therapy in the situation is a firm statement of **reassurance** that vestibular neuronitis, and most of the other acute vestibular disorders, are benign and self-limited conditions. The physician can tell the patient that the nervous system eventually adapts to an imbalance between the two vestibular end organs, and the vertigo ultimately stops. Even in disorders that permanently destroy one vestibular apparatus, the vertigo will diminish after several days as the brain begins to adapt. Such assurances greatly alleviate the patient's anxiety.

B. **Labyrinthitis**

1. **Bacterial (suppurative) labyrinthitis.** An active bacterial infection of the labyrinth (*suppurative labyrinthitis*) can occur in association with meningitis, mastoid disease, or middle ear disease with fistula. Severe vertigo, nausea, and vomiting are present, along with marked hearing loss. Fever, headache, or pain may or may not be present. *This is a potentially devastating disease.* Prompt diagnosis and administration of the appropriate antibiotics are the cornerstones of effective therapy (see Chap. 8).

2. **Viral labyrinthitis.** So-called viral labyrinthitis presents as a sudden onset of vertigo with some degree of hearing loss. Otoneurologic testing (calorics, electronystagmography, audiology) reveals a **peripheral lesion** (see sec II). Some cases have occurred in association with mumps and measles, leading to postulation of a viral etiology; however, in most cases the true etiology and pathology remain obscure. It seems appropriate to consider vestibular neuronitis and viral labyrinthitis in the same category. The vestibular symptoms and reduced caloric response usually return to normal spontaneously. **Treatment** is symptomatic, as outlined for vestibular neuronitis (see sec **III.A.2**). In

some cases the hearing loss persists and the disease progresses to recurrent episodes of vertigo, tinnitus, and hearing loss (see sec **III.E**).

C. Benign positional nystagmus and vertigo (Barany's vertigo)

  1. **Description.** Benign positional vertigo is probably the **most common vestibular syndrome** seen in clinical practice. Patients with this disorder do not have vertigo while sitting or standing still, but develop vertigo on turning the head into a particular plane. This commonly occurs when the patient is lying in bed and rolls over into the vulnerable position, at which time the room begins to spin. Benign positional vertigo occurs in middle age, perhaps somewhat more commonly in women.

  2. **Distinction from positional vertigo of central disorders.** Positional vertigo can also occur in a variety of conditions including serious brainstem disorders (e.g., multiple sclerosis, infarct, tumors) and drug intoxications (e.g., alcohol, barbiturates). The Nylen-Barany maneuvers help distinguish benign positional nystagmus from more ominous central conditions (see Table 4-1). In benign positional nystagmus there is a **latency period** of several seconds before the vertigo and nystagmus appear, and the nystagmus and vertigo are **transitory** and disappear on repetition of the provocative maneuver. These features clearly indicate a benign peripheral vestibular disorder and make further neurological investigation unnecessary. Some cases of benign positional vertigo follow head and neck injury (especially after temporal bone fracture), but in most instances the etiology is unknown.

  3. **Treatment.** Benign positional vertigo is generally self-limited, with disappearance of vertigo and nystagmus in a few weeks or months. Symptomatic treatment with one of the **anti–motion sickness drugs** (see Table 4-3) is often tried but is seldom of great benefit. Deliberately carrying out those movements that **provoke vertigo** will eventually "fatigue" the symptomatic response; some suggest that a remission of symptoms in benign positional vertigo can be accelerated by head exercises of this type, but this is uncertain. A few patients may experience symptomatic improvement by wearing a **soft cervical collar**—presumably the collar limits head movement so that the patient will be less likely to place his head in the provocative posture. As with vestibular neuronitis, the most important aspect of therapy is often **reassurance** to the patient that the condition is self-limited and does not represent a life-threatening illness.

D. Posttraumatic vertigo. Trauma to the head and neck is followed by vertigo in 25–50% of cases. The more severe the head injury and the closer the trauma to the labyrinth, the more likely is posttraumatic vertigo to occur. (It should be remembered that transient autonomic disturbances, such as palpitations, flushing, and sweating, also occur after head trauma and can produce lightheaded and "dizzy" sensations other than vertigo.) The posttraumatic vertigo syndromes fall into two main categories.

  1. **Acute posttraumatic vertigo.** Vertigo, nausea, and vomiting may begin acutely after head injury, due to sudden unilateral vestibular paresis (labyrinthine concussion).

    a. **Symptoms.** The **vertigo is constant.** There is **spontaneous nystagmus** with the rapid component beating away from the affected side; **loss of balance**; and **past-pointing** toward the affected side. The symptoms and signs are aggravated by rapid head motion and worsened with the affected side down.

    b. **Treatment** with one of the anti–motion sickness drugs (see Table 4-3) is often effective in diminishing the unpleasant symptoms. For the acute episode, scopolamine 0.6 mg PO or parenterally is often most efficacious. For more long-term oral therapy, both meclizine and dimenhydrinate have been widely used. The symptoms spontaneously improve over the first few days and then more gradually over the ensuing weeks. In most instances the patient is asymptomatic within 1 to 3 months.

2. **Posttraumatic positional vertigo.** The second syndrome is the development after head trauma of positional vertigo that may not begin until a few days or weeks after the injury. Positional vertigo often appears as the constant vertigo resolves.

   a. **Symptoms.** The symptoms are identical to those outlined for benign positional nystagmus and vertigo (see sec **III.C.1**). It is thought that in most cases the symptoms are due to labyrinthine rather than brainstem injury. Longitudinal fractures of the temporal bone are often associated with positional nystagmus.

   b. **Prognosis.** Posttraumatic positional vertigo usually resolves within 6 months, but in some cases the condition may become permanent. If the vertigo is not gone after 2 years, it will usually be permanent. In some rare cases when the disability is great, unilateral vestibular destruction or denervation of the affected side may be indicated to relieve symptoms.

E. **Meniere's disease**

1. **Description.** Some clinicians use the term *Meniere's disease* to describe any case of recurrent episodes of vertigo. However, true Meniere's disease occurs much less commonly than vestibular neuronitis or benign positional vertigo, and it also carries a much less favorable prognosis. Therefore, the diagnosis of Meniere's disease should be reserved for the specific clinical syndrome described below.

   Meniere's disease commonly has its onset in the third or fourth decade. The typical **signs** and **symptoms** of Meniere's disease include episodes of nausea and vertigo, tinnitus, a sensation of fullness or pressure in the ear, and fluctuating hearing loss. The tinnitus, pressure, and hearing loss often gradually build up before the attack of vertigo. The acute vertigo with nausea and vomiting usually lasts only a few hours, after which the patient makes a prompt recovery and regains otologic function. Some patients complain of constant instability between spells of vertigo.

   The **course of the disease** is characterized by remissions and relapses. Early in the disease there are often sporadic episodes of low-tone sensorineural hearing loss, with hearing returning to normal between attacks. As a result of multiple attacks, hearing loss becomes progressively worse, with some spontaneous fluctuations. In a few cases there may initially be a fluctuating hearing loss without vertigo, or vertigo without hearing loss, making correct clinical diagnosis very difficult. Meniere's disease is usually unilateral, but bilateral involvement occurs in up to 30% of cases. After 5 years of unilateral Meniere's disease, the likelihood of involvement of the second ear is markedly reduced.

2. **Differential diagnosis**

   a. All patients with clinical signs and symptoms of Meniere's disease should be evaluated to exclude the possibility of a **cerebellopontine angle tumor** (e.g., acoustic schwannoma). A battery of audiologic tests (pure tone audiometry, speech discrimination, SISI, tone decay) is helpful in distinguishing Meniere's disease from retrocochlear lesions (see Table 4-2). Skull x-rays and polytomograms of the internal auditory meatus also should be obtained routinely to evaluate possible asymmetry, which often occurs due to bony erosion by acoustic schwannoma. In cases in which a cerebellopontine angle tumor is even remotely suggested, further studies (e.g., CT scan, contrast studies) are indicated.

   b. **Congenital syphilis** can produce symptoms that mimic Meniere's disease. The onset of hearing difficulty is often delayed to middle age in cases of congenital syphilis; therefore, all patients with symptoms suggesting bilateral Meniere's disease also should be evaluated by the syphilis fluorescent antibody absorption test.

c. A small number of patients with symptoms of Meniere's disease will have **hypothyroidism** or **adrenal insufficiency** as an underlying disorder. Endocrine function should be evaluated, as hormonal replacement occasionally can ameliorate the labyrinthine symptoms in cases of myxedema.

3. **Treatment.** The basic pathologic change in many cases of Meniere's disease is hydropic degeneration within the endolymphatic scala—hence the term *endolymphatic hydrops.* Although theories abound, the true mechanism underlying these pathologic changes remains unclear. In view of this uncertainty regarding the pathogenesis, together with the unpredictable clinical course (which may include prolonged spontaneous remissions), it is not surprising that it has been difficult to formulate or evaluate a rational pharmacologic program for the treatment of Meniere's disease. One recent study found that all forms of treatment, including placebos, resulted in approximately two-thirds of patients being temporarily relieved of their symptoms. Unfortunately, *the only rational medical treatment for acute exacerbations of Meniere's disease is symptomatic therapy with one of the anti–motion sickness drugs* (see Table 4-3).

A low-sodium diet and the use of diuretics (e.g., thiazides or acetazolamide) have been advocated in Meniere's disease, based on the theory that these might correct an alleged fluid imbalance in the inner ear. The physiologic rationale for this therapy has never been demonstrated, and the popularity of diuretic–low-salt therapy has justifiably declined. Attention has recently been focused once again on diet, with allegations that food allergies may produce symptoms of Meniere's disease. The published data favoring this concept are at best anecdotal. In the past, a variety of vitamins, coenzymes, bioflavinoids, and trace elements have been advocated for treating Meniere's disease. Despite initial enthusiasm for all these agents, controlled studies indicated that they are not superior to placebo. Vasodilators, including nicotinic acid, isoxsuprine, papaverine, intravenous histamine, and betahistine, have been advocated for acute exacerbations of Meniere's disease. This therapy has been based on the questionable concept of "angiospastic vascular change" or "labyrinthine ischemia" as the underlying pathophysiologic factor in this disease. None of these agents is superior to placebo, and all are potentially toxic. The use of vasodilators is not recommended for Meniere's disease or other labyrinthopathies.

4. **Surgery for intractable disease.** Some patients with Meniere's disease will have recurrent uncontrollable and disabling attacks of vertigo. In these severe refractory cases, surgery may be necessary. When there is no useful hearing remaining in the diseased ear, a **destructive labyrinthectomy** is indicated to relieve symptoms. If some useful hearing remains in the diseased ear, a selective procedure such as **ultrasound labyrinthectomy** or **endolymphatic shunt** can be performed. Ultrasound labyrinthectomy relieves the vertigo in about 80% of patients, with only about a 10% chance of surgery-induced hearing loss. Endolymphatic shunt and sacculotomy operations stop the hearing loss and vertigo in about two-thirds of patients. **Streptomycin ablation** of the vestibular labyrinths is effective in abolishing vertigo in patients with persistent bilateral disease.

Symptoms often return several years following ultrasound labyrinthectomy, endolymphatic shunt, or streptomycin treatment.

F. **Congenital syphilis**

1. **Description.** Symptoms typical of Meniere's disease can occur in patients with late congenital syphilis, in whom onset of deafness is often delayed until middle age. Treponemal organisms can persist in the temporal bone, causing a chronic inflammatory process that results in labyrinthitis with endolym-

phatic hydrops and degeneration of the membranous labyrinth. The course is progressive, with ultimate involvement of both ears. The diagnosis is confirmed by obtaining a positive syphilis fluorescent antibody absorption test. It has been estimated that as many as 7% of patients presumed to have Meniere's disease actually have congenital syphilis. *All* patients suspected of having bilateral Meniere's disease should be evaluated for the possibility of occult syphilis.

2. **Treatment.** The generation time of the spirochete in late syphilis is quite prolonged, and long-term antibiotic therapy is important. Penicillin alone brings about significant improvement in only about 25% of cases, while penicillin plus prednisone (to reduce inflammation) results in improvement in about 50% of cases. Thus, this combined therapy seems to offer the best chance of benefit. The risks of penicillin and steroid therapy must be weighed against the disability produced by progressive discriminatory hearing loss. **Typical treatment regimens** include:

   a. **Benzathine penicillin** 2.4 million units IM once a week for 3 months, along with prednisone 60 mg every other day, or

   b. **High-dose ampicillin** 1.5 gm PO QID for 2 months, along with prednisone 60 mg every other day.

G. Acoustic schwannoma and other cerebellopontine angle tumors

1. **Description**

   a. **Schwannomas**—tumors of Schwann cells—commonly arise from the eighth cranial nerve in the internal auditory canal. Patients usually present with progressive unilateral hearing loss and/or tinnitus. Most patients do not complain of vertigo but rather of a dizzy feeling described as dysequilibrium, or imbalance. Later, ipsilateral facial hypalgesia, diminished corneal reflex, decreased taste, facial weakness, and ataxia occur as the tumor extends out of the internal auditory meatus.

   b. **Meningiomas** and other neoplasms also may occur in the cerebellopontine angle and produce similar symptoms. If these tumors are diagnosed early, they can be cured surgically. If the diagnosis is delayed until the tumor is large (> 2 cm), surgical cure becomes more difficult or impossible.

2. **Evaluation.** Unresectable acoustic schwannomas are often fatal. Therefore, all patients with unilateral sensorineural hearing loss, including patients who seem to have Meniere's disease, should undergo evaluation to exclude the possibility of an acoustic schwannoma. As a general rule, any vestibular abnormality in combination with sensorineural hearing loss places the patient into the "highly suspicious" category.

   a. Thorough **neurologic examination,** including testing corneal reflexes and testing taste over the anterior two-thirds of the tongue, is valuable for uncovering early signs of an enlarging cerebellopontine angle tumor.

   b. The **audiologic battery** is useful in distinguishing cochlear disease from retrocochlear lesions, such as acoustic schwannoma (see Table 4-2). Classic findings in retrocochlear lesions include poor speech discrimination in relation to pure tone threshold; no recruitment; tone decay; and poor short increment sensitivity.

   c. About 80–90% of patients with acoustic schwannoma have **reduced caloric response** on the side of the lesion as measured by electronystagmography (ENG).

   d. **Polytomography** of the internal auditory meati has an excellent chance of detecting a significant asymmetry. **CT scan** with contrast enhancement will reveal the presence of many cerebellopontine angle tumors. Finally, when the index of suspicion warrants further evaluation, a **positive contrast study** of the posterior fossa is more sensitive than pneumoencephalography or arteriography for demonstrating small acoustic schwannomas.

3. **Treatment.** For details on the treatment of acoustic schwannomas and other cerebellopontine angle tumors, see Chapter 11.

H. Brainstem ischemia

1. Description

a. **Vertigo** is the most frequent symptom in patients with vertebro-basilar disease and transient episodes of brainstem ischemia; it will be the only symptom of transient brainstem ischemia in about 20% of cases.

b. The **other signs** and **symptoms** of brainstem ischemia that most frequently follow are dysarthria, facial numbness, ataxia, hemiparesis, diplopia, and other visual disturbances. Decrease in hearing is rare in brainstem vascular disease, but it can occur with occlusion of the anterior inferior cerebellar artery (which usually supplies the inner ear by giving rise to the internal auditory artery).

c. It is extremely important to distinguish patients with episodes of transient brainstem ischemia from patients with "benign" disorders, such as vestibular neuronitis, in order to initiate therapy to avert a serious brainstem stroke (see Chap. 10).

d. The hallmark of transient brainstem ischemia is the **absence of signs of residual damage between attacks.** However, careful neurologic examination during or after an attack of vertigo can reveal subtle signs—such as a mild Horner's syndrome, skew deviation, internuclear ophthalmoplegia, or vertical nystagmus—that clearly localize the abnormality to the brainstem and not to the vestibular apparatus. Positional nystagmus is often elicited in patients with brainstem ischemia. The Nylen-Barany maneuvers may be helpful in distinguishing brainstem from vestibular disorders (see Table 4-1).

2. **Treatment.** The treatment of transient brainstem ischemia is reviewed in Chapter 10. Other disorders affecting the brainstem, such as multiple sclerosis (Chap. 13) and tumors (Chap. 11), also commonly produce vertigo or dysequilibrium.

I. **Drug-induced vertigo.** Intoxication with a variety of agents can produce vertigo and other labyrinthine symptoms (Fig. 4-3).

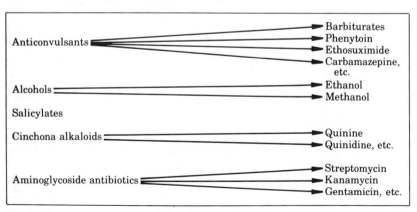

Fig. 4-3. Common causes of drug-induced vertigo.

1. **Anticonvulsants.** Most of the commonly used **anticonvulsant drugs** (e.g., phenobarbital, phenytoin, ethosuximide, and carbamazepine) will produce vestibulo-ocular signs (e.g., nystagmus, vertigo) and ataxia as blood levels approach the toxic range. Similar symptoms are a frequent feature of **alcohol intoxication.** In both instances, the vertigo and ataxia will disappear if the drugs are withheld, thereby allowing the blood levels to fall below the toxic range.

2. **Salicylates.** Tinnitus and vertigo are among the earliest signs of salicylate intoxication. Hearing loss may also occur, and its severity seems to be closely correlated with the blood salicylate level. When these symptoms appear in patients receiving chronic large doses of salicylates, it is an indication for discontinuing or reducing the dosage. The vestibular symptoms and hearing loss are reversible within two or three days after withdrawal of the drug.

3. **Aminoglycosides. Labyrinthine damage** is sometimes a serious complication of therapy with aminoglycoside antibiotics (e.g., streptomycin, amikacin, gentamicin, kanamycin, neomycin). About 75% of patients receiving 2 gm of streptomycin per day for over two months will develop some evidence of vestibular damage. Reducing the dose to 1 gm per day decreases the incidence to 25%.

   a. Initial symptoms are usually **nausea, vertigo,** and **dysequilibrium.** This is followed by a compensatory phase in which the imbalance is latent and appears only when the patient closes his eyes. The toxic effects of streptomycin and gentamicin are greater on the vestibular than on the auditory function of the eighth cranial nerve. Kanamycin and neomycin have greater toxic effects on auditory function than on vestibular function: a high-pitched tinnitus accompanied by high-frequency hearing loss occurs earliest, followed by impairment in lower sound ranges and difficulty in comprehending conversation.

   b. There is no specific **treatment** for the labyrinthine damage. Symptoms may begin to abate within a few days of stopping the antibiotic therapy; however, full recovery may take over a year, and some patients will have residual impairment of function.

   c. Several **precautions** can prevent serious aminoglycoside ototoxicity. The **total daily dose, duration of therapy,** and **drug blood levels** should be closely monitored. This is especially important in patients in whom there is renal insufficiency that interferes with the excretion of these drugs. All patients receiving aminoglycoside antibiotics should have frequent evaluation of their vestibular and auditory function. The medication should be stopped when impairment first appears.

IV. HYPERVENTILATION SYNDROME AND PSYCHOGENIC DIZZINESS

A. **Hyperventilation syndrome.** A surprisingly high proportion of patients who come to the physician complaining of dizziness suffer from episodes of the hyperventilation syndrome. **Anxiety** or related emotional disturbance triggers the attacks.

   1. **Description.** Hyperventilation results in hypocapnia, alkalosis, increased cerebrovascular resistance, and decreased cerebral blood flow. The patient complains of an **ill-defined lightheadedness,** often in association with circumoral or digital paresthesias, breathlessness, sweating, trembling, palpitations, and panic ("acute anxiety attack"). Of great aid in diagnosis, as well as in therapy, is the demonstration to the patient that the symptoms can be reproduced by voluntary hyperventilation for 3 minutes.

   2. **Treatment. Prophylactic therapy** of the hyperventilation syndrome is based on the reassurance to the patient that these attacks do not represent a serious or life-threatening illness. **Acute episodes** of hyperventilation syndrome can

be terminated by having the patient breathe into an oxygen rebreathing mask without turning on the oxygen (thereby allowing rebreathing of exhaled carbon dioxide and preventing the hypocapnia and alkalosis).

B. Psychogenic dizziness

1. **Description.** Some patients with neuroses or psychoses complain of dizziness that does not fit any recognizable condition such as vertigo, syncope, or dysequilibrium and is not reproduced by any of the maneuvers in the dizziness simulation battery. Dizziness is a symptom in over 70% of patients with **anxiety neurosis** and in over 80% of patients with **hysterical neurosis.** The dizziness in these patients has often been present for years and may be continuous rather than episodic. Many of these patients equate dizziness with loss of energy, difficulty concentrating, and mental fuzziness.

2. **Management**

    a. The management of patients with psychogenic dizziness is based on **reassurance.** Patients often resent the implication that their syndrome may be psychological, so it is insufficient merely to tell the patient that there is nothing wrong physically—the patient will continue to worry about serious medical illness and will go "doctor-shopping." Therefore, the physician should describe the psychiatric syndrome to the patient in lay terms. Such an explanation relieves many patients and makes them receptive to further reassurances.

    b. The **minor tranquilizers** of the benzodiazepine family (e.g., diazepam, chlordiazepoxide, oxazepam) may be useful in treating anxiety symptoms. However, drugs that are subject to misuse, such as the shorter-acting barbiturates, should be avoided in patients with anxiety or hysterical neuroses. When **depressive symptoms** are prominent, the tricyclic antidepressant agents are often helpful in relieving symptoms.

SELECTED READING

Brand, J. J., and Perry, W. L. M.   Drugs used in motion sickness—a critical review. *Pharmacol. Rev.* 18:895, 1966.

Drachman, D. A., and Hart, C. W.   An approach to the dizzy patient. *Neurology* 22:323, 1972.

Fields, W. S., and Alford, B. R. (Eds.).   *Neurologic Aspects of Auditory and Vestibular Disorders.* Springfield, Ill.: Thomas, 1964.

Roydhouse, N.   Vertigo and its treatment. *Drugs* 7:297, 1974.

Weiss, A. D.   Neurologic aspects of the differential diagnosis of vertigo. *Ann. Otol. Rhinol. Laryngol.* 77:216, 1968.

Weiss, A. D.   Central vestibular diagnosis—neurologic examination. *Ann. Otol. Rhinol. Laryngol.* 82:852, 1973.

Wolfson, R. J. (Ed.).   Symposium on Vertigo. *Otolaryngol. Clin. North Am.* 6:1, 1973.

5
Backache

I. **GENERAL APPROACH TO THE PATIENT WITH BACKACHE.** Backache is an extremely common symptom with many possible causes. Proper therapy, therefore, depends heavily on making the correct diagnosis. All patients complaining of backache should have the following **minimum evaluation:**

A. **History,** with special reference to:

1. **Location** of the pain

2. **Radiation** of the pain

3. **Body position** that brings exacerbation or relief

4. **Trauma**

5. **Litigation**

6. **Drugs** used for pain, and amounts required for relief

7. **Malignancy**

B. **Physical examination,** with special reference to:

1. Signs of **systemic infection**

2. Signs of **occult malignancy**

3. Local **tenderness,** or tenderness in sciatic notch

4. **Muscle spasm**

5. **Range of motion**

6. **Straight-leg raising**

7. **Rectal examination** (prostate sphincter tone)

C. **Neurologic examination,** with special reference to:

1. **Affect** and mood

2. **Muscle weakness,** atrophy, or fasciculations

3. **Sensory loss** including the perineum

4. **Reflexes** (deep tendon, abdominal, anal, cremasteric)

D. **Laboratory**

1. **X-ray** (posteroanterior, lateral, and oblique)

2. **CBC** and **ESR**

3. **Serum,** for:

a. Creatinine

b. Ca^{++}

c. Po_4

d. Alkaline phosphatase

e. Uric acid

f. Acid phosphatase (men only)

g. Fasting blood sugar

E. **Further studies** (e.g., bone scan, 2-hour postprandial blood sugar, and myelography) depend on the results of the above screening procedure. Usually this thorough basic evaluation will reveal the cause of the pain, and one can categorize the problem into one of the following diagnostic groups:

II. DISC SYNDROMES

A. **Pathophysiology.** The **intervertebral disc** serves the dual purpose of articulation, allowing flexibility of the spine, and cushioning, acting as a shock absorber to prevent damage to the bones.

   1. **Herniation,** or **rupture,** of an intervertebral disc refers to protrusion of the nucleus pulposus along with some part of the anulus into the spinal canal or intervertebral foramen. Because the anterior longitudinal ligament is much stronger than the posterior longitudinal ligament, disc herniation almost always occurs in a posterior or posterolateral direction. The material usually bulges as a solid mass and retains continuity with the body of the disc, although at times fragments may protrude through the posterior longitudinal ligament, break off, and lie free in the spinal canal.

   2. Some controversy exists concerning the **factors that lead to rupture** of the intervertebral disc. Many cases can be related to trauma, either acute severe injury or, more commonly, repeated minor injuries secondary to bending and lifting. Another contributing factor seems to be the degenerative changes in the disc that occur with aging: shrinkage of the nucleus pulposus and thickening of the anulus fibrosus. Disc herniation occurs most commonly in the lumbar region, followed next in frequency by cervical disc rupture. Thoracic disc herniation is distinctly uncommon.

B. **Lumbar disc herniation**

   1. **Clinical description.** Lumbar disc herniation is most common in adult white males, reaching a peak incidence in the fourth and fifth decades. It seems to occur more frequently in those whose occupation involves bending and lifting. Because the posterior longitudinal ligament in the lumbar region is stronger in its central portion, protruded discs tend to occur in a posterolateral direction, with compression of the nerve roots.

      a. **Areas affected**

         (1) The **last two lumbar interspaces** (L4-5 and L5-S1) are most commonly affected, particularly L5-S1. L3-4 is the next most common site. Rupture of higher lumbar discs is rare and almost always the result of massive trauma.

         (2) Because of the anatomic relationships in the lumbar spine, a protruding disc usually compresses the nerve root emerging one level below it. The most common disc syndromes of **nerve root compression** are presented in Table 5-1. However, this anatomic arrangement is by no means invariable. Thus, although the nerve roots affected by a disc can be clinically identified, the exact level of the protruded disc cannot always be localized with great certainty.

         (3) If there is a **free disc fragment,** it usually affects the root emerging above the herniated disc.

      b. **Development of symptoms.** More than half of the patients will date their symptoms to some type of trauma, either a hard fall or a twisting or bending stress.

         (1) The **initial complaint** is usually a dull, aching, often intermittent low back pain of gradual onset, although at times the pain is of sudden onset and severe. This pain is felt to be secondary to stretching of the posterior longitudinal ligament, since the disc itself probably pos-

Table 5-1. Symptoms and Signs in Lateral Rupture of Lumbar Disc

Disc	Root	Pain and Paresthesias	Sensory Loss	Motor Loss	Reflex Loss
L3-4	L4	Anterior surface of thigh, inner surface of shin	Anteromedial surface of thigh, extending down along shin to inner side of foot	Quadriceps	Knee jerk
L4-5	L5	Radiating down outer side of back of thigh and outer side of calf, and across dorsum of foot to great toe	Usually involves outer side of calf and the great toe	Extensor hallucis longus; less commonly, muscles of dorsiflexion and eversion of foot	None
L5-S1	S1	Radiating down back of thigh and outer side and back of calf, to foot and the lesser toes	Almost always involves outer side of calf, outer border of foot, and the lesser toes; less commonly, the back of the thigh	Gastrocnemius, and occasionally muscles of eversion of foot	Ankle jerk

sesses no pain fibers. Characteristically the pain is **aggravated** by activity or exertion, and by straining, coughing, or sneezing. It is usually **relieved** by lying on the unaffected side with the painful leg flexed. Often there is reflex spasm of the paravertebral muscles that causes pain and prevents the patient from standing fully erect.

(2) Course of symptoms. After a variable period of time, an aching pain begins in the buttocks and posterior or posterolateral aspect of the thigh and leg on the affected side, usually termed **sciatica.** This is often accompanied by numbness and a tingling that radiates into the part of the foot served by the sensory fibers of the affected root. These symptoms may be elicited by **Lesegue's test:** straight-leg raising with the patient lying prone. In the normal patient, the leg can be raised to almost 90 degrees without pain, while in the patient with sciatica, characteristic pain is produced by elevations of 30–40 degrees. Eventually, loss of sensation, muscle weakness, and loss of reflexes may ensue (see Table 5-1).

(3) In the uncommon situation where a **midline disc protrusion** occurs in the presence of a narrow spinal canal in the lumbar region, **cauda equina compression** may result, with paraparesis and loss of sphincter tone. A pseudoclaudication syndrome has been described, with pain in the legs on exertion, secondary to intermittent compression of the nerves of the cauda equina. The pathophysiology is possibly ischemia.

2. Diagnostic tests

a. Routine x-rays of the spine (including oblique projections) are performed when disc disease is suspected. This is useful in ruling out congenital anomalies or deformities, involvement of the spine with rheumatic diseases, and metastatic or primary tumors. In the case of disc disease, the x-rays may be normal or may show degenerative changes with narrowing of the intervertebral space and osteophyte formation.

b. Serum levels of calcium, phosphate, alkaline and acid phosphatase, and glucose should be ascertained in every case, since metabolic bone disease, metastatic tumors to the spine, and diabetic mononeuritis may all imitate intervertebral disc disease.

c. Lumbar puncture. Although the cerebrospinal fluid may show mildly elevated protein in the presence of disc disease, lumbar puncture usually adds little to the diagnostic evaluation. If a complete spinal block is present, the protein may be very elevated with an abnormal Queckenstedt maneuver.

d. Neurophysiologic studies. Electromyography (EMG) may be normal in disc disease, or fibrillation potentials and positive sharp waves may be seen in muscles innervated by the affected root after a delay of a few weeks. EMG may at times be useful in differentiating root compression from peripheral neuropathy, since with root compression, conduction in the motor system is usually normal even in the presence of fasciculations and fibrillations, and sensory conduction is unimpaired. The Hoffmann (H) reflex may be delayed or absent.

e. Myelography. When the diagnosis of a disc syndrome is certain, and one is not concerned about the possibility of a cauda equina tumor or some other abnormality, myelography need not be performed unless surgery is contemplated. When this is the case, myelography is carried out to determine the level of disc protrusion.

f. Discography has not been found to be particularly helpful in evaluating disc disease, since the results are often difficult to interpret. Further, it has been suggested that the procedure itself may produce damage to the intervertebral disc.

3. Treatment

  a. Conservative treatment. The **majority of patients respond** to conservative therapy and do not require surgery.

    (1) In patients with **mild symptoms,** suggest:

      (a) Ways to avoid bending or straining; instruct the patient in this as well as in proper posture.

      (b) Resting in bed when pain is present, and avoidance of painful activities.

      (c) Application of heat to the low back area.

      (d) Analgesics as necessary.

      (e) Exercises designed to strengthen the erector spinae and abdominal muscles.

      (f) A **lumbar corset,** to prevent excessive motion of the lumbar area.

    (2) In patients with **severe incapacitating pain:**

      (a) Strict **bed rest** on a firm bed, in whatever position is most comfortable.

      (b) Supporting boards underneath the mattress are useful to provide a firm surface.

      (c) Analgesics are given during this period, as are **antispasmodic agents,** such as diazepam.

      (d) If the symptoms remit, activities are gradually increased after a week or so, and the patient is then treated as in the case of mild symptoms.

      (e) Pelvic traction has *not* been generally found to be effective except to help enforce strict bed rest.

    (3) Conservative therapy **should not be abandoned** until a trial of strict bed rest for 3–4 weeks has failed.

  b. Surgery. *Surgery is more likely to be successful when there are objective signs of neurologic impairment.* Surgery produces good to excellent results in approximately two-thirds of the cases; half of the remaining are improved. The **usual indications** for surgery are:

    (1) The most common indication for surgery is **failure to respond to conservative therapy.** The decision for surgery in this case must be made by the patient, with the guidance of the physician. Surgery is usually elected when the pain is severe, incapacitating, and unrelieved by conservative therapy, although at times the frequency of recurrences of less severe pain may lead some patients to choose surgery.

    (2) Surgery **without delay** is mandated in the uncommon situation in which a **midline disc compresses the cauda equina,** with pareparesis and sensory loss in the legs along with loss of sphincter control.

    (3) When **nerve root compression is associated with motor loss,** especially quadriceps weakness or foot-drop, surgery is usually indicated. Occasionally, mild weakness may remit with conservative therapy.

  c. Chemonucleolysis. Injection of the disc with chymopapain has been offered as a treatment for herniated discs and has met with some success in mild disc syndromes. However, chymopapain is no longer available in the United States for this purpose, thus eliminating this form of therapy for the present time.

C. Cervical disc herniation

1. **Clinical description.** Cervical disc rupture often follows a traumatic event after a variable period of time, but it frequently occurs without any preceding traumatic event.

   a. **Areas affected.** Cervical disc protrusion most commonly occurs at the C5-6 or C6-7 levels. In contrast to the lumbar region, the cervical posterior longitudinal ligament is weaker in its central portion, so the herniations may be midline posterior, compressing the cord, or posterolateral, with root compression. **Signs of cord compression** include spastic pareparesis and posterior column sensory loss in the legs, hyperactive leg reflexes, and bilateral Babinski responses. Table 5-2 summarizes the **root syndromes** resulting from cervical disc rupture.

   b. **Development of symptoms.** Symptoms usually begin with recurrent attacks of **pain** in the posterior cervical area, often accompanied by **muscle spasm** in the paravertebral muscles. Later the pain begins to radiate into the ipsilateral arm, with numbness and tingling in the distribution of the particular root involved. As with lumbar disc disease, the symptoms are usually aggravated by coughing, straining, or sneezing.

2. **Diagnostic tests and treatment.** The same guidelines for diagnostic evaluation presented for lumbar disc herniation (see sec **II.B.2**) apply in general to cervical disc disease as well. Oblique cervical spine x-rays are especially important, as are flexion-extension views, and polytomography may be helpful. The measures for **conservative therapy** of cervical disc include cervical traction in addition to the others outlined in the lumbar disc section (sec **II.B.3.a**). A soft cervical collar may be helpful. With regard to **surgery,** the previously mentioned indications for surgery for lumbar disc disease (see sec **II.B.3.b**) apply to cervical disc disease as well, but one should bear in mind that **cervical cord compression** can occur and requires **early surgery.**

D. Thoracic discs

1. **Clinical description.** This is the rarest type of disc protrusion, accounting for less than 1% of all herniated discs.

   a. **Areas affected.** The **lower four thoracic interspaces** are most frequently involved, with T11-12 being most commonly affected. Because the extradural space is narrower in the thoracic region than in any other area of the spine (and because the majority of the disc protrusions are central), **cord compression** is more likely to occur than in the other disc syndromes.

   b. **Development of symptoms.** At times the onset of symptoms is acute or subacute and associated with trauma, but **the majority have a chronic course** unassociated with trauma. Initially **back pain** is the most common symptom, occurring in the thoracic, lumbar, or sciatic region. Again, the pain is often aggravated by coughing, sneezing, or straining. Symptoms of **cord compression,** when they occur, arise from pressure on the cord or compromise of the arterial supply to the cord. **Paraplegia** may occur suddenly. When the herniation is lateral, the **root compression** may mimic pleurodynia, angina, or visceral pain, depending on the level.

2. **Diagnostic tests.** The diagnostic evaluation proceeds according to the guidelines in the section on lumbar discs (see sec **II.B.2**). Thoracic disc disease is more likely to be associated with **intervertebral disc calcification** than the

Table 5-2. Symptoms and Signs in Lateral Rupture of Cervical Disc

Disc	Root	Pain and Paresthesias	Sensory Loss	Motor Loss	Reflex Loss
C4-5	C5	Neck, shoulder, upper arm	Shoulder	Deltoid, biceps	Biceps
C5-6	C6	Neck, shoulder, lateral aspect of arm, and radial aspect of forearm to thumb and forefinger	Thumb, forefinger, radial aspect of forearm, lateral aspect of arm	Biceps	Biceps, supinator
C6-7	C7	Neck, lateral aspect of arm, and ring, and index fingers	Forefinger, middle finger, radial aspect of forearm	Triceps, extensor carpi ulnaris	Triceps, supinator
C7-T1	C8	Ulnar aspect of forearm and hand	Ulnar half of ring finger, little finger	Intrinsic muscles of the hand, wrist extensors	None

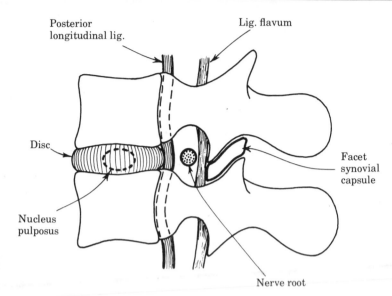

Fig. 5-1. The normal disc. The normal disc is composed of the central nucleus pulposus (a fibrogelatinous fluid), the cartilaginous plates covering the vertebral body surfaces, and the anulus fibrosus, which surrounds the nucleus pulposus and provides the bulk of the disc. The anterior and posterior longitudinal ligaments cover the respective surfaces of the disc.

other disc syndromes are, although the calcified interspace may not be the disc that has ruptured. If there are any signs of spinal cord involvement, **myelography** should be performed promptly, and usually films must be taken with the patient lying supine.

3. **Treatment.** Many patients with root compression alone will respond to **conservative treatment** (see sec **II.B.3**). However, when cord dysfunction is present, one must proceed with **surgery.** This is technically the most difficult area for back surgery, because of the narrow canal and the usual central herniation. Surgical results are probably best with the anterior transthoracic or transpleural approach.

III. DEGENERATIVE DISEASE OF THE SPINE (SPONDYLOSIS)

A. **Pathophysiology.** With advancing age, degenerative changes take place in the spine consisting of dehydration and collapse of the nucleus pulposus and bulging in all directions of the anulus fibrosus. The anulus becomes calcified, and hypertrophic changes occur in the bones at the margins of the vertebral bodies, creating lips or spurs (osteophytes) (Figs. 5-1 and 5-2). With narrowing of the intervertebral space, the intervertebral joints may become subluxated and compromise the intervertebral foramina, which may also be encroached upon by osteophytic processes.

B. **Clinical description**

1. **Root compression** indistinguishable from that produced by disc protrusion may occur, although the pain is usually less prominent with spondylosis.

2. **Dysesthesias** without pain may be present in the distribution of the roots affected, and corresponding muscle weakness and reflex changes may occur.

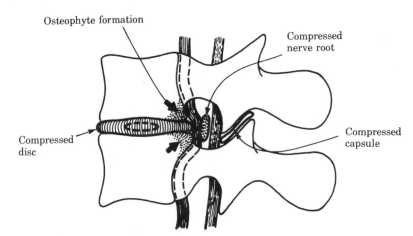

Fig. 5-2. Degenerative changes of the spine

These are more likely to be symptomatic in the cervical region, but they may occur in the lumbar area as well.

3. The **osteophyte formation** occurring in the more central portion of the vertebral body may **compress the spinal cord** in the cervical region or, the cauda equina may be compressed in the lumbar area in the presence of a narrowed canal **(lumbar stenosis).** In the cervical region this produces spastic pareparesis, often with posterior column sensory loss, hyperactive reflexes in the legs, and bilateral Babinski responses. Depending on the level, the arms may or may not be involved. An interesting situation often arises when the C5-6 interspace is involved: the biceps reflex is diminished because of root compression, and the triceps reflex is hyperactive because of cord compression. In the case of lumbar involvement, symptoms of cauda equina compression with paraparesis and sensory loss in the legs, along with loss of sphincter control, may result. A curious pseudoclaudication (or neurologic claudication) syndrome may also occur in which the patient notes back and leg pain on standing or walking; the pain is relieved by lying down.

C. **Diagnostic tests and treatment.** The work-up should proceed in the same manner as for disc disease, and conservative therapy is carried out in an identical fashion (see sec **II.B.2** and **3**). The **indications for surgery** also are the same as for disc disease: evidence of spinal cord compression, muscle weakness, or intractible pain. Surgery is a procedure to enlarge the intervertebral foramina, in the case of root compression, or a laminectomy to enlarge the spinal canal when the cord is compressed.

IV. SPONDYLOLYSIS AND SPONDYLOLISTHESIS

A. **Pathophysiology. Spondylolisthesis** is forward displacement of one vertebral body onto the vertebral body below it. This most commonly occurs in conjunction with **spondylolysis,** a condition in which the posterior portion of the vertebral unit is split so that there is loss of continuity between the superior and inferior articular processes (Fig. 5-3). This is believed to result from fracture of the neural arch shortly after birth, although it rarely becomes symptomatic until later in life; the average age of patients seeking treatment is 35 years. The most common site of involvement is the last lumbar vertebra (L5), which subluxates onto the sacrum. Less commonly, spondylolisthesis may occur secondary to degenerative disease of the spine; this usually involves L5 or L4.

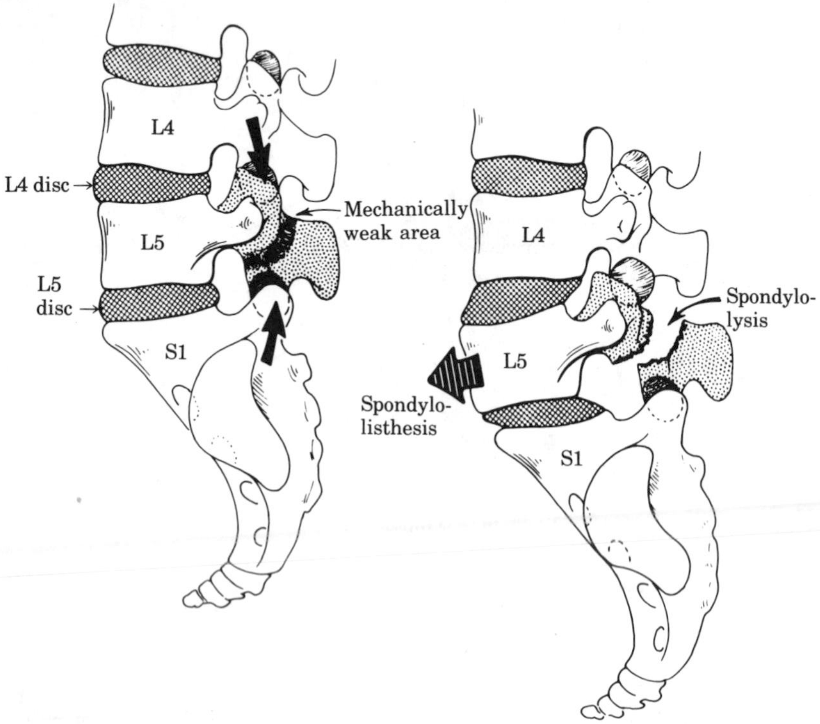

Fig. 5-3. Mechanism of spondylolysis. The pincer effect of the adjacent facets on the interposed isthmus is demonstrated with ultimate spondylolisthesis due to the restraining mechanism of the posterior articulation that is being detached.

B. **Clinical description.** The most common symptom is **low back pain,** usually beginning early in life and gradually worsening, that is accentuated by extension movements. However, the pain may begin abruptly in association with an injury. **Leg pain** from compression of the nerve roots is less common. With severe deformity, the cauda equina may be compressed.

C. **Treatment. Conservative therapy** consists of restriction of activity and institution of flexion exercises. A corset may be beneficial to provide stability to the spine. As the patient grows older, if conservative therapy has failed to halt progression of the condition, operative intervention (spinal fusion) is usually indicated.

V. NEUROLOGIC COMPLICATIONS OF DISEASES INVOLVING THE SPINE

A. **Ankylosing spondylitis.** Early in the course of ankylosing spondylitis there is low back pain. In a small percentage of patients this may radiate in a sciatic distribution, but neurologic findings are rare. Uncommonly, **compromise of the cauda equina** may occur, but this usually appears late in the course of the disease at a time when it has become inactive; it progresses insidiously, with muscle wasting, pain, and sensory loss in the legs, along with loss of sphincter control. Treatment is symptomatic.

B. **Rheumatoid arthritis** may result in serious neurologic complications from involvement of the cervical spine. The characteristic deformity is subluxation of one vertebra onto another. The most common situation is **atlantoaxial subluxation,** which may result in spinal cord compression. Another common site for subluxation is C3-4. Pain without cord compression is more likely to occur with atlantoaxial subluxation, while painless cord compression is more common at C3-4. These complications of rheumatoid arthritis generally occur only as a consequence of longstanding severe disease.

Treatment involves immobilization of the affected joint. This can be accomplished temporarily with **a hard four-post collar,** but definitive therapy requires **spinal fusion** at the involved interspace.

C. **Paget's disease** (osteitis deformans). Paget's disease often produces **back pain** but only rarely produces neurologic complications from involvement of the spine. However, many well-documented cases of **cord compression** have been reported. Compression may occur from narrowing of the spinal canal by hypertrophic bone, with subsequent direct compression, or from interference with the arterial supply to the cord. Cord compression may also result from vertebral collapse with dislocation of the vertebral bodies. There is no specific treatment for the back pain of Paget's disease, so **therapy** consists of palliation with back brace and analgesia.

D. **Metastatic disease** frequently causes **back pain** by involvement of vertebrae or spinal roots. It may produce **spinal cord compression** either because of collapse of extensively replaced vertebral bodies or by extramedullary (intradural or extradural) metastatic deposits. Plain x-rays of the spine may show evidence of metastatic disease. However, even when plain x-rays are normal, a bone scan is useful for diagnosis in cases of unexplained back pain. Lung, breast, and prostate cancer are the most frequent tumors producing back pain.

Treatment of the primary tumor and/or local radiation therapy to the involved vertebrae are useful palliative measures and often provide excellent **relief of pain.** *Spinal compression is an emergency* often requiring prompt myelography and surgical decompression, though some cases may be treated successfully with steroids and radiation therapy.

E. **Metabolic bone diseases** (e.g., osteoporosis, hyperparathyroidism, osteomalacia) frequently cause **back pain** but rarely produce neurologic deficits by spinal cord or root compression. **Treatment** is of the underlying condition if that is possible (i.e., discontinue steroids, give vitamin D and calcium, treat malabsorption or renal failure, remove parathyroid adenomas, etc.). Table 5-3 summarizes the differential diagnosis of various metabolic bone diseases that may present with back pain, based on serum Ca^{++}, PO_4, and alkaline phosphatase testing. If

Table 5-3. Differential Diagnosis of Various Bone Diseases that May Cause Back Pain

Disease	Serum Ca^{++}	Serum PO_4	Serum Alkaline Phosphatase
Hyperparathyroidism	↑	↓	N
Osteoporosis (primary or two degrees to steroid excess, hyperthyroidism, or acromegaly)	N or ↓	N	N
Osteomalacia			
Vitamin D lack or resistance	↓	↑	↑
Chronic renal failure	↓	↑	N or ↑
Malabsorption	↓	↓	↑
Malignancy with osseous metastases	↑	N	↑

no specific treatment is possible (e.g., as in postmenopausal osteoporosis), then palliative measures such as a back brace and analgesics are used.

VI. **SPINAL EPIDURAL ABSCESS** is a purulent infection of the epidural fat pad. It is thought that all cases are preceded by **vertebral osteomyelitis.** The infection usually reaches the vertebra via hematogenous spread from a distant infection, though direct spread from local skin infection is known to occur. The disease is rare, but when it occurs it is usually associated with **severe back pain** and almost always with **local tenderness.** Spinal epidural abscess may cause **spinal compression.** Myelography is required for diagnosis, and **treatment** consists of surgical removal of the abscess and four to six weeks of intravenous antibiotic therapy.

VII. **PSYCHIATRIC CAUSES OF BACK PAIN.** In cases of chronic back pain in which the neurologic examination is normal and categorization into any of the previously discussed syndromes is not possible, **depression** is a common finding. Such patients should not be treated with analgesics or other modes of therapy meant for specific backache syndromes. Tricyclic antidepressants may be useful. (See Chap. 9 for details.)

Back pain also may be seen in the context of various **characterologic diseases.** The prognosis in these cases is less favorable than in depression, and there is no effective therapy, though psychotherapy may meet with limited success. Analgesics (particularly opiates) should be avoided, since drug dependency is a very common complication in these patients. (Such patients often fail to have relief of their back pain while litigation is pending.)

SELECTED READING
Cailliet, R. *Low Back Pain Syndrome,* 2nd ed. Philadelphia: Davis, 1968.
Feldman, F., and Seaman, W. B. The neurological complications of Paget's disease in the cervical spine. *Am. J. Roentgenol.* 105:375, 1969.
Matthews, W. B. The neurological complications of ankylosing spondylitis. *J. Neurol. Sci.* 6:561, 1968.
Smith, P. H., Benn, R. T., and Sharp, J. Natural history of rheumatoid cervical luxations. *Ann. Rheum. Dis.* 31:431, 1972.
Wylie, W. G. The occurrence in osteitis deformans of lesions of the central nervous system with a report of four cases. *Brain* 46:336, 1923.
Youmans, J. R. *Neurological Surgery,* Volume I. Philadelphia: Saunders, 1973.

6   Raymond J. Fernandez and Martin A. Samuels

Epilepsy

Epilepsy may be defined as *a state of recurrent seizures*. Since seizures are due to aberrant electrical activity in virtually any part of the cerebral cortex (and perhaps even in the cerebellum and subcortical structures), one may expect that nearly every conceivable form of human experience could be caused by seizure discharges. However, although this is literally true, generally the term *epilepsy* (or *seizure disorder*) is used to characterize relatively stereotyped recurrent attacks of involuntary experience or behavior.

I. **CLASSIFICATION.** Many efforts have been made to classify the epilepsies using various parameters: etiology, symptomatology, duration, precipitating factors, post-ictal phenomena, and aura. The most useful of these classifications with regard to therapy utilizes the **clinical symptomatology** of the seizures; this mode of classification also permits differentiation of true epilepsies from similar yet clinically distinct conditions.

A. **Classification of epilepsies**

1. **Generalized**

   a. **Petit mal**

   b. **Grand mal**

      (1) Intermittent convulsions

      (2) Status epilepticus

   c. **Myoclonic epilepsy**

      (1) Infantile spasms

      (2) Childhood myoclonic epilepsy (late-onset myoclonic epilepsy)

   d. **Febrile seizures**

2. **Focal** (partial)

   a. **Simple symptoms**

      (1) Motor

      (2) Sensory

      (3) Autonomic

   b. **Complex symptoms** (psychomotor or temporal lobe)

      (1) Automatism

      (2) Psychic phenomena

3. **Neonatal**

B. **Classification of paroxysmal conditions resembling epilepsy**

1. Narcolepsy

2. Migraine

3. Paroxysmal abdominal pain

4. Breath-holding spells

5. Hypercyanotic attacks

6. Cardiovascular syncope

7. Hysteria

8. Malingering

9. Trigeminal neuralgia (tic douloureux)

10. Paroxysmal vertigo

C. **Management according to types of seizure patterns.** Since **patients often have more than one type of attack,** it is preferable to characterize an individual patient by the pattern of various types of seizures he experiences. Therapy may then be initially aimed at the predominant form of epilepsy seen in that particular patient, remembering that combinations of various therapeutic regimens are often necessary when control of different types of seizures in the same patient is required.

Within a single attack, however, it is most useful diagnostically and therapeutically to classify the seizure based on its initial manifestations, if that is possible. Thus a focal motor seizure that becomes generalized should be considered a focal rather than a generalized attack.

II. **EVALUATION OF THE PATIENT WITH EPILEPSY.** Epilepsy is only a symptom caused by excessive neuronal discharges. The precise cellular mechanism involved remains obscure and will not be discussed herein; it is sufficient to state that this symptom can be produced by protean abnormalities both in and out of the nervous system. The major categories of these are as follows.

A. **Genetic and birth factors**

1. Genetic influence (idiopathic, cryptogenic, essential)

2. Congenital abnormalities (including chromosome abnormalities)

3. Antenatal factors (infections, drugs, anoxia)

4. Perinatal factors (birth trauma, asphyxia neonatorum, infections)

B. **Infectious disorders**

1. Meningitis

2. Epidural or subdural abscess

3. Brain abscess and granuloma

4. Encephalitis

C. **Toxic factors**

1. Inorganic substances (e.g., carbon monoxide)

2. Metallic substances (e.g., lead, mercury)

3. Organic substances (e.g., alcohol)

4. Drugs and drug withdrawal

5. Allergic disorders (injection or ingestion of foreign protein)

D. **Trauma or physical agents**

1. Acute craniocerebral injuries

2. Subdural or epidural hematoma and effusion

3. Posttraumatic meningocerebral cicatrix

4. Anoxia or hypoxia

E. **Circulatory disturbances**

1. Subarachnoid hemorrhage

2. Sinus thrombosis

3. Encephalomalacia (thrombosis, embolus, hemorrhage)

4. Hypertensive encephalopathy

5. Syncope

F. Metabolic or nutritional disturbances

1. Electrolyte and water imbalance (hyponatremia, hypocalcemia, water intoxication, dehydration)

2. Carbohydrate metabolism (hypoglycemia, glycogen storage disease)

3. Amino acid metabolism (e.g., phenylketonuria)

4. Fat metabolism (e.g., lipid storage diseases)

5. Vitamin deficiency or dependency (e.g., pyridoxine dependency)

G. Neoplasms

1. Primary intracranial (astrocytoma, other gliomas, meningiomas)

2. Metastatic (breast, lung, melanoma)

3. Lymphoma and leukemia

4. Blood vessel tumors and vascular malformations

H. Heredofamilial

1. Neurofibromatosis

2. Tuberous sclerosis

3. Sturge-Weber syndrome

I. Febrile seizures

J. Degenerative diseases

K. Unknown causes

III. DIAGNOSTIC APPROACH. The diagnosis of epilepsy rests mainly on the **history**; it must be considered in any patient who suffers from recurrent attacks of relatively stereotyped involuntary behavior or experience. Particular diagnostic points relative to each of the types of seizures will be mentioned in the subsections in each category; however, the following general points apply broadly in the diagnosis of epilepsy.

A. Electroencephalogram (EEG). *There is no diagnostic test that will reliably either diagnose or exclude epilepsy.* The EEG is often normal even in a patient with a known seizure disorder, and, conversely, an abnormal EEG in the absence of symptoms does not automatically indicate treatment for seizures.

It is relatively unusual for seizure activity to be recorded during an EEG. Therefore, the usefulness of the test is largely dependent on interictal abnormalities, particularly when focal or lateralized slow waves are observed—a finding which suggests that a localized abnormality is responsible for the epilepsy. **In questionable cases,** in which the clinical diagnosis is in doubt, various activation procedures may be utilized (e.g., hyperventilation, photic stimulation, and sleep) to exacerbate an underlying abnormality not recognizable on the ordinary tracing.

B. Etiology. Once the diagnosis of epilepsy is made, a search for the etiology should ensue. The diagnostic course to be followed will vary depending on the type of seizure disorder identified and the age of the patient.

1. Patient history. In order to place the patient into the proper category, it is necessary to obtain a careful history from both the patient and someone who has witnessed the seizure or seizures.

  a. **Focality of seizures.** Important historic points derive from whether the seizures are generalized from their onset or have some focal quality. **If they are focal,** it must be determined whether the symptoms are simple movements and elementary sensations, or whether they are complex, such as automatic movements, psychic phenomena (e.g., déjà vu, *jamais vu,* or paranoid or hostile feelings), or gustatory or olfactory hallucinations.

  b. **Family history.** The family history may reveal relatives with epilepsy or with diseases associated with seizures.

  c. **Past medical history.** The patient's past medical history may give a clue concerning remote infections, such as meningitis or encephalitis, or a history of stroke or head trauma may be elicited, either of which may be epileptogenic.

  d. **Pregnancy history.** The history of the patient's mother's pregnancy, labor, and delivery should be reviewed for evidence of complications known to be associated with epilepsy in later life. Most notable among these are:

   (1) **CNS birth injuries** (mechanical, hypoxic, and hemorrhagic);

   (2) **CNS infections** (intrauterine and neonatal); or

   (3) **Metabolic insults** (e.g., symptomatic hypoglycemia).

 2. **A general physical examination** may reveal a medical illness that may be associated with seizures. Special care should be taken in examining the **skin,** since neuroectodermal disorders (e.g., tuberous sclerosis, neurofibromatosis, and Sturge-Weber syndrome) can be diagnosed in this way.

 3. **The neurologic examination** may show some lateralizing or localizing abnormality that would lead one to investigate more fully for an underlying cause for a patient's epilepsy.

  Once the patient has been categorized with regard to the predominant type of epilepsy from which he is suffering, further investigation and treatment may be considered.

IV. GENERALIZED SEIZURES

A. Petit mal

 1. **Description.** Petit mal epilepsy is manifested by **brief attacks of loss of awareness ("absences"),** sometimes associated with 3/sec minor motor activity, with exactly 3/sec generalized spikes and slow waves seen on EEG.
  Petit mal seizures usually begin when the patient is between 4 and 8 years of age. Most seizures are simple absence attacks, in which the patient does not lose body tone and does not fall. The attacks are usually 5–10 seconds in duration and rarely exceed 30 seconds. Minor motor activity is occasionally seen, usually facial twitching and, less often, automatisms, such as lip-smacking and repetitive swallowing. Sometimes these automatisms are suggestive of psychomotor (temporal lobe) epilepsy, but there is no aura and no postictal state, and the patients quickly return to normal activity. The patients themselves are rarely aware of these attacks, so the history must be obtained from an observer.

 2. **Diagnosis.** This form of epilepsy is unique in that *the clinical seizures and the EEG are of equal diagnostic importance.* **The EEG** shows a highly characteristic, generalized 3/sec spike and slow wave pattern. An **activation procedure,** particularly hyperventilation, is often required to bring out the abnormality. In the classic case, no further diagnostic evaluation is necessary.

 3. **Prognosis.** Most cases of classic petit mal epilepsy will **resolve spontaneously** by the time the person enters the third decade of life. However, **some**

cases will evolve into generalized grand mal seizure patterns. Four factors are associated with a **good prognosis** (cases that do not satisfy these four criteria will be less likely to show disappearance of the seizures and are more likely to evolve into other forms of epilepsy in later life):

a. Onset between the ages of 4 and 8 years and normal intelligence.

b. No other seizure type present.

c. Easy control with a single drug.

d. Classic, precisely 3/sec generalized spikes and slow wave pattern on EEG, without other EEG abnormalities.

4. **Treatment** (Table 6-1)

a. **Ethosuximide.** The treatment of choice in petit mal epilepsy is **ethosuximide** (Zarontin) 20–40 mg/kg/day, divided into two or three doses. The **dosage** usually begins with 20 mg/kg/day and is increased gradually at weekly intervals until the seizures are controlled or the patient develops gastrointestinal upset, ataxia, or severe drowsiness. The patient can be followed clinically for **toxicity,** and/or the serum levels of ethosuximide can be measured (therapeutic range = 40–80 μg/ml). *Ethosuximide has the tendency to evoke grand mal seizures*; if this occurs, **phenobarbital** or **phenytoin** (Dilantin) may be added (Table 6-2). Some neurologists begin all petit mal patients prophylactically on phenytoin or phenobarbital.

b. **Clonazepam (Clonopin).** There is evidence that clonazepam may be very useful in the treatment of petit mal epilepsy; eventually it may become a first-line drug for this condition. At present, however, it should be reserved for cases not controlled with ethosuximide. The drug has the advantage of having **very few side effects,** the most notable of which is **sedation.** Dosage of clonazepam is 0.01–0.03 mg/kg/day PO initially, divided into two or three doses, increasing slowly to 0.1–0.2 mg/kg/day.

c. **Oxazolidinediones.** If control cannot be obtained with ethosuximide or clonazepam, or if unacceptable toxicity is encountered, one of the oxazolidinediones may be utilized. Of the two available preparations, **paramethadione** (Paradione) is slightly less likely to produce side effects than is **trimethadione** (Tridione), but the former is often less effective. Despite the chemical similarity of the two drugs, failure of a patient to respond to one does not preclude possible use of the other. The same principle holds for the tendency to produce side effects.

The most common **side effects** are **sedation** and **photophobia.** However, the most important possible **complications** are nephrotic syndrome, neutropenia, aplastic anemia, exfoliative dermatitis, and hepatitis. These seem to be idiosyncratic but usually are reversible on discontinuation of the drug. The patient should be screened quarterly with complete blood count, urinalysis, and liver function tests, since development of these toxicities is an absolute contraindication to the continued use of oxazolidinediones.

These drugs also should be **discontinued** if a dermatitis develops, and they are **contraindicated in pregnancy.** They may produce grand mal seizures, but these often can be treated with concomitant use of phenytoin, phenobarbital, primidone, or carbamazepine without discontinuance of the oxazolidinedione.

d. **Succinimides other than ethosuximide.** The next two drug choices for control of petit mal epilepsy, as listed in Table 6-1, are succinimide derivatives, closely related to ethosuximide, namely **methsuximide** (Celontin) and **phensuximide** (Milontin). Both are given in dosages of

Table 6-1. The Treatment of Generalized Petit Mal Epilepsy*

Choice	Drug	Preparation	Dose	Route
1	Ethosuximide (Zarontin)	250 mg capsules; 50 mg/ml syrup	20 mg/kg/day, divided into two to three doses, increasing to a maximum of 40 mg/kg/day	PO
2	Clonazepam (Clonopin)	0.5, 1.0, 2 mg tablets	0.01–0.03 mg/kg/day increasing to 0.1–0.2 mg/kg/day, divided into three doses	PO
3	Trimethadione (Tridione)	150 mg tablets; 300 mg capsules; 40 mg/ml solution	20–40 mg/kg/day, divided into three doses (maximum, 2.4 gm/day)	PO
4	Paramethadione (Paradione)	150 and 300 mg capsules; 300 mg/ml solution	20–40 mg/kg/day, divided into three doses (maximum, 2.4 gm/day)	PO
5	Methsuximide (Celontin)	150 mg capsules; 300 mg capsules	5–20 mg/kg/day, divided into three doses (maximum, 1.5 gm/day)	PO
6	Phensuximide (Milontin)	250 mg capsules; 500 mg capsules; 60 mg/ml suspension	5–20 mg/kg/day, divided into three doses (maximum, 1.5 gm/day)	PO
	Acetazolamide (Diamox)†	125 mg tablets; 250 mg tablets	10–25 mg/kg/day, divided into three doses (maximum, 1 gm/day)	PO
	Sodium valproate (Depakene)‡	250 mg tablets; 60 mg/ml syrup	10–20 mg/kg/day divided into 3 doses	PO

*Concomitant use of phenytoin or phenobarbital is often necessary to control associated grand mal convulsions.
†This drug may be added to any of the above preparations, but is of little use alone.
‡Exact place in the sequence of drug choices not yet known.

Table 6-2. The Treatment of Generalized Grand Mal Convulsions and Focal Epilepsy

Choice	Drug	Preparation	Dose	Route
1*	Phenytoin (Dilantin)	30 and 100 mg capsules; 50 mg tablets; 6 mg/ml suspension; 25 mg/ml suspension; 250 mg ampules	5 mg/kg/day given one to three times per day (adults usually require 200–400 mg per day). Loading dose of 15 mg/kg may be given as rapidly as 50 mg/min	PO IV
2*	Phenobarbital (Luminal)	15, 30, 60, and 100 mg tablets; 4 mg/ml elixir	1–5 mg/kg/day, divided into two to three doses (adults usually require 60–120 mg/day)	PO IM IV
3	Primidone (Mysoline)	50 and 250 mg tablets; 25 mg/ml suspension	10–25 mg/kg/day, divided into two to three doses (adults usually require less, only 300–1000 mg/day)	PO
4	Carbamazepine (Tegretol)	200 mg tablets	7–15 mg/kg/day, divided into two to three doses (adults usually require 200–800 mg/day)	PO
5	Mephobarbital (Mebaral)	30, 50, 100; 200 mg tablets	2–10 mg/kg/day, divided into two to three doses (adults usually require 200–600 mg/day)	PO
6	Mephenytoin (Mesantoin)	100 mg tablets	5–10 mg/kg/day, given one to three times per day (adults usually require 200–600 mg/day)	PO
	Sodium valproate (Depakene)†	250 mg tablets; 60 mg/ml syrup	10–20 mg/kg/day divided into 3 doses	PO

*May reverse choices 1 and 2 in infants and children.
†Exact place in the sequence of drug choices not yet known. It is probably less effective for focal than for generalized seizures.

5–20 mg/kg/day PO, divided into two or three doses, and both have toxic potential similar to that of ethosuximide, except for the fact that methsuximide does not seem to have the same tendency to produce grand mal seizures as the rest of the succinimide drugs do.

The succinimides and oxazolidinediones may be used together in extreme circumstances, but it is recommended that they not be used concomitantly, since the tendency for bone marrow toxicity may be partially additive.

e. **Acetazolamide.** Acetazolamide (Diamox) is of limited value alone but **is often of some use in combination with another anticonvulsant.** Added to any of the above anticonvulsants, it occasionally improves seizure control. The dosage is 10–25 mg/kg/day PO, divided into three doses.

f. **A ketogenic diet** has been found to help control petit mal seizures, but its use is **reserved for difficult-to-control cases,** since the diet is unpleasant and difficult for the patient to maintain.

B. **Intermittent grand mal**

1. **Description.** Grand mal tonic-clonic convulsive epilepsy is defined as *recurrent episodes of sudden loss of consciousness, with associated major motor activity.* Grand mal tonic convulsions or clonic convulsions or both are characterized by sudden loss of consciousness in which the entire body usually becomes rigid in extension. The patient falls to the ground, sometimes with a cry, and may urinate and be temporarily apneic. Following a period of tonic rigidity, clonic jerking of the face, trunk, and limbs ensues. The rate of clonic jerking gradually decreases, and finally the patient becomes limp and comatose. Consciousness gradually returns, often associated with a postictal state of confusion, headache, and drowsiness. Patients may display various combinations of these components: they may have purely tonic or purely clonic attacks, or any combination thereof.

Although many patients describe a prodromal period of irritability that varies from a few minutes to several days before an attack, generalized grand mal epilepsy does not have a true aura, as may be seen in focal seizures. Because of the apoplectic nature of the attacks, these patients—unlike patients with petit mal epilepsy—are subject to serious injury during an attack due to compression fractures of vertebrae, caused by the intense muscle contraction, or to accidents consequent to the sudden loss of consciousness. The eyes may rove aimlessly during an attack or may be tonically deviated first to one side during the attack and then to the opposite side postictally.

2. **Differential diagnosis**

a. **Age range/incidence.** A family history of epilepsy is common and the hereditary nature of this condition is generally recognized. True grand mal convulsive epilepsy usually begins before the age of 30 years. The vast majority of these patients will have idiopathic epilepsy and will respond readily to treatment with one or two drugs. Between the ages of 30 and 60 years, the most common cause of grand mal convulsions is still idiopathic epilepsy, although the risk of intracranial tumor is significantly higher than in the younger age groups. Over the age of 60 years, the onset of grand mal convulsions most likely represents cerebrovascular disease (usually postcerebral embolus), but tumor and idiopathic epilepsy remain important diagnoses as well. At no time in life does the onset of grand mal convulsions primarily suggest brain tumor, although incidence of brain tumor peaks in middle life, and this diagnosis should certainly be excluded.

b. **Primary vs. secondary grand mal diagnosis.** *It is very important to attempt to* **rule out focal epilepsy** *that has spread to become generalized* (secondary grand mal epilepsy) as the cause of what is apparently primary grand mal epilepsy. Primary grand mal epilepsy is very likely to be either idiopathic or metabolic whereas focal epilepsy, with or without spread to grand mal convulsions, represents focal brain disease and thus may have a graver prognosis.

It should be kept in mind that **the history is often insufficient** to definitely rule out focal epilepsy with spread, so many cases of what are apparently generalized grand mal convulsions are in fact focal seizures with spread. Because these cases carry a more ominous prognosis with respect to focal brain disease, whenever the history is vague, one should assume that there is a possibility of focal seizures and act accordingly (that is, carry out a more vigorous evaluation, as outlined in sec **V.A**).

In cases of classic generalized grand mal convulsive epilepsy, when there is no question of a focal onset and no focal characteristics of the seizures on the EEG, the prognosis is good, because it is likely that the diagnosis will be idiopathic epilepsy, which can be controlled with drugs easily. Often seizures that begin in the second or third decade become less frequent and even stop entirely, allowing total discontinuation of anticonvulsant medications. Patients with idiopathic grand mal convulsions may experience exacerbation of their seizures with metabolic stresses, such as drug withdrawal, fever, hypoglycemia, and hyponatremia, all of which can produce grand mal convulsions in nonepileptic people.

Most patients who suffer their first seizure should be hospitalized for the initial evaluation, since no predictions concerning etiology, future course, or facility of control can be made on one isolated examination. **Routine studies** on all patients who have suffered their first grand mal convulsion should include the following:

(1) A careful **neurologic examination** should be aimed primarily at determining whether any focal or lateralizing aspects of the seizure state can be found either ictally or postictally.

(2) Complete blood count.

(3) Serum electrolytes (Na, K, Cl, CO_2).

(4) Blood urea nitrogen (BUN).

(5) Serum calcium.

(6) Blood sugar.

(7) Liver function tests (serum glutamic oxaloacetic transaminase, alkaline phosphatase, total bilirubin).

(8) Skull x-rays.

(9) Chest x-rays.

(10) Lumbar puncture for cerebrospinal fluid (especially if infection, degenerative disease, or intracranial hemorrhage is suspected):

   (a) Cell count

   (b) Glucose

   (c) Protein

   (d) Syphilis serology

(11) **Toxic screen** and **blood alcohol levels** are obtained if the degree of drug ingestion or withdrawal cannot be ascertained from the history.

(12) During a generalized grand mal convulsion, the **EEG** shows generalized spikes. Postictally, it is generally slow; and interictally, the EEG may be totally normal. If an abnormality is seen, care is taken to exclude a focal or lateralizing abnormality, either ictally or postictally. However, if there is a nonfocal, nonlateralizing EEG, the prognosis is good.

(13) Computed tomography (CT) of the brain (especially if hemorrhage, degenerative disease, or major structural abnormality is suspected).

3. **Treatment** (Table 6-2)

a. **Phenytoin.** The cornerstone of treatment of generalized grand mal convulsions is phenytoin (Dilantin) and phenobarbital. Both are excellent anticonvulsants, so the decision of which to use as a first choice must be made according to the individual patient.

(1) Indications. Most neurologists would agree that phenytoin is the single most effective anticonvulsant. Its major advantage over phenobarbital is that it does not produce drowsiness, even in overdosage and, practically speaking, will never produce a fatal overdose when taken PO. Furthermore, sudden stoppage of phenytoin will not produce withdrawal seizures, which may occur with the discontinuance of long-term barbiturates. Although seizures may recur if phenytoin is stopped, this is merely an exacerbation of the underlying epilepsy and is not a withdrawal phenomenon.

Phenytoin has little or no value as an illicit street drug, and thus the physician can be relatively confident that the patient will not sell this medication and will not take it himself unless it is prescribed. It can be given to patients in any age group, and it is well absorbed from the gastrointestinal tract, making oral use efficient and practical. It can also be given IV, making it particularly useful in status epilepticus (see sec **IV.C** on generalized grand mal status epilepticus). IM injection is possible, but it is not recommended, since blood levels resulting from this route are unpredictable. Its **major disadvantage** is its production of unsightly hirsutism and gingival hypertrophy [see sec **IV.B.3.a.(3)**].

(2) Administration. Therapeutic serum levels of $10–20$ μg/ml correlate well with the anticonvulsant properties of phenytoin. When given at 5 mg/kg/day (about 300 mg/day in an average adult), it takes 5 to 15 days to reach the therapeutic range. However, if a loading dose of 15 mg/kg (about 1000 mg in an average adult) is given PO, the therapeutic range can be reached within a few hours. Since the biological half-life of phenytoin is usually about 24 hours, the drug only needs to be given once per day. If given IV, the therapeutic range can be reached in minutes.

Thus **dilantinization** should be considered much in the same way as digitalization. The rate at which a patient is dilantinized depends on the clinical situation. The therapeutic range can be reached in as little as 20 minutes or as long as 15 days. Obviously, the number of dose-related side effects will increase with the speed at which the patient is dilantinized, so the general rule of thumb is to proceed as slowly as is clinically safe. For example, if the patient has had only one seizure and will be in the hospital for several days for initial evaluation and observation, 5 mg/kg/day is administered PO (about 300 mg/day in an average adult), and therapeutic effects are expected in about 5 days. However, some patients have excessive phenytoin metabolism, in which case the therapeutic effects may not be demonstrated for as long as 2 weeks.

On the other hand, if the patient has had several seizures or if he or she cannot be hospitalized for some reason, one might wish to administer 15 mg/kg in the first 24 hours (about 1000 mg in an average adult), perhaps in three doses. The entire loading dose can be given at once if even more rapid dilantinization is desired. The latter method would result in therapeutic levels in perhaps 5 or 6 hours. Various approaches to dilantinization are outlined in Table 6-3.

It is not necessary to follow frequent serum phenytoin measurements, since the following **clinical signs** are readily available to evaluate the approximate phenytoin levels.

Table 6-3. Various Methods of Dilantinization

Therapeutic Range* Reached (after initial dose)	Rate of Administration	Route	Comment
20 minutes	1000 mg at 50 mg/minute in adults (10–15 mg/kg at 25 mg/min in children)	IV	Always with pulse, BP, and respiration monitored. Given by syringe. Not mixed in bottle
4–6 hours	1000 mg stat in adults; then 300 mg/day (about 15 mg/kg stat in children; then 5 mg/kg/day)	PO	Local gastric upset is common. Give with meals or milk
24–30 hours	300 mg every 8 hours for three doses; then 300 mg per day in adults (5 mg/kg every 8 hours for three doses; then 5 mg/kg in children)	PO	Mild ataxia is common initially
5–15 days	300 mg/day in adults (5 mg/kg/day in children)	PO	No unusual side effects

*The therapeutic range is 5–20 μg/ml of serum.

(a) **Nystagmus** develops when the phenytoin level is about 10–20 μg/ml. It is very common to see bilateral horizontal nystagmus on lateral gaze (and occasionally even vertical nystagmus) when phenytoin levels are in the therapeutic range.

(b) **Ataxia** develops when the level is about 30 μg/ml.

(c) **Lethargy** develops when it reaches about 40 μg/ml. The development of frank ataxia should warn the physician that the dosage should be decreased.

(3) **Side effects.** The side effects of phenytoin are protean, but fortunately the most serious ones are infrequent and are usually reversible. The untoward effects can be divided into three categories: local, idiosyncratic, and dose-related.

(a) **Local side effects.** The only local side effect is **gastric upset,** which can usually be relieved if phenytoin is taken with meals or milk.

(b) **Idiosyncratic side effects.** Several idiosyncratic effects are seen, many of which require discontinuation of the drug. For example, **dermatitis** may develop with fever and eosinophilia. A **lupuslike syndrome** occasionally occurs, with positive antinuclear antibodies and lupus erythematosus cell preparation; and occasional **blood dyscrasias** occur, including leukopenia, agranulocytosis, thrombocytopenia, aplastic anemia, and pseudolymphoma.

If any of these complications occur, phenytoin is discontinued in favor of another anticonvulsant, usually phenobarbital. **Gingival hypertrophy** and **hirsutism** are common side effects of phenytoin, and although they are not in themselves contraindications to the use of the drug, they may be sufficiently bothersome cosmetically to indicate replacement of phenytoin by another anticonvulsant.

Many neurologists use phenobarbital as the first-choice anticonvulsant in young patients for this reason alone.

(c) Dose-related side effects. A number of dose-related side effects also exist, including **cerebellar ataxia** and **nystagmus,** as mentioned previously; a **megaloblastic anemia** due to interference with folic acid and vitamin B_{12} metabolism; **low-protein-bound thyroxine** due to competitive binding of phenytoin to the thyroid-binding globulin; and **hypocalcemia,** with **osteoporosis** and **elevated serum alkaline phosphatase.** The latter effect is probably caused by phenytoin's effects on the liver, which accelerates vitamin D metabolism, producing a relative deficiency of vitamin D. It has been reported that long-term phenytoin use occasionally may be associated with cerebellar degeneration and polyneuropathy.

Many of these side effects can be treated without stopping the phenytoin by lowering the dosage if it is above therapeutic range; administering folate, vitamin B_{12}, or vitamin D when indicated; and by recognizing that an apparently low T_4 only represents an artifactual lowering of T_4 binding to thyroid-binding globulin.

(4) Drug interactions. Many commonly used drugs interfere with the metabolism of phenytoin, thus elevating its blood level. If frequent clinical examinations are done to monitor the blood level of phenytoin, the dosage can be lowered until the proper therapeutic range is reached for a particular patient. Serum levels of phenytoin may be helpful, but they are not necessary in this regard.

Drugs known to elevate the blood level of phenytoin or to increase the risk of toxic side effects are as follows:

(a) Isoniazid (INH)

(b) Coumarin anticoagulants

(c) Disulfiram (Antabuse)

(d) Chloramphenicol (Chloromycetin)

(e) Benzodiazepines (Librium, Valium, Serax, Clonopin)

(f) Methylphenidate (Ritalin)

(g) Phenothiazines

(h) Estrogens

(i) Ethosuximide (Zarontin)

(j) Phenylbutazone (Butazolidin)

(k) Alcohol

b. Phenobarbital is a barbiturate and has potent anticonvulsant properties. Whether it is as effective as phenytoin is a moot question. It is certainly either the first or second choice in the treatment of generalized grand mal convulsions.

(1) Indications. Phenobarbital may be used as the first-choice anticonvulsant in infants and young children and in adolescents to avoid the negative cosmetic effects of phenytoin and in patients who experience idiosyncratic side effects as a result of taking phenytoin. Furthermore, it may be combined with phenytoin in patients who have reached therapeutic levels of phenytoin, but whose seizures have not been controlled.

The drug has the advantage of **easy administration** by means of PO, IM, or IV routes, with **very few side effects** other than sedation.

Furthermore, it is the least expensive anticonvulsant. However, as mentioned previously, **overdosage** of phenobarbital can cause fatal respiratory depression. The drug also can produce dependency and, if suddenly withdrawn, may produce a withdrawal syndrome similar to delirium tremens, with agitation, fever, and seizures.

Although phenobarbital is less likely to produce a withdrawal syndrome than are shorter-acting barbiturates, it certainly may do so in some patients. Also, barbiturate withdrawal seizures can be the most refractory type of epilepsy to treat. They usually respond only to large doses of barbiturates, being extraordinarily refractory to other anticonvulsants.

Phenobarbital may be sold illicitly, and it may be used by psychologically unstable individuals to commit suicide. However, in reliable persons in whom good medical follow-up is available, phenobarbital is a safe, inexpensive, and effective anticonvulsant.

(2) Administration. The required dosage of phenobarbital is less predictable than that of phenytoin. Children require 3–5 mg/kg/day (the serum therapeutic range is 20–50 μg/ml), whereas adults usually require proportionally less, about 60–120 mg/day. The biological half-life of phenobarbital is even longer than that of phenytoin (about 96 hours) and thus, theoretically, it can be given less frequently. However, the sedative effects of the drug usually preclude giving the entire daily dose at one time. Thus it is generally necessary to administer it in two or three divided doses.

There is no limiting factor to increasing the dosage of phenobarbital, except sedation, and often much higher dosages than have been recommended are required to control seizures. The use of phenobarbital for continuous seizures is slightly different and is covered in the section on grand mal status epilepticus.

(3) Side effects. The major contraindication of phenobarbital is that it produces **sedation** when it is given in the anticonvulsant therapeutic range. Usually this effect will decrease as the patient becomes tolerant to the drug, but sometimes it does not. In patients in whom the sedative effects are tied closely to the anticonvulsant effects, phenobarbital sometimes cannot be used. Fortunately, this situation is rare. Furthermore, as the patient becomes tolerant to the sedative property of phenobarbital, he or she also may become tolerant to the anticonvulsant properties, in which case the dosage must be increased, producing drowsiness again. Usually, the drowsiness decreases after a few days or weeks, and the potent anticonvulsive effects remain. In **children,** the drug may cause paradoxical hyperactivity and irritability, which may require that it be discontinued.

Rarely, phenobarbital may produce a megaloblastic anemia, similar to that produced by phenytoin. This effect is responsive to folate or vitamin B_{12}, but sometimes this therapy results in exacerbation of seizures, requiring that another anticonvulsant be used. Relative vitamin D deficiency and osteomalacia may also be seen with phenobarbital use, but less frequently than with phenytoin.

c. Primidone (Mysoline) is closely related chemically to phenobarbital, but it will occasionally help to control grand mal convulsions when phenobarbital fails.

(1) Indications. Primidone may be used alone, but more often it is used in combination with phenytoin when phenobarbital fails. Phenobarbital and primidone are rarely used in combination because of their close chemical relation.

(2) Administration. The usual dosage for children under 6 years old is

10–25 mg/kg/day, divided into two or three doses. Again, adults require proportionally lower dosages, usually in the range of 300–750 mg/day.

Children should be started on 50–100 mg/day, and the dosage gradually increased until either seizure control or unacceptable sedation occurs. Adults should be started at low dosages (50–125 mg/day), which can be gradually increased to the therapeutic range. Primidone can only be given PO.

(3) Side effects. The major side effect is **sedation,** which may be severe and less likely to disappear with time as it does with phenobarbital. This can be avoided sometimes by beginning with a low dosage and gradually increasing it to the therapeutic range (10–25 μg/ml).

A syndrome of **vertigo** with **cerebellar ataxia** may develop in the first few days of therapy, but this generally resolves spontaneously. An **allergic rash** rarely develops, but when it does, primidone should be replaced with another anticonvulsant. A **megaloblastic anemia** may also develop occasionally, most often due to folate deficiency, but occasionally this is caused by vitamin B_{12} deficiency. This can be treated with folate or vitamin B_{12} or both without discontinuing the medication.

Primidone has the same potential for **tolerance** and **withdrawal** as phenobarbital does, and its ability to produce **life-threatening respiratory depression** in overdosage is the same as with other barbiturates.

d. Carbamazepine (Tegretol) is a dibenzazepine derivative, which is related structurally to imipramine (Tofranil).

(1) Indications. Carbamazepine is well established in the treatment of neuralgic pains (e.g., tic douloureux) but it is also a potent anticonvulsant. It is very effective for the control of grand mal seizures. In fact, the drug may be more effective than primidone, but because of its graver, although rare, side effects, it is regarded as the fourth-choice drug in the treatment of grand mal convulsions.

(2) Administration. Dosage in children under 1 year old is 50–100 mg/day; in children between 1 and 6 years old, 150–300 mg/day; and in patients over 6 years old, 200–800 mg/day, given PO in two or three doses. Barring abnormalities in the blood count or liver function tests, the dosage may be gradually increased until either unacceptable sedation or control of seizures occurs.

A serum carbamazepine test is available, and the therapeutic range is 4–6 μg/ml. Carbamazepine may be used alone or in combination with either phenytoin or phenobarbital or both, or primidone. However, it is very rare that three drugs are required to control ordinary generalized grand mal convulsions.

A summary of the common drug combinations used to treat grand mal convulsions is given in Table 6-4.

(3) Side effects include allergic skin rashes, sedation, dry mouth, gastrointestinal upset, cholestatic jaundice, aplastic anemia, and pancytopenia. Furthermore, **teratogenic effects** have been seen in animals given carbamazepine, although this has not been seen in humans. As a result, patients should be followed closely with quarterly complete blood counts and liver function tests, and the drug should be discontinued if any abnormalities are noted. **Carbamazepine should be avoided in pregnancy if possible.**

Most of these side effects have been reversible; but irreversible, fatal blood dyscrasias have occurred although very rarely.

Table 6-4. Common Drug Regimens for Generalized Grand Mal
Convulsions and Focal Epilepsy

Choice	Drugs
1*	Phenytoin (Dilantin)
2*	Phenobarbital (Luminal)
3	Phenytoin plus phenobarbital
4	Phenytoin plus primidone (Mysoline)
5	Carbamazepine (Tegretol)
6	Phenytoin plus carbamazepine
7	Phenobarbital plus carbamazepine
8	Primidone plus carbamazepine
9	Phenytoin plus phenobarbital plus carbamazepine
10	Phenytoin plus primidone plus carbamazepine

*Choices 1 and 2 may be reversed if specifically indicated (such as in children and adolescents).

    e. Miscellaneous drugs. Occasionally drugs related to phenytoin or phenobarbital are useful when their parent compounds fail or are poorly tolerated. Mephobarbital (Mebaral) 2–10 mg/kg/day and mephenytoin (Mesantoin) 5–10 mg/kg/day are used most commonly for this purpose. The side effects are similar to those of their parent compounds. A new drug, sodium valproate (dipropylacetate) has been reported to be effective in all varieties of epilepsy, although less so in focal seizures. The dosage is 10–20 mg/kg/day PO (600–1200 mg in an average adult). The effective plasma level is probably about 50–100 μg/ml. The drug appears to be safe and effective but its exact place in the standard treatment protocol for epilepsy is yet to be determined. At present it is reserved for resistant cases. The drug interferes with platelet function, and signs of hemorrhagic disease, including petechiae, epistaxis, and prolonged bleeding after surgery have been seen. Severe hepatotoxicity has also been reported as a complication of the use of sodium valproate.

  4. Pregnancy. The question of how to manage epilepsy in the pregnant patient is difficult. However, there are some general principles to guide the physician.

    a. The **effect on the fetus** of most anticonvulsants is not known. In most cases, experimental evidence is not available. The use of anticonvulsants has been associated with a slightly increased incidence of serious congenital anomalies, but human studies are always limited by the fact that epilepsy itself may have similar effects. Because of the lack of evidence for safe use of most anticonvulsants, it is recommended that *as many anticonvulsants as possible be discontinued in pregnancy, particularly in the first trimester.*

    b. Generalized **petit mal seizures** and **focal epilepsy** probably have no adverse effect on the mother or fetus, and thus anticonvulsants may be discontinued easily in most of these patients for the duration of the pregnancy. However, if petit mal or focal seizures are overwhelmingly disabling or dangerous to the patient, then the risk to the patient must be weighed against the unknown risk to the fetus.

    c. Generalized grand mal convulsions may, in themselves, be a danger to the fetus by producing hypoxia. *It is generally agreed that frequent grand mal convulsions during pregnancy are dangerous to the fetus.* Thus one might attempt to decrease anticonvulsants during pregnancy. However, if the seizures cannot be controlled, it is reasonable to use whatever anticonvulsant is required, since the risk to the fetus is probably greater with multiple grand mal convulsions than it is with any of the anticonvulsants.

5. **Drug withdrawal seizures.** Seizures may occur as part of the withdrawal syndrome from many drugs, the most common and important of which are **alcohol** and **barbiturates.** If they are only caused by withdrawal from these agents they should be primary, generalized grand mal convulsions. However, if there appears to be a focal aspect to the seizure or a postictal state in a patient suspected of withdrawing from drugs, the possibility of focal brain disease must be raised, and the diagnosis of simple drug withdrawal seizures cannot be made.

In general, these seizures are treated acutely, just as any other form of generalized grand mal convulsions. There are, however, many commonly held misconceptions about this type of seizures, which the following points may help to clarify.

a. Phenytoin is useful in treating both alcohol and barbiturate withdrawal seizures, acutely and prophylactically. However, long-term anticonvulsant treatment with phenytoin or any other drug is often unsatisfactory, since patients rarely continue their medications faithfully when taking drugs or alcohol. Thus most neurologists only use phenytoin when necessary to control severe convulsions, but not on a long-term basis. In the case of alcohol withdrawal seizures ("rum fits"), paraldehyde, which may be used for the control of other aspects of the withdrawal syndrome, is often helpful in preventing severe convulsions as well.

b. Barbiturates in very large doses (sometimes more than 1 gm of phenobarbital) may be necessary to control severe barbiturate withdrawal seizures. In these cases, other anticonvulsants, including phenytoin, are of little value. One can only suspect such a situation by obtaining a history from the patient's friends or relatives. Short-acting barbiturates, such as secobarbital, are more likely to produce a withdrawal syndrome than long-acting agents, such as phenobarbital. However, **all barbiturates can produce withdrawal seizures.** When administering barbiturates in doses higher than about 250 mg in acute situations, preparations should be made to perform endotracheal intubation if necessary.

c. When faced with a known barbiturate addict who has discontinued use of the drugs abruptly, it is usually wise to administer barbiturates prophylactically to prevent withdrawal seizures, and then gradually taper the drug over several days or weeks.

The level of the patient's tolerance can be judged clinically by administering secobarbital (Seconal) 200 mg PO and observing for nystagmus and cerebellar ataxia ½ hour later. If no toxicity is noted, secobarbital 100 mg can be administered every ½ hour until nystagmus or cerebellar ataxia is noted. The total dose administered may be considered the addict's daily maintenance dose. This dose can then be tapered by 50–100 mg every other day to withdraw the drug completely and safely.

d. In most cases of alcohol withdrawal seizures (and many cases of barbiturate withdrawal seizures as well), the illness is self-limited and does not require anticonvulsant therapy.

C. **Continuous grand mal convulsions** (convulsive grand mal status epilepticus)

1. **Description.** Generalized grand mal status epilepticus is defined as either *continuous grand mal convulsions* or *convulsions that are so frequent that each attack begins before the postictal period of the preceding one ends.* For example, the patient's motor movements may be continuous or stop intermittently. In the latter case, the patient may respond to stimuli or even follow simple commands, but before regaining total consciousness, another seizure may intervene.

2. Diagnosis. The diagnosis of generalized grand mal status epilepticus is not difficult. The patient exhibits tonic and/or clonic movements of all limbs, which are often associated with a conjugate deviation of the eyes (although the eyes may be seen to rove or to show clonic movements in one direction at one moment and in the opposite direction at another). The direction of deviation of the eyes in generalized status epilepticus is not usually of lateralizing value in determining a possible focus from which the attack may have precipitated.

Without a history from an observer of the onset of the seizures, there is no way to be sure whether the seizures were caused by continuous, primary, generalized grand mal epilepsy, or whether they are the result of spread from an attack of focal epilepsy. Since the latter holds a graver prognosis with respect to the underlying disease process that could have precipitated the attack (i.e., it implies focal brain disease), it is assumed that there is a focus until proved otherwise. In this way a serious focal brain lesion will not be overlooked, such as subdural hematoma, which may appear as continuous, generalized grand mal epilepsy.

3. Prognosis. *The outlook for grand mal status epilepticus depends on the underlying disease.* If, as is often the case, the patient is a known epileptic who has either stopped his anticonvulsant medications and/or was ingesting alcohol or taking drugs that he recently discontinued, then the prognosis is good. If the status epilepticus is the first manifestation of generalized grand mal convulsive epilepsy, then the prognosis is good again. If the underlying disease process is inherently benign and reversible, such as hypoglycemia, hypocalcemia, or drug or alcohol withdrawal, and it is diagnosed and treated properly and rapidly, then the prognosis is the same as for the underlying disease that led to the metabolic or chemical imbalance. If, however, status epilepticus was precipitated by severe head trauma, with brain contusion or subdural hematoma, or if the continuous seizures are the manifestation of a brain tumor or encephalitis, then the prognosis is considerably worse.

The status epilepticus, itself, may have grave consequences as a result of the hypoxia, acidosis, fractured vertebrae, and myoglobinuria that may result in the occasional patient with severe apnea and extreme muscle damage as a result of the seizure activity per se. However, if the patient is observed in a controlled environment, none of the latter difficulties should result.

In every patient with continuous grand mal convulsions, the following evaluation should be performed.

a. A **careful history** (from friends or relatives) and **physical examination** should be aimed at:

(1) Signs of head trauma.

(2) CNS infection.

(3) Drug intoxication.

(4) History of epilepsy and anticonvulsant use.

(5) Any evidence of focal characteristics of the seizures themselves.

(6) Recent surgery (e.g., thyroid or parathyroid surgery that might predispose a patient particularly to hypocalcemia).

(7) A history or physical signs of insulin use might lead one to consider hypoglycemia as a major possibility.

b. An ECG, if technically possible (sometimes it can be done interictally), may show a long QT interval, which is evidence of possibly significant hypocalcemia.

c. Before therapy is initiated, blood is drawn and sent to the laboratory for:

(1) Complete blood count.

(2) Serum glucose.

(3) Serum calcium.

(4) Serum sodium.

(5) When specifically indicated, serum and urine may be sent for toxic screen, and serum is sent for anticonvulsant levels.

    d. Nearly all patients in grand mal status epilepticus are febrile, so this alone is not an indication to do a lumbar puncture. Lumbar puncture is technically difficult in a convulsing person, and it should not be done until after the seizures are controlled unless strong indications are present (e.g., historic or physical evidence of possible bacterial meningitis).

4. Treatment of patients without history of seizures (Tables 6-5 and 6-6)

    a. When to treat. *Seizures rarely require emergency intervention.* Continuous focal seizures of any type and continuous, generalized petit mal seizures are not emergencies and should not be treated as such. A great deal of harm can be done by overdosing patients in an attempt to control these types of seizures with aggressive anticonvulsant therapy.

        Continuous, generalized grand mal tonic convulsions or clonic convulsions or both comprise the only variety of seizures that requires deliberate, relatively rapid therapy on an emergency basis. And even in this situation, *termination of the seizure within seconds or minutes is rarely required and should only be sought when the seizure activity has resulted in severe hypoxia or acidosis, which in turn threatens the patient's life.*

        Treatment of grand mal status epilepticus in patients who do not have a history of epilepsy or life-threatening acidosis or hypoxia is as follows.

    b. General measures

        (1) The patient is placed in the prone position, preferably with the head down to prevent aspiration, until full consciousness is regained.

        (2) Care is taken to maintain an adequate airway. Usually this can be accomplished with an oral airway, but occasionally endotracheal intubation is required.

Table 6-5. Treatment of Childhood Generalized Grand Mal Status Epilepticus (under 18 years of age)*

	Drug	Dose	Route	Rate
Step 1†	Glucose	1–2 ml/kg of 50% dextrose	IV	Rapid (push)
Step 2a	Phenobarbital	5–10 mg/kg	IV	Over minutes
Step 2b	Phenobarbital	5–10 mg/kg (maximum, 20 mg/kg)	IV	Every 10–15 minutes
Step 3	Phenytoin	10–15 mg/kg	IV	25 mg/minute
Step 4	Paraldehyde	Up to 2.5 ml/kg of 5% solution	IV	Slow drip
Step 5	Diazepam	Up to 10 mg	IV	Over minutes
Step 6	Pancuronium	1–5 mg	IV	Rapid (push)
Step 7	General anesthesia	—	—	—

*A reasonable amount of time should elapse between steps to assess drug action.
†If the course of treatment is interrupted at any point by life-threatening hypoxia or acidosis, proceed immediately to step 4, 5, or 6.

Table 6-6. Treatment of Adult Generalized Grand Mal Status Epilepticus
(in patients over 18 years old)*

	Drug	Dose	Route	Rate
Step 1†	Thiamine	100 mg	IV	Rapid (push)
	Glucose	25–50 gm	IV	Rapid (push)
Step 2	Phenytoin	1000 mg	IV	50 mg/min
Step 3a	Phenobarbital	90–120 mg	IV or IM	—
Step 3b	Phenobarbital	30–60 mg	IV or IM	Every 10–15 minutes to total dose of 500 mg
Step 4	Diazepam	Usually 5–10 mg	IV	Over minutes
Step 5	Pancuronium	1–5 mg	IV	Rapid (push)
Step 6	General anesthesia	—	—	—

*A reasonable amount of time should elapse between steps to assess drug action.
†If the course of treatment is interrupted at any point by life-threatening hypoxia or acidosis, proceed immediately to step 4 or 5.

(3) The patient is placed in a safe environment with padded bed rails but is not restrained, since most intraictal injuries are caused by restraint in abnormal postures.

(4) **After blood is drawn for initial chemical studies,** drug therapy is initiated [Tables 6-5 (children) and 6-6 (adults)].

c. **Drug therapy**

(1) **Thiamine.** In adults, thiamine 100 mg IV is always given before glucose to protect the patient against an exacerbation of Wernicke's encephalopathy, a relatively common disease among patients with status epilepticus.

(2) **Glucose.** All patients should receive glucose (25–50 gm by rapid IV infusion in adults and 1–2 ml/kg of 50% dextrose by IV infusion in children).

(3) **NaCl.** In patients with seizures thought to be secondary to hyponatremia (serum sodium is usually lower than 120 mEq/L), hypertonic (3%) sodium chloride should be given by slow IV drip. These patients are usually resistant to conventional anticonvulsant therapy.

In most cases, this diagnosis is not recognized until the serum sodium level is available; however, a history of compulsive water drinking, head trauma (causing the syndrome of inappropriate antidiuretic hormone), or hyponatremia in the past may raise a suspicion of this diagnosis. Note that hypertonic saline infusions are dangerous and should be reserved for severely ill patients with strongly suspected or proved hyponatremia. In these patients an attempt should be made to correct only half the calculated sodium deficit with 3% saline, which should be sufficient to terminate the seizures. The rest of the deficit can be corrected by restricting free water intake and waiting for diuresis to occur.

The formula for calculating the required sodium infusion is:

$$\text{mEq Na}^+ \text{ required} = (\text{desired serum Na} - \text{patient's serum Na}) \times (0.6 \times \text{patient's weight in kg})$$

(4) **Calcium.** In patients with hypocalcemia, one or two ampules of calcium gluconate, depending on the patient's size (90 mg of elemental calcium per ampule), should be given IV over a 5–10 minute period. In patients with an unknown etiology in which the suspicion of hypocalcemia is high (i.e., long QT interval on ECG or recent history of thyroid or parathyroid surgery), calcium should be given also, even before the serum calcium levels are available.

(5) **Phenytoin** (Dilantin) is a very effective anticonvulsant, particularly in adults. In addition to having a higher therapeutic index than other anticonvulsants, it has the additional advantage of having very little effect on the EEG. Also, it does not complicate the subsequent evaluation of the seizure disorder. Furthermore, phenytoin, even at high dosages, has little or no effect on the patient's level of consciousness, thus allowing full neurologic evaluation once the seizures have stopped.

Levels of phenytoin in the patient's serum correlate with its **clinical effectiveness.** Given IV (15 mg/kg, or about 1000 mg in adults, over 20 minutes), therapeutic levels of 10–20 μg/ml can be reached within a few minutes. Thus initial anticonvulsant therapy for generalized grand mal status epilepticus should be IV phenytoin, as already described.

This injection is given preferably by a physician, and **blood pressure, respiratory rate,** and **ECG are monitored** during the injection, since occasional fatalities have been reported due to hypotension, heart block, and respiratory depression during excessively rapid phenytoin injections. **Phenytoin should be given undiluted** since the drug may precipitate out in intravenous solutions.

IV phenytoin is **relatively contraindicated** in patients with known heart disease, particularly where conduction abnormalities are known to be part of the disease process. The injection itself requires up to 20 minutes, after which the patient should be observed for 20 or 30 minutes. Most seizures will improve significantly or stop during this time.

(6) **Phenobarbital** is generally considered the next choice for control of generalized grand mal status epilepticus. However, in children, pediatric neurologists consider phenobarbital to be the first-choice drug, rather than the second, hoping that phenytoin will not be needed either acutely or chronically.

Phenobarbital should be given **IV** if possible (5–10 mg/kg in children and 90–120 mg in adults), either as the initial drug or as the second-line drug if phenytoin fails to control the seizures. This may be repeated every 10–15 minutes in slightly different dosages (5–10 mg/kg in children and 30–60 mg in adults) to a maximum dose of about 20 mg/kg in children and 500 mg in adults.

Respiratory depression is common with barbiturates, particularly when given IV; and then they should be given only when the facilities are available for emergency endotracheal intubation. In patients who received phenobarbital as the first-line drug, phenytoin may be used as the second (as already outlined).

(7) **Diazepam** (Valium) is a benzodiazepine derivative that possesses some anticonvulsant activity; and recently it has gained a great deal of popularity in the treatment of continuous generalized convulsions. Although it will nearly always stop the muscular movement, it will less often actually control the epileptic discharges seen by EEG. Furthermore, since its action is brief, it should never be given alone but always in combination with a long-acting anticonvulsant such as phenytoin. However, there are some situations in which this sequence

is not effective or the patient is severely apneic or hypoxic and, as a result, enough time cannot be allowed for the conventional anticonvulsants to work. In this rather unusual circumstance, diazepam may be very useful (up to 10 mg by slow IV infusion) to control clinical seizure activity. Thus use of this drug should be reserved for this unusual situation and that of partially treated epilepsy (mentioned in the next section), since production of coma may make neurologic evaluation of the patient extremely difficult. Endotracheal intubation is very often required at this stage and hypotension is a frequent problem.

(8) **Paraldehyde** is useful in controlling refractory forms of generalized grand mal status epilepticus, particularly in children. However, because of the technical difficulties in giving larger amounts of the drug (it may produce cold abscesses when given IM and will dissolve plastic tubing or syringes when given IV), most neurologists use it only to treat small children, who require very small amounts of the drug. In this case the drug can be diluted considerably in saline and given IV without danger of dissolving the plastic tubing.

A 5% solution of paraldehyde in saline, up to 2.5 ml/kg, is given IV by a slow drip at a rate that is titrated to control the seizures. However, respiratory depression can occur, as with barbiturates, so the drug should only be given under careful observation with facilities for artificial respiration at hand.

(9) **Pancuronium** (Pavulon) is a neuromuscular blocking agent that has no anticonvulsant properties. It is used only for continuous generalized convulsions when all other measures have failed and/or the patient is suffering the effects of excessive muscular movement, apnea, or life-threatening acidosis. The dosage is 1–5 mg by rapid IV infusion, after which the patient must be intubated and placed on a respirator. This drug is rarely required.

(10) **General anesthesia** is the last resort for the control of grand mal status epilepticus. In addition to controlling the muscular movements, it also acts as an anticonvulsant and will terminate the most resistant forms of status epilepticus. Long-acting anticonvulsants should always be given before general anesthesia is administered.

5. **Treatment of patients with known epilepsy.** When faced with a patient in continuous generalized grand mal convulsions, who is a known epileptic on treatment, it is often difficult to determine initially whether the patient has been taking his or her medications faithfully and has suffered some intercurrent illness precipitating status epilepticus, or whether the patient's status is a result of discontinuation of anticonvulsants, possibly coupled with barbiturate withdrawal seizures. Thus in this case serum samples are drawn immediately and are sent to the laboratory for the usual studies (as outlined previously) as well as for anticonvulsant levels. However, the results may take many hours or days to obtain.

a. **Diazepam.** Often a limited trial of diazepam is useful in this circumstance (up to 5 mg by slow IV infusion). If the patient has some anticonvulsant in his or her serum (perhaps slightly below the therapeutic range), then diazepam will often control the seizures enough so that a history can be obtained from the patient or the anticonvulsant levels can be determined by the laboratory.

b. **Other anticonvulsants.** If diazepam fails to abort the seizures, then **phenytoin** and **phenobarbital** may be used as outlined previously, as long as preparations have been made for endotracheal intubation if the patient experiences respiratory depression. **Overdosage** of phenytoin may be associated with heart block or respiratory depression, so careful monitoring of the ECG should be maintained, and phenytoin should be discontinued if any conduction abnormalities are noted. Also, phenytoin should probably not be given to patients with possible therapeutic levels of phenytoin already in their systems unless facilities are available for temporary cardiac pacemaking.

D. Myoclonic epilepsy. The term *myoclonus* is used to describe several different types of abnormal involuntary movements characterized by single or repetitive jerks of a body part. The phenomenon of myoclonus may be a symptom of a disease that involves numerous parts of the nervous system. However, some types of myoclonus are associated with paroxysmal discharges of the EEG, suggesting that it is epileptic in nature. Other types have no associated EEG abnormality, and these are not generally felt to be epileptic in nature. The latter variety includes many **biochemical disorders,** such as uremia and hepatic failure; nocturnal myoclonus, occurring as a person is about to fall asleep; myoclonus seen in some spinal cord lesions; and palatal myoclonus, which is thought to be caused by disease of the central tegmental tract of the brainstem. Action myoclonus, seen occasionally as a sequel to hypoxic brain damage or encephalitis, sometimes has associated EEG spikes and sometimes does not.

Two particular varieties of myoclonus are associated with EEG abnormalities and are thought to be epileptic in the usual sense of the word. These are infantile spasms and childhood (late-onset) myoclonic epilepsy.

1. Infantile spasms

    a. Description. Infantile spasms are defined as *massive flexor* (rarely extensor) *spasms of the extremities and trunk that begin in infancy, usually between the ages of 4 and 9 months,* and are associated with hypsarrhythmia.

    There are two varieties of infantile spasms. The so-called cryptogenic variety occurs with a normal past history. That is, there is a normal pregnancy, delivery, and normal child development until the onset of seizures. The patient's development usually regresses rapidly thereafter. The so-called symptomatic variety may be caused by perinatal hypoxia, mechanical trauma, congenital infection, developmental anomalies of brain (particularly lissencephaly), various aminoacidurias (particularly phenylketonuria), or neuroectodermal disorders (e.g., tuberous sclerosis). These patients are delayed developmentally even before the onset of the seizures. Both types are characterized by generalized flexor spasms of the neck, trunk, and extremities. The attacks occur in bouts several times a day, occurring sometimes as often as 50 times per day, often during periods of drowsiness.

    b. Diagnosis. The diagnosis depends on the characteristic appearance of spells in an infant between the ages of 4 and 9 months, although occasionally the onset can be earlier or later (up to 2 years). The EEG shows an abnormality that is referred to as hypsarrhythmia (generalized asynchronous spikes and high-voltage slow, sharp activity), which is highly characteristic of this disorder. Diagnostic evaluation should include a search for a metabolic, infectious, or structural abnormality, which may be the cause of the spasms.

    c. Prognosis. The prognosis with infantile spasms is poor, particularly if there is an earlier onset and if there is delayed development prior to the onset of the seizures. Most patients die in childhood due to complications of the chronic, underlying neurologic disease.

    d. Treatment (Table 6-7)

        (1) Adrenocorticotrophic hormone (ACTH) may have some effect on the course of infantile spasms in that it may control the seizures and improve the EEG transiently. However, there is no evidence that

Table 6-7. Treatment of Infantile Spasms

Choice	Drug	Preparation	Dose	Route
1	ACTH	ACTH for parenteral injection	30 units, divided into one to two doses for 4–6 weeks	IM
2	Clonazepam (Clonopin)	0.5, 1.0, 2.0 mg tablets	0.01–0.03 mg/kg/day, divided into three doses, increasing by 0.25–0.5 mg every 3 days to a maintenance dosage of 0.1–0.2 mg/kg/day	PO
3	Diazepam (Valium)	2, 5, and 10 mg tablets; 0.4 mg/ml syrup	1–2 mg every 3 hours	PO
4*	Ketogenic diet			
5†	Acetazolamide (Diamox)	250 mg tablets	10–25 mg/kg/day, divided into three doses	PO

* A ketogenic diet may be used with any of choices 1, 2, or 3, but it is of little use alone.
† Acetazolamide may be used with any of choices 1, 2, or 3, but it is of little use alone.

treatment with ACTH will alter the ultimate outcome. ACTH, 30 units per day, divided into one to two doses may be given IM for 4–6 weeks.

(2) **Clonazepam** (Clonopin), a benzodiazepine derivative that is related to diazepam, has recently been shown to be useful in the treatment of various types of myoclonus. It is started at 0.01–0.03 mg/kg/day PO and is gradually increased to 0.1–0.2 mg/kg/day, divided into three doses.

(3) **Diazepam** (Valium) is occasionally effective in infantile spasms in dosages of about 1–2 mg PO every 3 hours.

(4) **A ketogenic diet** is often used in combination with any of these drugs.

(5) **Acetazolamide** (Diamox) may also be used in combination with any of the therapies discussed.

2. **Childhood myoclonic epilepsy** (late-onset myoclonic epilepsy)

   a. **Description.** Childhood myoclonic epilepsy refers to a group of conditions characterized by myoclonic attacks, usually beginning in the second year of life and often associated with other seizure types and an abnormal EEG. Myoclonic epilepsy of childhood may be either primary (cryptogenic) or secondary to a variety of degenerative disorders.

   In the primary variety, patients are usually normal at birth and for the first year of life. Usually during the second year, they begin having multiple types of seizures, among which are jackknife spasms, salaam attacks (outward thrusts of the arms and flexion at the waist), akinetic (drop) attacks as well as ordinary grand mal convulsions, and absence attacks that strongly resemble petit mal epilepsy clinically. In the secondary type, the clinical presentation varies depending on the underlying condition.

   b. **Diagnosis.** The diagnosis of idiopathic myoclonic epilepsy of childhood is suggested strongly in a 1- to 3-year-old child who develops multiple seizure types, among which are forms of myoclonic epilepsy (as already described) and intellectual deterioration. The EEG is usually grossly abnormal, with spikes, polyspikes, and areas of atypical (i.e., other than 3/sec) spikes and slow wave patterns (Lennox-Gastaut syndrome). The diagnosis of primary myoclonic epilepsy of childhood depends on the exclusion of secondary myoclonic epilepsy due to:

      (1) Lafora's disease, which is inherited as a recessive trait. Intracytoplasmic glycoprotein inclusions are seen in neurons as well as other cells widely distributed both inside and outside the nervous system;

      (2) Lipidoses involving neurons (e.g., Batten's disease, juvenile Tay-Sachs disease); or

      (3) Various degenerative diseases of the nervous system (e.g., SSPE).

   It is important to make the diagnosis of an inherited myoclonic epilepsy so that genetic counseling may be provided. It is often necessary to resort to brain biopsy in cases of late-onset myoclonic epilepsy to clarify the diagnosis.

   c. **Prognosis.** In general, the prognosis for the primary variety of late-onset myoclonic epilepsy is poor. Some patients, however, seem to progress very slowly or even to level off for long periods; and treatment is, by and large, more satisfying in this condition than in the infantile forms. In the secondary forms, the prognosis depends on the underlying illness.

   d. **Treatment** (Table 6-8)

      (1) **Phenytoin** and **phenobarbital** are used either singly or in combina-

Table 6-8. Treatment of Childhood (Late-Onset) Myoclonic Epilepsy

Choice	Drug	Preparation	Dose	Route
1	Phenobarbital (Luminal)	15, 30, 60, and 100 mg tablets; 5 mg/ml elixir; injectable	3–5 mg/kg/day, divided into two to three doses	PO, IM
2	Phenytoin (Dilantin)	30 and 100 mg tablets; 6 mg/ml suspension; 20 mg/ml suspension; 250 mg/ampules	5 mg/kg/day, divided into one to three doses	PO
3	Clonazepam (Clonopin)	0.5, 1.0, 2 mg tablets	0.01–0.03 mg/kg/day, increasing to 0.1–0.2 mg/kg/day	PO
4	Ethosuximide (Zarontin)	250 mg capsules; 50 mg/ml syrup	20 mg/kg/day, divided into two to three doses, increasing to 40 mg/kg/day	PO
5	Carbamazepine (Tegretol)	200 mg tablets	7–15 mg/kg/day, divided into two to three doses	PO
6	Acetazolamide (Diamox)	250 mg tablets	10–25 mg/kg/day, divided into three doses	PO
7	Ketogenic diet			
8	Dextroamphetamine (Dexedrine)	5, 10, 15 mg capsules; 1 mg/ml elixir	5–40 mg/day, divided into two to three doses	PO
	Sodium valproate (Depakene)*	250 mg tablets; 60 mg/ml syrup	10–20 mg/kg/day divided into 3 doses	PO

* Exact place in the sequence of drug choices not yet known.

tion, since grand mal convulsions are usually a major part of late-onset myoclonic epilepsy.

(2) **Clonazepam** and **diazepam** may be useful to control the myoclonus (see sec **IV.D.1.d.(2), (3)**, infantile spasms).

(3) **Ethosuximide** may be useful, particularly if an important component of atypical petit mal epilepsy is seen either clinically or on EEG.

(4) **Carbamazepine** is sometimes of limited use in these patients.

(5) **Acetazolamide** and a **ketogenic diet** are often added to these drugs and may be particularly useful in this type of seizure disorder.

(6) **Dextroamphetamine** (Dexedrine) 5–40 mg/day, divided into two to three doses PO, is often useful, both for the seizures and to counteract the sedative effects of the multiple anticonvulsants, which are often used in an attempt to control the extraordinarily difficult type of seizure disorder.

3. Febrile seizures

1. **Description.** Febrile seizures are defined as *brief generalized seizures in a child, usually between the ages of 6 months and 5 years, who is febrile prior to the seizure in the absence of central nervous system* (CNS) *infection.*

   If the definition of febrile seizures is strictly followed, then it is possible to separate out a group of children who have a better prognosis than most.

   a. The child should be between 6 months and 5 years of age.

   b. There should be a clear history of fever prior to the onset of the seizure.

   c. The spell itself should be apoplectic in onset with absolutely no focal characteristics.

   d. It should be short, usually less than 10 minutes in duration.

   e. There should be no Todd's (postictal) paralysis, and the EEG should be normal 2 weeks after the seizure (often normal within 24 hours).

   f. Usually such seizures are over by the time the family can bring the child to the emergency room, and therapy is rarely required.

   g. Lumbar puncture should be normal, free of any evidence of infection.

   h. Routine laboratory studies, including electrolytes, CBC, calcium, phosphate, magnesium, and BUN are all normal.

   i. In situations in which the possibility of lead poisoning exists, a lead level may also be determined.

   If all these criteria are satisfied, then the patient with febrile seizures has an excellent prognosis. Although there is a 50% chance of a recurrence with fever in the future, most patients will have no future seizures after the age of 5 years. If, however, all these criteria are not strictly satisfied, febrile seizures cannot be diagnosed properly, and the prognosis will vary, depending on the patient's underlying condition. Most spells that do not quite fit these criteria will be idiopathic convulsions exacerbated by fever, which is a common occurrence. Thus whenever these criteria are not strictly satisfied, a more complete evaluation of the patient must be done to search for an underlying cause of the seizure disorder other than fever. If none is found, then the diagnosis is idiopathic epilepsy, and anticonvulsants should be started as described in sec **IV.C.** and Table 6-2.

2. **Treatment** (Table 6-9). By definition, very little or no therapy is required to control a single febrile convulsion.

   a. **Control of fever.** Control of fever with either aspirin (60 mg/year of age to maximum of 300 mg every 4 hours either PR or PO) or tepid baths is adequate in most cases.

Table 6-9. Treatment of Febrile Convulsions

Choice	Agent	Dose	Route	Rate
Acutely				
1	ASA	60 mg/year of age to a maximum of 300 mg every 4 hours	PO PR	
and/or				
1	Tepid baths			
2	Phenobarbital	5 mg/kg	IV	Over minutes
Prophylactically				
1	Phenobarbital	3–5 mg/kg/day, divided into two to three doses	PO	

b. **Phenobarbital.** Occasionally one dose of phenobarbital 5 mg/kg given slowly IV is required.

c. **Prophylactic therapy.** In patients with recurrent febrile seizures, prophylactic therapy with phenobarbital is indicated. Most of these patients will no longer require anticonvulsant therapy after the age of 5 years.

V. FOCAL EPILEPSY

A. **Description.** Focal epilepsy refers to seizures that arise from a particular focal region of the brain. A focal seizure may:

1. Remain focal;

2. Spread to involve neighboring regions of cortex (jacksonian seizure); or

3. Proceed to a generalized convulsion.

B. **Diagnosis.** In any of these cases it is the onset of the spell that determines whether it is a focal seizure. Since any area of the cerebral cortex may be involved with focal epileptic discharges, nearly every variety of human experience can initiate a seizure. In fact, often the nature of the behavior or the experience that precedes a generalized convulsion gives a clue to the focus from which the seizure emanated.

The disturbance of cortical function that precedes a generalized convulsion is referred to as the **aura.** By definition, an aura occurs only in focal epilepsy and is of strong differential value in diagnosing a patient who has had a generalized convulsion. Thus an aura rules out primary, generalized grand mal epilepsy and confirms the diagnosis of focal epilepsy with spread to a secondary generalized convulsion. A postictal (Todd's) paralysis also suggests a focal seizure. *This distinction is crucial, since focal epilepsy represents focal brain disease, whereas generalized epilepsy does not.*

In focal epilepsy a careful search for the underlying disease process always should be made. A history of the exact nature of the focal seizures or the aura of secondary generalized seizures may provide valuable information regarding the location of the abnormality. A focal or lateralizing EEG abnormality may also be helpful.

Focal seizures are usually divided into two major categories: those with simple and those with complex symptoms.

1. **Simple symtoms** refer to elementary sensations, simple movements, or speech disturbances. These disturbances may be the motor, sensory, or au-

tonomic. Examples of focal motor seizures are localized, repetitive movements of a body part, masticatory movements, vocalization, adversive postures, or tonic postures. Sensory seizures may be somatic, visual, auditory, gustatory, vertiginous, or abdominal, and autonomic attacks may initiate nausea, vomiting, or diaphoresis. Aphasic attacks of various types are also well known as manifestations of focal epilepsy, originating in speech areas. These seizures are thought to originate in the areas of cortex, which are known to subserve movement or sensation for the particular body parts involved. The cortical representation of autonomic functions is less well understood, and the question of whether subcortical structures might be the source of these spells is raised.

2. **Complex symptoms** refer to apparently integrated purposeful activity, with amnesia and psychic phenomena, such as hallucinations, déjà vu (factitious familiarity with an unfamiliar environment), jamais vu (factitious unfamiliarity with a familiar environment), paranoid feelings, forced thinking, and affective disturbances. This group of disorders has been referred to as *psychomotor epilepsy,* which is thought to arise from abnormalities in the temporal lobes. Most cases of **temporal lobe epilepsy** begin between the ages of 10 and 30 years. Cases that begin after the age of 30 years should raise the question of brain tumor, primary or secondary.

In younger children, temporal lobe epilepsy may be difficult to distinguish from petit mal seizures. However, the presence of an aura and postictal confusion in the former often helps to make the distinction clinically. The EEG is often helpful, particularly if it shows the typical 3/sec spikes and slow wave pattern of classic petit mal epilepsy. A normal EEG interictally is of no help in making the distinction.

C. Evaluation

1. A careful history and physical examination with special reference to evidence of **old strokes, birth injury, congenital anomalies, remote infections, head trauma, cranial surgery,** and **neoplasm** (particularly carcinoma of the breast, lung, colon, melanoma, and renal cell carcinoma).

2. EEG (If the routine EEG is normal, activation procedures may be used, including sleep, hyperventilation, and photic stimuli. Occasionally special recording methods are used, such as nasopharyngeal leads, in an attempt to record abnormalities in the temporal lobes—areas that are far from the standard scalp electrodes).

3. Computed tomography of the brain (CT scanning) using contrast material (if the routine study is normal) to highlight neoplastic tissue.

4. Technetium pertechnitate scan if CT scanning is not available.

5. Lumbar puncture, with special reference to cell count, cytology, syphilis serology, and protein.

6. Chest x-ray.

7. Skull x-ray.

8. Complete blood count.

9. Erythrocyte sedimentation rate.

10. Stool guaiac.

11. Serum electrolytes.

12. Serum calcium and phosphate.

13. Liver function tests (SGOT, total bilirubin, and alkaline phosphatase).

14. Urinalysis.

15. BUN and serum creatinine.

16. Blood sugar.

17. Further studies, including pneumoencephalography (PEG) or arteriography, may be required if the screening studies discussed are abnormal, requiring further evaluation of a particular part of the nervous system.

  In children with focal epilepsy, there is less likelihood of a serious underlying brain disease than in adults, and thus the evaluation is sometimes less extensive. If the evaluation is negative, then treatment may be begun, but careful, frequent follow-up examinations are necessary, since the primary disease process may only become obvious some time after the epilepsy begins.

D. Prognosis. The **outlook** depends on the underlying condition; even if the primary disease is benign (e.g., mesial temporal sclerosis) or no primary disease can be found (idiopathic focal epilepsy), these seizures are generally much more difficult to treat than generalized epilepsy. In the case of psychomotor epilepsy, interictal behavioral abnormalities are a common accompaniment of the disease. Whether these psychiatric syndromes (e.g., schizophrenialike illness sometimes seen in patients with temporal lobe epilepsy) are due to the same primary disease that caused the epilepsy is unknown at the present time. However, it is generally agreed that *anticonvulsants have little or no effect on the interictal behavior disorders seen in these patients.* Many require antipsychotic drugs for the control of these disorders, and the prognosis for a normal life in these patients is poor. In focal seizures with simple symptoms, there is no concomitant psychiatric illness, but the seizures themselves may be very difficult to control without reaching drug toxicity.

E. Treatment

1. Medical. The drug treatment of focal epilepsy is the same as that for generalized grand mal convulsions (Tables 6-2 and 6-4). The only difference in the therapy is that multiple drugs are required more often to control focal seizures than to control generalized convulsions. However, vigorous treatment with multiple drugs often leads to respiratory depression and other iatrogenic difficulties in the management of focal seizures.

  An important principle of treatment is that *focal epilepsy, even when continuous (focal status epilepticus), is not an emergency and should not be treated as such.* It is also important to remember that control is difficult, and rapid control of focal phenomena is rarely, if ever, required. Thus one should proceed cautiously and methodically through the choices of drugs shown in Tables 6-2 and 6-4, making sure not to produce unacceptable side effects in an effort to control small focal abnormalities. The common drug combinations shown in Table 6-4 may be used in focal epilepsy in the same way as in generalized convulsions.

2. Surgical. Occasionally focal seizures are impossible to control medically, and surgical intervention is necessary. Some patients will improve with cerebellar stimulators, while others will require surgical removal of the offending focus. However, results in these extraordinarily severe cases are variable, so surgical treatment should be reserved for medical failures and should not be used as a first-line form of therapy. Exceptions to this rule are patients with focal epilepsy caused by a surgically removable tumor, arteriovenous malformation (AVM), or congenital anomaly.

  Some neurosurgeons believe that the behavioral abnormalities sometimes seen in temporal lobe epilepsy may be reversed by removal of the epileptogenic focus. However, this is not a generally accepted notion and, at present, only medically uncontrollable seizures are an indication for surgery.

VI. NEONATAL SEIZURES

A. Description. Neonatal seizures refer to seizure activity during the first 30 days of life.

  Unlike in the older patient, seizures in the newborn are often subtle and more difficult to diagnose. Common manifestations of neonatal seizures include:

1. Tonic eye deviation or rapid eye movements or both.
2. Repetitive eyelid blinking.
3. Facial grimacing.
4. Fragmentary clonic movements of single extremities.
5. Tonic posturing of a single extremity.
6. Apnea, often associated with other seizure activity but sometimes as the sole manifestation of the seizure.
7. Generalized tonic-clonic seizures, which occur but are uncommon.

B. Diagnosis. The diagnosis rests on the clinician's ability to recognize the symptoms, which are often only fragmentary movements that may be epileptic in nature. Treatment of the seizure itself is rarely an emergency unless respirations are compromised; it is more important to diagnose the patient's condition rapidly, so appropriate therapy can be initiated promptly. Speed is important because several types of neonatal seizures may result in irreversible cerebral damage.

1. The common causes of neonatal seizures are as follows:
   a. Central nervous system **birth injury** that is either:
      (1) **Hypoxic,** as can be seen in abruptio placentae, placenta previa, and fetal distress; or
      (2) **Mechanical trauma,** as can be found in large babies or infants delivered with mid or high forceps. The latter may develop subdural hematomas that can cause the seizures.
   b. **Metabolic abnormalities,** such as:
      (1) **Hypocalcemia,** which is the most common metabolic abnormality leading to neonatal seizures.
         (a) Early-onset hypocalcemia (within the first 3 days of life) is commonly seen in babies with low birth weights, in premature infants, and in babies who are small for their gestational age. There is often a history of pregnancy complicated by toxemia, perinatal distress, or mechanical birth trauma.
         (b) Late-onset hypocalcemia (after the third day of life) is thought to be due to the high phosphate load the infant receives in the first few days of life. The serum calcium level is usually below 7.5 mg/100 ml in both early and late-onset hypocalcemia.
      (2) **Hypomagnesemia** presents much the same picture as hypocalcemia and in the same high-risk groups, but it is less common. Hypomagnesemia and hypocalcemia may coexist, and both must be treated.
      (3) **Hypoglycemia** usually occurs within the first few hours of birth. In babies who are small for their gestational age, premature, have diabetic mothers, or are septic, one should suspect possible hypoglycemia. Many pediatricians will start early feedings or an IV glucose infusion as prophylaxis against hypoglycemia. Also, blood sugar should be monitored frequently in high-risk groups, since hypoglycemia can produce irreversible cerebral damage. It is obviously better to prevent neonatal hypoglycemic seizures than to treat them once they occur.
      (4) **Pyridoxine dependency** usually produces seizures within minutes or hours after birth.
      (5) Other metabolic abnormalities, including **aminoacidurias** and **drug withdrawal** (infants of addicted mothers), should be considered, but they are less common.

Table 6-10. Treatment of Neonatal Seizures*

Step*	Drug†	Dose	Route	Rate
1	Glucose	2–4 ml/kg of 25% dextrose	IV	Rapid (push)
2	Pyridoxine	50 mg	IV	Rapid (push)
3	Calcium	Up to 10 ml 10% calcium gluconate	IV	Over minutes
4	Magnesium	Up to 5 ml 3% MgSO₄	IV	Over minutes
5	Phenobarbital	10–20 mg/kg	IV	Over minutes
6	Phenytoin	10–15 mg/kg	IV	25 mg/minute
7	Paraldehyde	Up to 2.5 mg/kg of a 5% solution	IV	Slow drip
8	Diazepam	Up to 3 mg	IV	Over minutes
9	Pancuronium	1–2 mg	IV	Rapid (push)

*If the course of treatment is interrupted at any point by life-threatening hypoxia or acidosis, proceed immediately to step 7, 8, or 9.
†A reasonable amount of time should elapse between steps to assess drug action.

    c. Central nervous system infections, both intrauterine and postnatally acquired may produce seizures in the first month of life. The evaluation should include routine CSF examination and antibody titers for toxoplasmosis, rubella, cytomegalovirus, and herpesvirus.

    d. Developmental anomalies of many varieties may occur with seizures during the neonatal period.

  C. Treatment (Table 6-10). Once blood is drawn and sent to the laboratory for analysis, therapy is begun at once. The sequence shown in Table 6-10 is self-explanatory; however, it is extremely rare that one needs to progress beyond step 5 (phenobarbital). Also, if at any time this orderly process is interrupted by life-threatening acidosis or hypoxia, then paraldehyde, diazepam, or pancuronium is given immediately, and the patient is placed on artificial ventilation.

VII. PAROXYSMAL CONDITIONS RESEMBLING EPILEPSY. A number of paroxysmal disorders exist that may be related to epilepsy, either by virtue of their clinical similarity and possible confusions in diagnosis, or by virtue of their possible, although unproved, true epileptic nature. It is important to diagnose these syndromes correctly, since some have specific therapies of their own, a few of which may actually conflict with anticonvulsant therapy.

  A. Narcolepsy

    1. Description. Narcolepsy is defined as a group of disorders characterized by some or all the following characteristics:

      a. Sleep attacks (irresistable episodes of sleep).

      b. Cataplexy (sudden attacks of loss of postural tone sparing consciousness, often stimulated by emotional experiences, such as laughter, passion, or fear).

      c. Sleep paralysis (total paralysis that lasts a few minutes, usually on awakening from sleep but sometimes just before falling to sleep).

    d. Hypnagogic hallucinations (vivid visual or auditory hallucinations or both just as the person is falling asleep).

    e. The EEG may show the characteristic phenomenon of sleep-onset rapid eye movement (REM) sleep.

There are two types of **normal sleep.** The non-REM variety is characterized by four levels, defined by EEG patterns, corresponding roughly to the depth of sleep (I being the lightest; IV, the deepest). During non-REM sleep, body tone is maintained, and the person shifts postures frequently. The other variety, REM sleep, is characterized by total loss of tone in all muscles except the extraocular muscles and some muscles of the nasopharynx. An EMG (electromyograph) placed on these muscles will document this fact.

The EEG taken during REM sleep shows light sleep, which can only be distinguished from stage I non-REM sleep by placing EMG and ENG (electronystagmograph) leads over the extraocular muscles to document the characteristic rapid conjugate movement of the eyes.

Normally, when a person goes to sleep, he passes through at least one cycle of non-REM sleep (I through IV) before entering REM sleep. The relation between REM and non-REM portions of sleep changes with age: In infants, a large proportion of time is spent in REM sleep, but this decreases with age, and, in adults, only about 20% of the night is spent in REM sleep. It is during this portion that dreaming is thought to occur.

It is believed that control of the relation between the waking state with REM and non-REM sleep is mediated in part by the **reticular activating system** (RAS) in the brainstem.

The essential abnormality in narcolepsy is thought to be an underactive reticular activating system. Some patients with narcolepsy will slip uncontrollably from the waking state directly into REM sleep (so-called sleep-onset REM), and it is believed that, as a result of this process, the rest of the syndrome evolves. For example, **sleep paralysis** and **cataplexy** are merely components of the paralysis that occurs during normal REM sleep (as already noted); and **hypnagogic hallucinations** are merely dreams, normally occurring in the REM sleep state.

Patients with narcolepsy are most likely to fall asleep in situations that would normally produce drowsiness (i.e., postprandial and during boredom), presumably because of an underactive reticular activating system, and are unable to maintain the waking state under stress. Patients who have more severe narcolepsy will of course fall asleep at inappropriate times, such as while driving a car.

Studies of accident-prone drivers have revealed a much higher-than-expected number of narcoleptics. The relation between emotional experiences and cataplexy is unknown, but it is thought to be mediated through the reticular activating system also.

2. Diagnosis. The diagnosis depends on a characteristic history and the typical EEG pattern, although the latter will not occur in every episode of sleep. Thus a normal sleep EEG does not rule out narcolepsy. Conversely, sleep-onset REM, found incidentally in asymptomatic patients should not lead to treatment for narcolepsy. However, it should be considered in patients with hypersomnia, whether or not the other associated abnormalities are found. The EEG may be helpful if positive (i.e., if it shows sleep-onset REM); however, the diagnosis can be made legitimately with a normal EEG if the history is sufficiently characteristic.

It is possible to confuse narcolepsy with epilepsy, particularly if the sleep attacks come on very suddenly. However, a history of an irresistable tendency to sleep and the associated abnormalities should confirm the proper diagnosis by history alone.

The outlook for narcolepsy is generally good, and it usually responds dramatically to drug therapy.

3. Treatment. There is no single treatment for all the elements of narcolepsy. The individual patient must be treated for his or her predominant symptoms, sometimes combining drugs to attain adequate relief from the entire complex.

a. Sleep attacks, hypnagogic hallucinations, and sleep paralysis

(1) Amphetamines are known to suppress REM sleep. It is not known whether this characteristic of these agents is the reason for their effectiveness in narcolepsy. However, it is clear that amphetamines are often useful to control sleep attacks and are sometimes useful to control hypnagogic hallucinations and sleep paralysis.

Many problems are associated with **chronic use of amphetamines.** For example, many narcoleptics abuse these agents, constantly raising the dosage as their tolerance develops. Other patients find that under treatment they are less aware of an upcoming sleep attack, thus making them an even greater risk for accidents. Since amphetamines interfere with normal sleep, these patients often require increasingly higher doses during the day to protect against an even greater tendency for sleep attacks.

Side effects of amphetamine use include a syndrome of irritability, paranoid ideation, and psychosis. Furthermore, these agents are relatively contraindicated in patients with coronary artery disease and hyperthyroidism.

Despite these drawbacks, when used carefully, they are still the best treatment of the major manifestations of narcolepsy. Whichever amphetamine preparation is used, therapy should begin with low dosages and be gradually increased until a satisfactory therapeutic effect is obtained. Some commonly used agents are as follows:

(a) Methylphenidate (Ritalin) 20–200 mg/day PO, divided into two or three doses.

(b) Methamphetamine hydrochloride (Fetamin) 20–200 mg/day PO, divided into two or three doses.

(c) Dextroamphetamine sulfate (Dexedrine) 20–200 mg/day PO, divided into two or three doses.

(2) **Monoamine oxidase (MAO) inhibitors** often have a striking therapeutic effect. However, serious side effects, such as orthostatic hypotension, hypertension, edema, and impotence are common, requiring discontinuance of the medication in a large number of patients. They cannot be given in combination with dibenzepin derivatives (e.g., tricyclic antidepressants, doxepin, or carbamazepine), sympathomimetics (e.g., amphetamines), food with high tyramine content (cheese, sour cream, chianti wine, sherry, beer, pickled foods, etc.). Withdrawal of monoamine oxidase inhibitors may result in insomnia, hallucinations, and serious depression, with suicidal thoughts and severe anxiety. For this reason, they are only recommended when amphetamines cannot be used and the symptoms of narcolepsy are unbearable. Even then the drug should be administered only under strict supervision.

(a) Phenelzine sulfate (Nardil) 15–75 mg/day, divided into three or four oral doses.

b. Cataplexy

(1) **Tricyclic antidepressants.** Amphetamines and monoamine oxidase inhibitors have little effect on cataplexy. However, it has been shown that the tricyclic antidepressants may be particularly effective in the relief of this symptom. Furthermore, they are effective in much lower

dosages than are required for the treatment of depression, suggesting a separate mechanism for their effect in this syndrome.

(a) Imipramine (Tofranil) 50–100 mg/day PO, divided into one to three doses.

c. **Sleep attacks and cataplexy.** Theoretically, the combination of a tricyclic antidepressant and an amphetamine is dangerous, since the latter causes a release of catecholamines at the neuronal synapse; the former blocks reuptake of the catecholamine neurotransmitter. This combination could therefore produce hypertensive episodes, but actually one may generally use imipramine (25 mg three times per day) together with methylphenidate (5–10 mg three times per day) without difficulty and with good control of both sleep attacks and cataplexy. Tricyclic antidepressants should *not*, however, be used in combination with a monoamine oxidase inhibitor.

C. **Migraine** (see also Chap. 2). Because of its paroxysmal attacks of neurologic symptoms, usually followed by headache, migraine has some relation to epilepsy. However, the differential diagnosis between the two conditions is not usually difficult. In one situation, brainstem or basilar artery migraine, loss of consciousness may occur due to vasomotor changes consequent to transient brainstem ischemia, and this may imitate epilepsy. In some rare circumstances, the cerebral ischemia due to vasospasm may actually trigger bona fide convulsions, usually in a patient with known epilepsy. On the other hand, some patients with migraine have associated paroxysmal EEG abnormalities. Some of these patients experience relief of their headaches when treated with anticonvulsants, so a trial of phenytoin or phenobarbital is often warranted in these patients. (See Chapter 2 for the details of diagnosis and treatment of migraine.)

D. **Paroxysmal abdominal pain** ("abdominal epilepsy"). A syndrome of paroxysmal abdominal pain occurs in children for which no gastrointestinal or intra-abdominal cause can be found. Some of these patients will respond to conventional anticonvulsant therapy, which has led some to believe that this pain is caused by an epileptic syndrome. Thus in a child with recurrent seizurelike episodes of abdominal pain, in which a thorough medical evaluation has revealed no cause, it is probably reasonable to perform an EEG and conduct a therapeutic trial of phenytoin, phenobarbital, or some other relatively safe anticonvulsant.

E. **Breath-holding spells** usually begin during the first 2 years of life, but rarely before 6 months of age. A precipitating factor, such as fear, pain, anger, or frustration leads to a brief bout of crying, during which the breath is held in expiration. Cyanosis then develops, which may be followed by loss of consciousness and a brief generalized convulsion. The exact mechanism for this type of spell and its physiologic consequences are not known, but the brief convulsion that is sometimes seen is presumably caused by cerebral hypoxia.

Treatment consists of parental reassurance and practical advice on how to protect the child during a spell. There is no doubt that behavioral influences may lead to an increase in the frequency of spells, and parents should be advised of this possibility. While it is often difficult to do, parents should be advised to ignore the spells if possible.

It is important to distinguish between breath-holding spells and true epilepsy, because the prognosis and treatment differ. Anticonvulsants are not indicated in the treatment of breath-holding spells, and they are not effective in terminating the attacks. The spells almost always terminate by the age of 5 years, and they have no relation to the later development of epilepsy.

F. **Hypercyanotic attacks.** In patients with cyanotic, congenital heart disease, particularly tetralogy of Fallot, sudden episodes of increased cyanosis may occur followed by loss of consciousness and perhaps a convulsion. The mechanism for these attacks may be spasm of the already small infundibulum (right ventricular outflow tract). The pulmonary circulation, which is already compromised, is decreased further, and the blood becomes even more unsaturated with oxygen than it is normally. Then cerebral anoxia increases suddenly, and loss of consciousness and, possibly, convulsions result. The treatment is repair of the anomaly or at least surgical creation of an aortopulmonary shunt (Blalock-Taussig operation) until definitive repair is technically possible. No anticonvulsants are required. Treatment of the acute attack is administration of oxygen in as high a concentration as can be obtained.

G. Cardiovascular syncope. Syncope is loss of consciousness due to an acute decrease in cerebral blood flow. If it is prolonged, convulsions may occur, particularly in patients with known epilepsy. The causes of syncope are protean, but they must always be ruled out when the patient suffers from episodic loss of consciousness, with or without convulsions. It is important to make this distinction, because the treatment of cardiovascular syncope varies significantly from the treatment of epilepsy. In fact, phenytoin, the first choice anticonvulsant in most situations, is strongly contraindicated in syncope caused by heart block. Thus cardiovascular syncope must be carefully excluded before the patient is treated for epilepsy. The major causes of syncope are:

1. Heart block

2. Arrhythmias (usually ventricular tachycardia or ventricular fibrillation)

3. Carotid sinus hypersensitivity

4. Vasovagal attacks

5. Aortic stenosis

6. Asymmetric septal hypertrophy

The diagnosis is not so difficult to make if the attack is observed, since in cardiovascular syncope, there is hypotension, whereas epilepsy alone does not produce hypotension. The heart rate may be very slow (as in heart block, carotid sinus hypersensitivity, or vasovagal syncope) or very rapid and weak or absent altogether (as in tachyarrhythmias).

If an attack is not observed, then the differential diagnosis between cardiovascular syncope and epilepsy can be very difficult. Also, whenever there is doubt concerning the mode of onset of the attacks, particularly in elderly patients, cardiovascular syncope should be considered, and several days of halter ECG monitoring should be performed. This, of course, will not entirely rule out very infrequent arrhythmias or episodes of heart block, but it is the best procedure available.

Carotid sinus massage may be performed under controlled circumstances, and a detailed cardiologic evaluation is often useful to exclude significant aortic valvular disease or asymmetric septal hypertrophy. No anticonvulsant therapy is required and is, in fact, contraindicated in heart block.

H. Hysteria (see Chap. 9). Hysteria may present a difficult problem in two ways when it occurs in a patient with epilepsy.

1. **Hysterical hyperventilation** may result in loss of consciousness and tetany, simulating epilepsy. This condition can be remedied by using a rebreathing bag for acute therapy. It is not really an epileptic phenomenon.

2. **Hysterical seizures** may be very difficult to distinguish from true epilepsy. The normal EEG is of some help but, as stated previously, many patients with bona fide epilepsy display repeatedly normal EEGs, thus making this an inadequate criterion. An experienced clinician can sometimes distinguish a poor imitation of a true convulsion, but when the patient is able to imitate a convulsion accurately, there is no practical method of distinguishing hysterical attacks from real ones.

One helpful criterion is whether the patient is incontinent. It is said that all

Table 6-11. Common Toxicities and Recommended Monitoring for the Major Anticonvulsants

Drug	Plasma Half-life	Major Toxicity	Safety in Pregnancy	Therapeutic Range (Serum)	Monitor
ACTH		1. Glucose intolerance 2. Salt retention 3. Ulcer disease	Not safe		1. Stool guaiac every week 2. Electrolytes every week
Acetazolamide (Diamox)		1. Hyperchloremic acidosis 2. Gastrointestinal upset 3. Nephrolithiasis	Not safe		1. Electrolytes every 3 months 2. Serum calcium every 6 months
Carbamazepine (Tegretol)	12–30 hours (half-life falls if drug is used chronically)	1. Rash 2. Sedation 3. Dry mouth 4. Gastrointestinal upset 5. Jaundice 6. Aplastic anemia 7. Pancytopenia	Possibly dangerous; should be avoided if possible	$4-10\ \mu g/ml$	1. CBC every week for 2 months, then every 3 months 2. Liver function tests every 3 months
Clonazepam (Clonopin)		1. Sedation	Unknown		1. Clinical response 2. Level of consciousness
Dextroamphetamine (Dexedrine)		1. Agitation 2. Hypertension 3. Tachycardia 4. Angina pectoris 5. Tolerance 6. Withdrawal 7. Anorexia	Probably unsafe (avoid if possible)		1. Signs and symptoms of toxicity
Diazepam (Valium)	IV = 0.5–4 hours; PO = 24 hours	1. Sedation	Unknown		1. Clinical response 2. Level of consciousness

Drug	Onset	Side Effects		Therapeutic Level	Monitoring
Ethosuximide (Zarontin)	2–3 days	1. Gastrointestinal upset 2. Ataxia 3. Sedation 4. Grand mal seizures 5. Pancytopenia 6. Abnormal liver function tests	Unknown	40–100 μg/ml	1. CBC every 3 months 2. Liver function tests every 6 months
Mephenytoin (Mesantoin)		Same as phenytoin	Unknown	5–20 μg/ml	Same as phenytoin
Mephobarbital (Mebaral)		Same as phenobarbital	Unknown	20–50 μg/ml	Same as phenobarbital
Methsuximide (Celontin)		1. Gastrointestinal upset 2. Ataxia 3. Sedation 4. Pancytopenia 5. Abnormal liver function tests	Unknown	40–100 μg/ml	1. CBC every 3 months 2. Liver function tests every 6 months
Paraldehyde		1. Hepatic toxicity 2. Respiratory depression when given parenterally 3. Cold abscesses when given IM	Unknown		1. Liver function tests 2. Respiratory function
Paramethadione (Paradione)	12–24 hours	1. Photophobia 2. Sedation 3. Aplastic anemia and neutropenia 4. Nephrotic syndrome 5. Grand mal seizures 6. Dermatitis 7. Hepatitis	Possibly dangerous; should be avoided if possible	6–41 μg/ml	1. CBC every 3 months 2. Urinalysis every 6 months 3. Liver function tests every 6 months

(Continued)

Table 6-11 (Continued)

Drug	Plasma Half-life	Major Toxicity	Safety in Pregnancy	Therapeutic Range (Serum)	Monitor

Phenobarbital (Luminal)	2–6 days	1. Sedation
		2. Irritability (children)
		3. Ataxia
		4. Rash
		5. Megaloblastic anemia
		6. Osteomalacia
			Unknown	20–50 μg/ml	1. Level of consciousness
					2. Nystagmus
					3. CBC every 6 months
					4. Serum Ca^{++} every 6 months
					5. If anemic:
					  a. Vitamin B_{12}
					  b. Folate

Phensuximide (Milontin)		1. Gastrointestinal upset 2. Ataxia 3. Sedation 4. Grand mal seizures 5. Pancytopenia 6. Abnormal liver function tests	Unknown	40–80 μg/ml	1. CBC every 3 months 2. Liver function tests every 6 months

| Phenytoin (Dilantin) | 20–24 hours | A. Local
  1. Gastro-
    intestinal
    upset
B. Idiosyncratic
  1. Dermatitis
  2. Gingival
    hypertrophy
  3. Hirsutism
  4. Pseudolymphoma
  5. Leukopenia,
    thrombocy-
    topenia,
    agranulo-
    cytosis,
    aplastic
    anemia
  6. Lupuslike
    syndrome
C. Dose-related
  1. Cerebellar
    ataxia
  2. Folate and
    vitamin B_{12}
    deficiency;
    megaloblastic
    anemia
  3. Hypocalcemia
    and osteo-
    malacia
  4. Low bound
    thyroxine | Possibly dangerous; should be avoided if possible. | 5–20 μg/ml | 1. CBC every 6
   months
2. Calcium every 6
   months
3. Ataxia
4. Nystagmus
5. Lymph nodes
6. If anemic:
  a. Vitamin B_{12}
  b. Folate |

(Continued)

Table 6-11 (Continued)

Drug	Plasma Half-life	Major Toxicity	Safety in Pregnancy	Therapeutic Range (Serum)	Monitor

Primidone (Mysoline)	3–12 hours	1. Sedation
		2. Megaloblastic anemia
		3. Ataxia
		4. Rash
		5. Irritability (children)
			Unknown	7–15 μg/ml. Also: Serum phenobarbital level due to metabolism of primidone = 20–40 μg/ml	1. Level of consciousness
					2. Nystagmus
					3. CBC every 6 months
					4. If anemic:
					  a. Vitamin B_{12}
					  b. Folate

Trimethadione (Tridione)	12–24 hours	1. Photophobia 2. Sedation 3. Aplastic anemia-neutropenia 4. Nephrotic syndrome 5. Grand mal seizures 6. Dermatitis 7. Hepatitis	Dangerous; should be avoided	20–40 μg/ml	1. CBC every 3 months 2. Urinalysis every 6 months 3. Liver function tests
Valproate sodium (Depakene)	8–12 hours	1. Hepatic toxicity 2. Hemorrhagic tendency 3. Sedation 4. Nausea, vomiting	Unknown; large doses are teratogenic in animals; no malformation reported in humans	50–100 μg/ml	1. Liver function tests every 3 months 2. CBC every 3 months

persons are incontinent during a grand mal convulsion unless their bladders are empty. Thus if a patient has multiple attacks, he or she will certainly be incontinent during some of them, whereas many patients with hysterical seizures are not incontinent. However, this criterion is of no help in patients who are incontinent or in patients with hysterical attacks, which mimic petit mal or focal seizures, that do not show incontinence as a part of the bona fide seizure pattern.

I. **Malingering.** Seizures imitated by malingerers pose a problem similar to that of hysterical seizures. Imitations of generalized convulsions are very rarely associated with incontinence, even less so than in hysterical seizures. The only way to distinguish other forms of imitations is for the physician to use his or her experience with respect to the appearance of real epilepsy. However, even the most experienced observer can be misled, and occasionally malingerers are treated with anticonvulsants.

J. **Tic douloureux** (see Chap. 2). Trigeminal neuralgia and some other neuralgia-like syndromes have certain characteristics in common with epilepsy. They occur intermittently, usually with an apoplectic onset, and may respond to anticonvulsants, particularly phenytoin and carbamazepine. It is rare, however, that they actually pose a difficult differential diagnosis with true epilepsy.

K. **Paroxysmal vertigo** (see Chap. 4). Several syndromes of paroxysmal vertigo exist that may be confused occasionally with focal epilepsy, namely *benign positional vertigo* (Barany's vertigo), and *Meniere's syndrome*. Usually these two syndromes may be distinguished from epilepsy on the basis of history and physical examination. The former may have a clear history of positional exacerbation of vertigo, and the patient will experience vertigo and nystagmus if the head is positioned properly during the neurologic examination. The latter shows episodes of vertigo that are always associated with concomitant hearing loss in the affected ear. Although the hearing loss will fluctuate with the attacks of vertigo, over time decreased hearing will be noted, and this can be documented by neurologic examination and audiometry.

SELECTED READINGS

General
Gastaut, H., and Broughton, F. *Epileptic Seizures: Clinical and Electrographic Features, Diagnosis and Treatment.* Springfield: Thomas, 1972.

Kutt, H., et al. Usefulness of blood levels of antiepileptic drugs. *Arch. Neurol.* 31:283, 1974.

Lennox, W. G. *Epilepsy and Related Disorders.* Boston: Little, Brown, 1960.

Livingston, S. *Comprehensive Management of Epilepsy in Infancy, Childhood and Adolescence.* Springfield: Thomas, 1972.

Richens, A. Drug interactions in epilepsy. *Dev. Med. Child Neurol.* 17:94, 1975. ·

Robb, P. *Epilepsy: A Review of Basic and Clinical Research.* Bethesda: U. S. Department of Health, Education, and Welfare, 1965.

Schmidt, R. P., and Wilder, B. J. *Epilepsy* (Contemporary Neurology Series). Philadelphia: Davis, 1968.

Sutherland, J. M., Tait, H., and Eadley, M. J. *The Epilepsies: Modern Diagnosis and Treatment* (2nd ed.). Edinburgh: Livingstone, 1974.

Woodbury, D. M., Penry, J. K., and Schmidt, R. P. *Antiepileptic Drugs.* New York: Raven Press, 1972.

———— Drugs for epilepsy. *Med. Lett. Drugs Ther.* 18:25, 1976.

———— Sodium valproate: A new anticonvulsant. *Med. Lett. Drugs Ther.* 19:93, 1977.

Petit Mal Epilepsy
Browne, J. R., et al. Ethosuximide in the treatment of absence (petit mal) seizures. *Neurology* 25:515, 1975.

Holowach, J., et al. Petit mal epilepsy in children. *Pediatrics.* 30:893, 1962.

Livingston, S., et al.   Petit mal epilepsy. *J.A.M.A.* 194:227, 1965.
Livingston, S., Torres, I., Pauli, L. L., and Rider, R. V.   Petit mal epilepsy, *J.A.M.A.* 194:227, 1965.
Penry, J. K., and Dreyfus, F. E.   Automatisms associated with absence of petit mal epilepsy. *Neurology* 21:142, 1969.

Grand Mal Convulsions
Bell, D. S.   The dangers of treatment of status epilepticus with diazepam (Valium). *Br. Med. J.* 1:159, 1968.
Kutt, H., and McDowell, F.   Management of epilepsy with diphenylhydantoin sodium. *J.A.M.A.* 203:969, 1968.
Parsonage, M. J., and Norris, J. W.   Use of diazepam in treatment of severe convulsive status epilepticus. *Br. Med. J.* 3:85, 1967.
Wallis, W., Kutt, H., and McDowell, F.   Intravenous diphenylhydantoin in treatment of acute repetitive seizures. *Neurology* 18:513, 1968.

Myoclonic Epilepsy
Koskinremi, M., et al.   Progressive myoclonus epilepsy. *Acta. Neurol. Scand.* 50:307, 1974.
Lance, J. W., and Adams, R. D.   The syndrome of intention on action myoclonus as a sequel to hypoxic encephalopathy. *Brain* 86:111, 1963.
Mikkelsen, B., et al.   Clonazepam in the treatment of epilepsy. *Arch. Neurol.* 33:322, 1976.
Senton, D. W., and Patterson, P. R.   Infantile spasms. *Neurology* 12:351, 1962.

Febrile Convulsions
Dodge, P. R.   Febrile convulsions. *J. Pediatr.* 78:1083, 1971.
Millichap, J. G.   *Febrile Convulsions.* New York: Macmillan, 1968.
Millichap, J. G., Aledort, L. M., and Madsen, J. A.   A critical evaluation of therapy of febrile seizures. *J. Pediatr.* 56:364, 1960.
Prichard, J. S., and McGreal, D. A.   Febrile convulsions. *Med. Clin. North Am.* 42:379, 1958.

Focal Seizures
Falconer, M. A.   The pathologic substrate of temporal lobe epilepsy. *Guys Hosp. Rep.* 119:47, 1970.
Sumi, S. M., and Teasdall, R. D.   Focal seizures: A review of 150 cases. *Neurology* 13:583, 1963.
Williams, D.   Temporal lobe epilepsy. *Br. Med. J.* 1:1439, 1966.

Surgery
Falconer, M. A.   Reversibility by temporal lobe resection of the behavioral abnormalities of temporal lobe epilepsy. *N. Engl. J. Med.* 289:451, 1973.
Falconer, M. A., and Taylor, D. C.   Surgical treatment of drug-resistant epilepsy due to mesial temporal sclerosis: Etiology and significance. *Arch. Neurol.* 19:351, 1968.

Neonatal Seizures
Hopkins, I. J.   Seizures in the first week of life. *Med. J. Aust.* 2:647, 1972.
Keen, J. H.   Significance of hypocalcemia in neonatal convulsions. *Arch. Dis. Child.* 44:356, 1969.
Rose, A. L., and Lombroso, C. T.   Neonatal seizure states: A study of clinical, pathological and electroencephalographic features in 137 full-term babies with long-term follow-up. *Pediatrics* 45:404, 1970.
Volpe, J.   Neonatal seizures. *N. Engl. J. Med.* 289:413, 1973.

Narcolepsy
Hishikawa, Y., Ida, H., Nakai, K., et al.   Treatment of narcolepsy with imipramine and dismethylimipramine. *J. Neurol. Sci.* 3:453, 1966.

Kales, A., and Kales, J. D. Sleep disorders. *N. Engl. J. Med.* 290:487, 1974.

Murray, T. J., et al. Narcolepsy. *Can. Med. Assoc. J.* 110:63, 1974.

Parkes, J. D., et al. Narcolepsy and cataplexy: Clinical features, treatment and CSF findings. *Q. J. Med.* 43:525, 1974.

Wyatt, R. J., Fram, D. H., Buchbinder, R., et al. Treatment of intractable narcolepsy with a monoamine oxidase inhibitor. *N. Engl. J. Med.* 285:987, 1971.

Yoss, R. E., and Daly, D. D. Narcolepsy. *Med. Clin. North Am.* 44:953, 1960.

Yoss, R. E., and Daly, D. D. On the treatment of narcolepsy. *Med. Clin. North Am.* 52:781, 1968.

Zarcone, V. Narcolepsy. *N. Engl. J. Med.* 288:1156, 1973.

Paroxysmal Abdominal Pain

Livingston, S. Abdominal pain as a manifestation of epilepsy. *J. Pediatr.* 38:687, 1951.

Moore, M. F. Abdominal epilepsy. *J.A.M.A.* 222:1426, 1972.

Mulder, D., Daly, D., and Barley, A. Visceral epilepsy. *Arch. Intern. Med.* 93:481, 1954.

Breath-holding Spells

Gauk, E. W., Kidd, L., and Prichard, J. S. Mechanism of seizures associated with breath holding spells. *N. Engl. J. Med.* 268:1436, 1963.

Livingston, S. Breathholding spells in children: Differentiation from epileptic attacks. *J.A.M.A.* 212:2231, 1970.

Lombroso, C. T., and Lerman, P. Breath holding spells (cyanotic and pallid infantile syncope). *Pediatrics* 39:563, 1967.

Hypercyanotic Attacks

Brando, J. L., and Zion, M. M. The cyanotic (syncopal) attack in Fallot's tetralogy. *Br. Med. J.* 1:1323, 1959.

Morgan, B. C., Guntheroth, W. G., Bloom, R. S., and Fyler, D. C. A clinical profile of paroxysmal hyperpnea in cyanotic congenital heart disease. *Circulation* 31:66, 1965.

Cardiovascular Syncope

Hutchinson, E. C., and Stock, J. P. P. The carotid sinus syndrome. *Lancet* 2:445, 1960.

Shaysey-Schafer, E. P. The mechanism of syncope after coughing. *Br. Med. J.* 2:860, 1953.

Shaysey-Schafer, E. P. Syncope. *Br. Med. J.* 1:506, 1956.

Thomas M. Walshe

Brain Death

I. DEFINITION

A. Medical definition. The criteria for the diagnosis of death traditionally have been cessation of the circulation and asystole. In certain cases, however, the cardiorespiratory function can be maintained artificially while the brain is irreversibly destroyed.

1. The concept of **death defined by brain viability,** termed *brain death,* has developed in the past 15 years, following advances in resuscitation technology. Brain death often results from **acute anoxia,** such as in cardiorespiratory arrest or prolonged hypotension, which devastates the brain but spares the less sensitive organs so that they can be revived. **Brain tumor, trauma, cardiac arrest,** and **stroke** may cause complete destruction of the brain but allow artificial maintenance of the other organs.

2. The **pathology of brain death** (the so-called respirator brain) is widespread necrosis and edema without inflammatory reaction. Transtentorial (temporal lobe) and cerebellar tonsillar herniations occur. Brain swelling causes increased intracranial pressure and an absence of cerebral blood flow.

3. The **clinical recognition of brain death** has become important because the brain-dead cadaver provides high-quality organs for transplantation. Moreover, the high cost of supportive and resuscitative care makes it desirable to recognize the brain-dead patient as early as possible.

B. Legal definition. The law concerning death is based on *Black's Law Dictionary,* which states that death is ". . . *defined by physicians* as a total stoppage of the circulation of the blood and a cessation of the animal and vital functions consequent thereupon."

1. In 1970 the state of Kansas enacted legislation specifically providing that "A person will be considered medically and legally dead, if, in the opinion of a physician based on ordinary standards of medical practice, there is an absence of spontaneous brain function." This law also states that **cessation of cardiorespiratory function** can be used to define death.

2. In 1974 the California law was changed so that if brain function was absent, death had to be declared: "A person shall be pronounced dead if it is determined that the person has suffered total and irreversible cessation of brain function."

3. Currently **no other states have laws defining brain death.** However, some state medical societies have included brain death in a formal definition-of-death statement in an attempt to set the standard of medical practice for the state.

C. Other sanctions. The concept of brain death has been accepted by the Roman Catholic church and at the First World Meeting on Transplantation of Organs. At the twenty-second World Medical Assembly in the Declaration of Sydney, the physician was deemed responsible for the definition of death, and cerebral death was named as an acceptable basis. In 1973 the American Neurological Association accepted brain death as a definition of death.

II. CRITERIA

A. Exclusions

1. Before the criteria can be applied, the **diagnostic and therapeutic measures** needed to correct the underlying illness must be taken.

2. If there is suspicion of **intoxication with CNS depressants,** the diagnosis of brain death cannot be made.

   a. **Blood levels** of drugs do not always correlate with mortality in drug overdose.

   b. The signs suggesting brain death do not persist for more than 36 hours in most cases of uncomplicated drug intoxication. Careful neurologic observation reveals **gradually increasing reflex activity** in such cases, indicating improvement. Usually the earliest reflex to return is the pupillary light response. If the patient continues to improve, oculocephalic, corneal, and other reflexes return. The EEG may be isoelectric in some cases of drug overdose but usually shows fast activity superimposed on generalized slowing.

3. **Hypothermia** of less than 90°F (32°C) also precludes the application of the criteria for brain death. Hypothermia occurs in patients with brain death, but the temperature is usually higher than 90°F (32°C) and the hypothermia is not found initially.

4. **The concept of brain death is specific.** It does not apply to patients existing in a persistent vegetative state or to other severe degrees of brain damage. Decisions concerning these patients need to be based on other criteria, because the prognosis of such conditions is not clear-cut.

B. **Signs.** The criteria for brain death are not agreed on by all authorities, and there are several sets of established criteria. However, there is enough agreement to provide guidelines for the clinician. In addition to the findings listed in Table 7-1, a history that establishes the diagnosis of an untreatable structural brain lesion supports the diagnosis of brain death.

The first set of criteria for brain death were defined in 1968 by an ad hoc committee from Harvard Medical School. The Harvard criteria are quite rigid, and many patients who have brain death do not fulfill them. Another set of criteria, based on a large number of cases, was developed by the NIH Collaborative Study of Cerebral Survival. The following criteria are modified from these NIH criteria.

C. **Duration.** The diagnosis of brain death is usually not even considered for several hours after the onset of artificial support. The original ad hoc committee recommended that the signs should be consistent for 24 hours, but recent analysis of

Table 7-1. Criteria for Brain Death

Criteria	Comments
Unresponsiveness	No behavioral response to noxious stimuli. No reflex response, such as increased heart or respiratory rate, to noxious or other stimuli
Apnea	If necessary to prove apnea exists, removal from respirator for 1–2 min provides maximum stimulus by CO_2 retention if arterial P_{CO_2} is normal at start
Absent cranial reflexes	Fixed pupils and immobile eyeballs on ice water irrigation of auditory canals. Absent corneal reflex and pharyngeal reflexes. No spontaneous blinking, swallowing, or vomiting
Isoelectric EEG	Absent EEG activity occasionally occurs in patients who do not have brain death (e.g., patient with drug overdose). If EEG activity is present, diagnosis of brain death cannot be made.

brain death cases shows that over half the patients with proven brain death suffer cardiac arrest before the 24-hour waiting period is over. Therefore, if the signs are clear and there is *no suspicion of drug intoxication,* the diagnosis can be made several hours after onset. Making the diagnosis before cardiac decompensation and arrest occur provides highest-quality organs for transplantation.

D. **Reflex activity**

1. The **pupils are often dilated** but may be in midposition in brain death. The **most helpful reflex signs** in diagnosing brain death are fixed pupils and absent corneal, oculocephalic, and vestibular reflexes.

2. **Spinal cord reflex** activity persists in as many as two-thirds of patients with angiographically proved brain death. The presence of these reflexes indicates a functional spinal cord but does not exclude brain death. Although they are usually absent, the **deep tendon reflexes** may persist in brain death. Other spinal cord reflexes must be separated from decerebrate and decorticate postures, which would exclude the diagnosis of brain death.

3. The **snout reflex, jaw jerk, abdominal reflexes,** and **plantar responses** may also persist and are not indicative of survival.

E. **Electroencephalogram**

1. The **electroencephalogram** (EEG) is a very helpful test in the diagnosis of brain death. In the absence of drug intoxication, survival does not occur in patients who have an isoelectric EEG for 12–24 hours.

2. Because of the **high gains needed,** it is necessary to use leads to monitor external movement and the electrocardiogram. An electrode on the right hand serves to measure external movement; since there is no muscle activity, there will be no muscle artifact. The study is run at standard gains, and again at twice standard gains, for at least 30 minutes. Gains are turned to maximum for one or two minutes to assure the absence of brain waves. There should be no EEG responses to pain or other stimuli.

3. When **any brain wave is present,** the diagnosis of brain death **cannot** be made.

F. **Cerebral angiography.** Some European authorities think that cerebral arteriography to demonstrate absent cerebral blood flow is necessary for the diagnosis of brain death. However, an **angiogram is seldom necessary** when clinical observation and EEG are available. Funduscopy, which shows sludging of blood in the retinal veins ("boxcars"), is clinical evidence of absent cerebral blood flow.

G. **Physician responsibility.** The **psychosocial implications of death** are always difficult for both the physician and the patient's family. The difficulty is compounded in patients in whom there are superficial signs of survival.

1. Once the physician has determined the diagnosis, the meaning of **the syndrome is explained** carefully to the patient's family. To prevent confusion and misunderstanding, it is wise to ensure that the family realizes that the patient is dead before supportive therapy is stopped or organ donation is suggested.

2. The **clinical record** must reflect the decision-making process and should document the signs carefully. Two physicians, neither of whom is a member of the transplantation team, should agree on the diagnosis in the record.

III. SUMMARY

A. The diagnosis of brain death is made by a physician based on the observation of a number of **clinical signs** that indicate absent brain function.

B. **EEG** corroborates the diagnosis and is done when possible.

C. Documentation of **absent cerebral blood flow** is confirmatory but usually not necessary.

D. Death is declared and **documented in the record** before supportive therapy is stopped.

E. Careful **explanation to the family** is of paramount importance.

SUGGESTED READING

Ad Hoc Committee of Harvard Medical School. A definition of irreversible coma. *J.A.M.A.* 205:85, 1968.

Allen, N., Burkholder, J. D., Comiscioni, J., and Molinari, G. F. Predictive value of clinical criteria in cerebral death. (Abstr.) *Neurology* (Minneap.) 26:356, 1976.

Bates, D., Caronna, J. J., Cartlidge, N. E. F., Knill-Jones, R. P., Levy, D. E., Shaw, D. A., and Plum, F. A prospective study of nontraumatic coma: methods and results in 310 patients. *Ann. Neurol.* 2:211, 1977.

Becker, D. P., Cavett, M. R., Nelson, J. R., and Stern, W. E. An evaluation of the definition of cerebral death. *Neurology* (Minneap.) 20:459, 1970.

Bennett, D. R., Hughes, J. R., Korein, J., Merlis, J. K., and Suter, C. *Atlas of Electroencephalography in Coma and Cerebral Death.* New York: Raven, 1976.

Beresford, H. R. *Legal Aspects of Neurologic Practice.* Philadelphia: Davis, 1975. P. 106.

Bradac, G. B., and Simon, R. S. Angiography in brain death. *Neuroradiology* 7:25, 1974.

Fabro, J. A. Statutory definition of death. *N. Engl. J. Med.* 286:549, 1972.

Jennett, B. Resource allocation for the severely brain damaged. *Arch. Neurol.* 33:595, 1976.

Jorgensen, P. B., Jorgensen, E. O., and Rosenklint, A. Brain death: pathogenesis and diagnosis. *Acta Neurol. Scand.* 49:335, 1973.

Mills, D. H. Statutory brain death? *J.A.M.A.* 229:1225, 1974.

Mills, D. H. More on brain death. *J.A.M.A.* 234:838, 1975.

Mohandas, A., and Chou, S. N. Brain death: a clinical and pathological study. *J. Neurosurg.* 35:211, 1971.

Plum, F., and Posner, J. B. *The Diagnosis of Stupor and Coma.* Philadelphia: Davis, 1972. Pp. 223–240.

Pope Pius XII. The prolongation of life. *Am. Q. Papal Doctrine* 4:393, 1958.

Silverman, D. Cerebral death—the history of the syndrome and its identification. *Ann. Intern. Med.* 74:1003, 1971.

Silverman, D., Masland, R. L., Saunders, M. G., and Schwab, R. S. Irreversible coma associated with electrocerebral silence. *Neurology* (Minneap.) 20:525, 1970.

Snyder, B. D., Ramirez-Lassepas, M., Lippert, D. M. Neurological status and prognosis after cardiopulmonary arrest. 1. A retrospective study. *Neurology* 27:807, 1977.

Starr, A. Auditory brain-stem responses in brain death. *Brain* 99:543, 1976.

Walker, A. E. Cerebral Death, in T. N. Chase (Ed.), *The Nervous System,* New York: Raven Press, 1975. Pp. 75–88.

Walker, A. E., Didmond, E. L., and Moseley, J. The neuropathological findings in irreversible coma. *J. Neuropathol. Exp. Neurol.* 34:295, 1975.

PART II
NEUROLOGIC DISEASES

Infectious Diseases

I. BACTERIAL MENINGITIS

A. Making the diagnosis

1. **Necessity of rapid diagnosis.** Untreated bacterial meningitis is virtually 100% fatal within a matter of days. Furthermore, if therapy is delayed, the probability of a patient's escaping death or permanent disability diminishes rapidly. In general, the more acute the onset of symptoms and the more rapid the progression of the illness, the more urgent it is to initiate therapy.

2. **Indications for lumbar puncture (LP).** Because of the urgency of starting specific antibacterial therapy, it is imperative to examine a sample of cerebrospinal fluid (CSF) as soon as possible in every patient with suspected bacterial meningitis. Examination of the CSF is the only means of making a definite diagnosis and obtaining positive identification of the infecting organism.

   However, identification of an organism in a possible parameningeal or systemic source of infection is not adequate to guide the choice of appropriate antibiotic coverage and, in over 25% of cases, blood cultures will fail to yield an organism. Thus all material for bacteriologic examination should be obtained prior to beginning antibiotics if at all possible.

   a. **Risks of lumbar puncture.** Much is often made of the risks of lumbar puncture in the presence of increased intracranial pressure, especially if they are the result of a mass lesion. There are many instances of relatively stable patients who decompensate from herniation that is coincident with or shortly follows a lumbar puncture. Presumably, withdrawal of fluid from the lumbar space and, probably more important, the continuing leak of CSF through the dural defect that remains after removal of the needle may disturb intracranial pressure equilibrium in such a way as to allow herniation of brain substance downward through the tentorial notch or the foramen magnum. Although these risks are real, it cannot be stressed too strongly that more patients have been harmed by failure to perform a lumbar puncture, with resultant delay in the diagnosis and treatment of bacterial meningitis, than have been harmed by the performance of an unnecessary one.

   In uncomplicated bacterial meningitis, lumbar puncture is relatively safe. Therefore it should be performed immediately when a reasonable suspicion of bacterial meningitis arises. It is good practice in all cases of suspected meningitis, and absolutely essential in high-risk lumbar punctures, to have a secure IV in place when the puncture is performed and to be prepared to infuse hyperosmolar agents if necessary. When lumbar puncture is required in the presence of signs of a possible mass lesion, a hyperosmolar agent may be infused in advance.

   b. **Situations in which lumbar puncture is hazardous.** There are rare cases, which are similar to bacterial meningitis, in which lumbar puncture is unusually hazardous.

      (1) Patients with brain abscess may have a fever, an abnormal mental status, and meningismus. Brain abscess may be difficult to distinguish from bacterial meningitis if an adequate history is not available.

      (2) Brain tumors and other masses may also be associated with meningismus on occasion, and these patients are prone to various infections that may produce a fever.

(3) Certain complications of bacterial meningitis (e.g., cortical vein thrombosis with venous infarction, arterial infarction, subdural empyema, and subdural effusion) may also increase the risk of lumbar puncture.

c. Guidelines for performing lumbar puncture in hazardous situations. When the possibility of a mass lesion exists, several general principles are helpful:

(1) Seizures, including focal seizures, isolated cranial nerve palsies, focal neurologic signs of acute onset, and depressed mental status may all occur early in the course of bacterial meningitis in the absence of a mass lesion. These symptoms alone do not contraindicate lumbar puncture.

(2) Papilledema occurs rarely in bacterial meningitis and suggests the presence of a mass lesion.

(3) A clear history of a slowly progressive focal neurologic deficit that precedes the symptoms of bacterial meningitis suggests the presence of an abscess, tumor, subdural hematoma, or other mass lesion.

(4) Signs of progressive herniation comprise the only absolute contraindication to lumbar puncture.

d. Alternatives to lumbar puncture. If lumbar puncture is contraindicated in a particular clinical situation, there are a few alternatives.

(1) The lumbar puncture may be deferred while emergency radiologic studies are performed to confirm or exclude the presence of a mass lesion.

(2) In suspected supratentorial masses:

(a) Skull x-rays, to look for midline calcified pineal or erosion of the dorsum sellae, indicative of chronic, increased intracranial pressure.

(b) Echoencephalogram to demonstrate a midline third ventricle.

(c) CT scan.

(d) Angiography.

(3) In suspected infratentorial mass:

(a) CT scan.

(b) Angiography.

(4) In suspected acute hydrocephalus:

(a) CT scan.

(b) Angiography.

(c) Ventriculography.

(5) CSF may be obtained by a **ventricular tap** through an open fontanelle in an infant or by means of a burr hole in children and adults. This procedure may only be performed by an experienced neurosurgeon and carries its own high risks.

(6) In very rare instances, limited almost entirely to pediatric practice when the diagnosis of bacterial meningitis seems indisputable on clinical grounds, when the infecting organism may be predicted with a high degree of confidence, and when the patient is in the process of or appears to be at high risk of herniation, antibiotics may be started without obtaining a sample of CSF. In these instances a blood culture is taken to isolate an organism from the blood, and lumbar puncture is performed 8–24 hours after both antibiotics and antiedema therapy are initiated. By following this procedure the risk of lumbar puncture is lessened, but the CSF formula may still be purulent and allow the diagnosis to be confirmed. However, if the appropriate antibiotic is chosen, there is little chance of culturing an organism from the CSF.

3. Lumbar puncture technique

a. Preparing the patient

(1) A blood glucose is drawn within 15 minutes of beginning the procedure.

(2) The procedure is explained to the patient and all steps are described during the procedure to minimize the patient's anxiety. In high-risk lumbar punctures informed consent must be obtained from the patient or his or her family.

(3) Positioning the patient

(a) Whenever possible, the lumbar puncture is performed with the patient on his or her side with knees and hips flexed. The patient may be left relatively relaxed while being prepped and draped, and only when the physician is prepared to introduce the needle are the patient's hips and back maximally flexed.

(b) The patient's back is perpendicular to the bed. The L3–4 interspace is located at the level of the superior iliac crests, and any scoliosis or abnormalities of the spine are noted.

(c) If the puncture cannot be performed with the patient lying on his side, it may be done with the patient in a sitting position, leaning forward onto a table that is covered with a pillow. It is essential that the patient's spine be perfectly vertical. The CSF pressure cannot be accurately measured in this position and, if the intracranial pressure is elevated, there may be more risk of herniation if the tap is done while the patient is in the sitting position rather than the lying position.

(4) Preparing the skin

(a) Wash the patient's back with iodine-soaked sponges; begin at the site of the proposed puncture and wash in concentric circles. Wash with iodine two to three times, and then wash with alcohol-soaked sponges three times, taking care to wash off all the iodine.

(b) Change gloves before proceeding to avoid introducing iodine into the subarachnoid space on the lumbar puncture needle.

(c) Cover the patient with a sterile drape.

b. Introducing the needle

(1) Have all equipment for the puncture ready before introducing the needle (i.e., 20-gauge lumbar puncture needle, stopcock attached to a manometer and appropriately positioned, and three or four sterile tubes with stoppers).

(2) If the patient is alert, anesthetize the skin with a small wheal of Xylocaine or procaine at the exact site of the proposed puncture. The skin wheal is painful and should be raised slowly with an intradermal injection of 0.1–0.2 ml of anesthetic. A further 0.2–0.5 ml may be injected into deeper layers of the dermis, but there is no need to inject anesthetic deep into the muscle, because it is usually more painful than the single passage of a 20-gauge needle.

(3) Introduce a 20-gauge lumbar puncture needle with the stylus in place through the skin in the center of the skin wheal. Direct the bevel of the needle so its flat surface is parallel to the long axis of the patient's spine; hence the needle will spread, rather than cut, the dural fibers that run longitudinally. Direct the needle tip 10 to 15 degrees cephalad (more or less toward the umbilicus), and introduce the needle slowly but steadily until the needle is felt to pierce a tough membrane or is thought to be near the dura. At that point, the needle is introduced in steps of 2–3 mm, and the stylus is removed between each step to check for CSF return. Once CSF return is obtained, the needle is introduced 1–2 mm farther, and the bevel is turned perpendicular to the long axis of the spine. Care must be taken not to introduce the needle too far, because puncture of the venous plexus anterior to the cord is the most common cause of a "traumatic tap."

(4) If CSF return cannot be obtained at the L3–4 interspace, the L2–3 or L4–5 spaces may be tried. After repeated lumbar punctures, a patient may develop a persistent CSF leak, keeping CSF pressure so low that it will not flow through a 20-gauge needle unless the patient's head is elevated several inches.

(5) Each time the stylus is withdrawn, be ready to plug the stopcock and manometer into the needle as quickly as possible to minimize unnecessary CSF loss.

c. Collecting the CSF

(1) Measure the CSF pressure by allowing fluid to flow into the manometer. Evidence that the needle is properly positioned in the subarachnoid space includes good respiratory variation of the fluid level in the manometer and rapid fall of the fluid level after maneuvers that raise it (e.g., pressure on the patient's abdomen, turning the manometer and stopcock 90 degrees so it is parallel to the bed and fills with fluid, and pressure on the jugular veins in the neck [Queckenstedt's maneuver]). Be sure the patient is as relaxed as possible, with legs and hips slightly extended from the maximally flexed position when the pressure is measured.

(2) Collect the fluid into at least three sterile tubes. One scheme is as follows:

(a) Tube No. 1: Collect 2 ml for protein and glucose. This tube is centrifuged, and the sediment is used for microscopic examination.

(b) Tube No. 2: Collect 1–2 ml for culture and sensitivities.

(c) Tube No. 3: Collect 1 ml for cell count and 1 ml for serology.

(3) If the opening pressure (OP) is high, there is little advantage in collecting less fluid than has been suggested to minimize the chances of precipitating herniation. Much of the danger from the lumbar puncture is from leakage of CSF through the dural defect that is created by the needle.

(4) In virtually all cases of bacterial meningitis, the CSF pressure is found to be elevated. Thus the patient should be observed closely (no less often than every 15 minutes for the next 4 hours), and hyperosmolar agents are administered if the patient shows evidence of neurologic deterioration.

If the patient deteriorates during the performance of the lumbar puncture or is considered to be at a high risk of herniation, the stylet is replaced into the needle and the needle is left in place. Mannitol 1.0–1.5 gm/kg is infused over 20–30 minutes, and high-dose steroid therapy is begun with dexamethasone (Decadron) 10 mg given by rapid intravenous infusion. After the mannitol has been infused, the needle is withdrawn.

d. Withdrawal of the needle. Cases have been reported in which nerve roots were trapped by a lumbar puncture needle when the stylet was replaced; the root was avulsed as the needle was withdrawn. Therefore when the needle is withdrawn, the stylet should not be in place.

e. Examination of the CSF

(1) CSF formula

(a) The CSF formula in bacterial meningitis will be purulent (elevated cell count with predominant polymorphonuclear leukocytes and a low sugar) except in the following cases.

The meningitis has been "partially treated." Occasionally, early in overwhelming infection, especially with *Streptococcus pneumoniae,* there is poor polymorphonuclear response.

The patient is leukopenic or immunosuppressed. Certain bacteria and spirochetes may not produce a purulent profile (e.g., *Treponema pallidum, Leptospira* species, and *Listeria monocytogenes*).

(b) Other diseases in the differential diagnosis of a purulent CSF formula are listed in Table 8-1.

(2) Microscopic examination. The following examinations are performed, as indicated, on the sediment of fresh centrifuged CSF:

(a) Gram stain in all cases.

(b) Acid-fast bacilla (AFB) test. The greater the volume of CSF examined, the higher the yield of this procedure. Therefore the CSF sediment may be concentrated by allowing four to five drops of CSF to dry sequentially on one area of a slide.

(c) India ink preparation. This is not as good a screening test for *Cryptococcus* as Gram stain, in which the organisms appear as large gram-positive cocci. If the Gram stain suggests fungal infection, the India ink preparation is done to identify the organism.

(d) Wet smear for fungi and amebae.

(e) Examination of polymorphonuclear cells with **polarized light** to look for keratin fragments. These fragments indicate chemical meningitis, secondary to the spillage of the contents of a dermoid cyst or craniopharyngioma.

(3) Bacteriologic examination

(a) Routine cultures for bacteria. CSF is smeared on a blood agar plate or a chocolate agar plate or slant or is inoculated into a nutrient broth. It is essential to plant any or all these cultures as soon as possible after the lumbar puncture.

(b) If indicated, fluid may be cultured for mycobacteria, fungi, and amebae.

(4) Special studies

(a) Counterimmunoelectrophoresis and other tests for the identification of capsular antigens. Meningitis due to meningococcus, *Hemophilus influenzae,* and pneumococcus may be rapidly diagnosed, even in the absence of a positive Gram stain, by the documentation of the presence of specific capsular antigens in the CSF.

Table 8-1. The Cerebrospinal Fluid Formula

Purulent Profile	Lymphocytic–Low Glucose Profile	Lymphocytic–Normal Glucose Profile
Elevated WBC, predominantly polymorphonuclear leukocytes, low sugar, and high protein	Elevated WBC, predominantly lymphocytes, low sugar and high protein	Elevated WBC, predominantly lymphocytes, normal sugar, and high protein
Infectious		
Bacterial meningitis	Tuberculous meningitis	Viral meningitis or encephalitis
Viral meningitis in the early phase	Fungal meningitis	Bacterial meningitis in the resolving or partially treated phase
Embolic cerebral infarction with endocarditis	Bacterial meningitis that is either in the resolving or partially treated phase or with certain organisms (e.g., spirochetes, *Leptospira, Listeria monocytogenes*)	Parameningeal infections (e.g., intracranial abscess, sinusitis, mastoiditis, cortical vein thrombophlebitis)
Parameningeal infections (e.g., subdural empyema, brain abscess, cortical vein thrombophlebitis)	Viral meningitis	Fungal and tuberculous meningitis in the early phase
Tuberculous meningitis in the early phase		Parasitic infestation (e.g., toxoplasmosis, trichinosis)
Acute hemorrhagic leukoencephalitis		Polyradiculitis (Landry-Guillain-Barré syndrome)
		Postinfectious encephalomyelitis
		Active demyelinating diseases
Noninfectious		
Chemical meningitis (e.g., contrast media, detergents, keratin released from tumors, foreign agents)	Carcinomatous meningitis	
	Sarcoidosis of the meninges	
Behçets disease		
Mollaret's recurrent meningitis		

Source: adapted from Hyslop, N.E., Jr., and Swartz, M.N. Bacterial meningitis. *Postgrad. Med.* 58:120, 1975.

(b) **Serologic test for syphilis.** It is a good practice to perform a CSF serologic test for syphilis (STS) on all patients who receive a lumbar puncture for any reason.

(c) **Viral** isolation studies or viral antibody titers.

(d) **Serologic tests** for cryptococcal or coccidioidal antigen or antibody.

4. Additional studies

a. Once the presumptive diagnosis of bacterial meningitis has been made, the patient's overall medical status is reassessed to look for factors that may have predisposed the patient to the development of meningitis. These factors include:

(1) Recent head trauma with **skull fracture,** usually a basilar fracture, giving organisms access to the intracranial cavity.

(2) The presence of a "CSF leak," usually due to head trauma and involving a defect in the cribriform plate.

(3) Recent intracranial surgery.

(4) Meningomyelocele

(5) Immune deficiency status.

(6) The presence of a **parameningeal focus** of infection: sinus otitis (usually chronic), mastoiditis, osteomyelitis of the skull, occult brain abscess, and infected pilonidal sinuses.

(7) A source of systemic sepsis, especially endocarditis.

b. **Routine tests** in all patients with presumptive bacterial meningitis:

(1) **Hematologic**

(a) CBC.

(b) Examination of a peripheral blood smear.

(2) **Metabolic**

(a) BUN (or creatinine).

(b) Blood glucose.

(c) Electrolytes.

(d) Urinalysis (U/A).

(e) If nephrotoxic drugs are to be used, a baseline **creatinine clearance** (Cl_{cr}) is obtained.

(3) **Radiologic**

(a) Chest x-ray.

(b) Skull x-rays, with views of sinuses and the base of the skull.

(4) Blood, urine, and throat cultures.

c. **Special studies** for special circumstances:

(1) If there is evidence of a parameningeal focus of infection, special skull views, spine views, or polytones may be helpful.

(2) When there is evidence of a **CSF leak** and in all cases of **recurrent meningitis** without an obvious cause, radioactively labeled tracers or a dye solution may be injected into the subarachnoid space, and

pledgets are placed in the nasal cavity or ear canal. The pledgets are then examined over time to document CSF rhinorrhea or otorrhea.

In the past, it was widely believed that CSF rhinorrhea could be distinguished from a mucous discharge at the bedside by the use of Dextrostix, since the CSF glucose level is generally greater than 30, whereas there is a lower concentration of glucose in mucus. Experience has not proved this test to be entirely reliable, however.

(3) CT scanning, radionuclide brain scanning, and EEG are noninvasive techniques that may give data that will help locate a possible **brain abscess.**

(4) In **neonatal infections,** the mother is examined for signs of infection. Amnionitis, endometritis, maternal urinary tract infections (UTIs), and septicemia are known to predispose to neonatal meningitis. A knowledge of the identity and antibiotic sensitivity of maternal perinatal infections may help to determine the best therapy for the neonate.

B. The general medical care of a patient with bacterial meningitis

1. Systemic therapy

a. Shock

(1) Septic shock, if present, should be treated with volume replacement, pressors, and institution of antibiotic therapy as quickly as possible.

(2) Shock that is secondary to hemorrhagic infarction of the adrenals (Waterhouse-Friderichsen syndrome) is a much discussed, but rare, complication of meningococcal meningitis. It is associated with severe skin lesions in meningococcal disease. However, in a patient with bacterial meningitis and shock, emergency treatment with corticosteroids is warranted until the patient has stabilized and the medical situation is evaluated better.

b. Hydration. Because of the likely presence of brain swelling and increased CSF pressure in central nervous system infection, care is taken not to overhydrate the patient. If the patient is not hypotensive, approximately 1200–1500 ml half-normal saline is adequate daily fluid intake in adults, and about 1000 ml/sq m body surface area is adequate in children. The volume of fluid in which the antibiotics are administered and any oral intake are included in this total. These restrictions may be gradually relaxed as the patient's infection responds to therapy, especially if the CSF pressure is decreasing. Solutions that contain more than 50% "free water" (e.g., 5% dextrose in water) should not be administered except in small volumes when they are used to dissolve the antibiotics.

c. Fever. Salicylates, acetaminophen, and baths in tepid water may all be used to lower body temperature. The rectal temperature should not be allowed to exceed 103°F (40°C).

d. Isolation. Patients with meningococcal infections or meningitis of unknown etiology are placed under respiratory precautions for the first 24 hours of their antibiotic therapy, or until menigococcal disease is excluded. Precautions may be necessary in cases of bacterial infections that have broad drug resistance, so the organisms are prevented from spreading throughout a patient care area and infecting other susceptible patients.

2. Treatment of predisposing factors

a. Parameningeal infections are treated concurrently with meningitis, with surgical drainage if necessary.

    b. Foci of systemic sepsis are treated appropriately and may require more prolonged antibiotic therapy than the meningitis (e.g., SBE, osteomyelitis, and wound infection).

    c. Minor CSF leaks need not be repaired until after the CNS infection is clearly under control.

C. Antibiotic therapy

  1. General principles

    a. Patients are hospitalized for the entire course of treatment, and the entire course of antibiotics is administered parenterally.

    b. The minimum duration of antibiotic therapy necessary is unknown for each organism, but in meningitis with the common organisms (*S. pneumoniae, H. influenzae,* and *Neisseria meningitidis*), the practice is to treat at full dose of parenteral antibiotics for at least 10 days and at least 7 days after the patient becomes afebrile. If any surgery is performed near the end of therapy, the antibiotics are continued at least 72 hours after surgery. In infections with less sensitive organisms (e.g., enteric gram-negative organisms) or after trauma or surgery, when pockets of organisms can infect poorly perfused tissues, it is reasonable to prolong the duration of antibiotic therapy to 3 weeks or longer.

    c. The CSF is examined, in an uncomplicated case, 24–48 hours after the initiation of therapy and shortly after the antibiotics are stopped. When the patient is clearly responding to the therapy clinically, the 24-hour lumbar puncture may be deferred. The CSF cell-count differential, protein, and glucose are determined with each lumbar puncture, and the CSF is examined microscopically and cultured appropriately to document that it has been sterilized.

      In meningeal infections with organisms that are relatively sensitive to antibiotics with good CSF penetration (e.g., streptococcal species, *Neisseria,* and *H. influenzae*), the CSF should be sterile within 24 hours of beginning therapy, and the differential cell count should revert to one of lymphocytic predominance. (The CSF protein level is not an indication of adequacy of therapy and may continue to be high for 2–3 weeks. The CSF glucose may also be low for longer than 2 weeks despite curative therapy.) Other organisms, especially gram-negative rods other than *H. influenzae,* may continue to grow out of the CSF for as long as 72 hours after the initiation of therapy, and the infection may ultimately be cured. Persistence of the infecting organism in the CSF beyond the expected interval, however, may imply a need to change antibiotics or to add intrathecal antibiotics. It may also indicate the presence of an occult parameningeal focus of infection that continues to seed the CSF.

    d. Drug toxicity. In the treatment of bacterial meningitis, the highest doses of drugs that can be tolerated are generally used, and often the patients have underlying hepatic, renal, or hematologic disease. Therefore, the patient must be observed carefully for the development of drug toxicity.

  2. Pharmacology of antibiotics used in the chemotherapy of bacterial meningitis

    a. Chloramphenicol

      (1) Pharmacology

        (a) Half-life = 1½–3½ hours in serum.

        (b) CSF concentration is 30–80% of plasma concentration.

        (c) The drug is inactivated primarily in the liver by glucuronidation, and the inactive metabolites are excreted in the urine. Therefore the dose does not have to be decreased in renal failure but does in severe hepatic insufficiency and in neonates, in whom the glucuronidation reaction is not fully developed.

(2) Dosage

(a) Premature: 25 mg/kg/day IV divided into two doses at 12-hour intervals.

(b) Full term: 50 mg/kg/day IV divided into two doses at 12-hour intervals.

(c) Children: 100 mg/kg/day IV divided into four doses at 6-hour intervals.

(d) Adults: 4–8 gm/day IV divided into four doses at 6-hour intervals.

(3) Toxicity

(a) Hypersensitivity reaction: rash, fever, angioedema, stomatitis, and idiosyncratic bone marrow suppression with pancytopenia. The latter reaction occurs in less than 1/40,000, but it is always irreversible. Also, it is not related to the dose, but it occurs usually after prolonged exposure or on a second exposure.

(b) Dose-related and reversible **bone marrow suppression** occurs with plasma drug levels of 25 mg/ml or higher. The earliest signs are decreased reticulocyte count with vacuolization of early erythrocytic and myelocytic forms in the bone marrow. Recovery usually occurs about 12 days after the drug is stopped.

(c) Gray baby syndrome and **cardiovascular collapse** occur with excessive doses in premature infants and neonates with inadequate hepatic glucuronyl transferase activity.

(4) Precautions

(a) Bone marrow function must be checked frequently. CBC, differential, platelet count (or peripheral smear), serum iron, total iron-binding capacity (TIBC), and reticulocyte count should be checked three times weekly. The first sign of bone marrow suppression is increased serum iron, with increased saturation of TIBC.

(b) Extreme care must be used in giving the drug to children less than 1-month old.

(c) If used in combination with penicillin, the first dose of penicillin is given at least ½ hour before the first dose of chloramphenicol, and succeeding doses of the two drugs should not be given within ½ hour of each other.

b. The penicillins

(1) Penicillin G

(a) Pharmacokinetics. Penicillin G is excreted by the kidney primarily, and partially in bile. The half-life is approximately ½ hour in adult serum but is 3 hours in neonates who are less than 1 week old. The half-life increases in renal failure.

CSF levels in normal infants are below the therapeutic range; in meningitis, CSF levels are variable, ranging between 10 and 30% of the serum level.

(b) Dosage

Neonates: 50–100,000 units/kg/day IV divided into two doses.

Infants: 250,000 units/kg/day IV divided into four to six doses.

Children: 12×10^6 units/day divided into six doses.

Adults: 24×10^6 units/day IV, given as 2×10^6 units every 2 hours.

Renal failure ($Cl_{cr} < 10$ ml/min).

In children, same doses as above.

In adults, 2×10^6 units every 4 hours IV.

(c) Toxicity

Hypersensitivity reactions: rash, fever, eosinophilia, angioedema, anaphylaxis, serum sickness, and encephalopathy. **Seizures** can occur with high doses or intrathecal use.

Penicillin G is available as a sodium or potassium salt, and it may create a significant **salt load** in infants or in renal failure.

(d) Precautions. The potassium salt contains 1.7 mg $K^+/10^6$ units.

(2) Ampicillin

(a) Pharmacokinetics

Half-life = 1½ hours in serum.

Ampicillin is excreted primarily by the kidneys. Therefore the dose must be reduced in renal failure.

CSF penetration is comparable to that of penicillin G.

(b) Dosage

Neonates: 50–100 mg/kg/day IV divided into two doses 12 hours apart.

Two weeks to 2 months: 100–200 mg/kg/day IV divided into three doses 8 hours apart.

Over 2 months: 300–400 mg/kg/day IV divided into four doses six hours apart.

Adults: 8–12 gm/day IV divided into four doses 6 hours apart.

Renal failure in adults: 2–3 gm given at the following intervals:

Cl_{cr}	Dose Interval
80	Every 6 hours
50–80	Every 6 hours
10–50	Every 9 hours
10	Every 12 hours

(c) Toxicity. Hypersensitivity reactions are the same as with penicillin G. Ampicillin rash does not necessarily represent hypersensitivity and, in itself, does not prevent continuation of the drug, its future use, or the use of other penicillins.

(3) Oxacillin

(a) Pharmacokinetics

Oxacillin is excreted by the kidneys and liver.

Half-life = 30–60 minutes.

CSF penetration is the same as with penicillin G.

(b) Dosage

Week 1:   50–100 mg/kg/day IV divided into two to three doses.

Weeks 2 to 4:   100–200 mg/kg/day IV divided into two to three doses.

Infants and children: 200 mg/kg/day IV divided into four to six doses.

Adults: 12 gm/day IV divided into four to six doses.

Renal failure: Same dose that would be given on the every-6-hour schedule; given every 8 to 12 hours if the Cl_{cr} is less than 10.

(c) Toxicity. Same as ampicillin and penicillin G, plus interstitial nephritis.

(4) Nafcillin

(a) Pharmacokinetics.

90% is excreted in bile.

Half-life ≃ ½ hour.

CSF levels are the same as with penicillin G.

(b) Dosage. The same as for oxacillin. Double the interval between doses if the Cl_{cr} is less than 10.

(c) Toxicity

Hypersensitivity reactions.

Interstitial nephritis.

(5) Carbenicillin

(a) Pharmacokinetics

Half-life ≃ 1 hour.

Carbenicillin is excreted by the kidney.

CSF levels are similar to those with penicillin G.

(b) Dosage

Neonates: 400 mg/kg/day IV divided into four doses.

Infants: 400–600 mg/kg/day IV divided into 6 to 12 doses.

Adults: 24–36 gm/day IV, given as 2–3 gm IV every 2 hours.

Severe **renal failure** (Cl_{cr} < 10 ml/min):   2 gm IV every 8 to 12 hours.

(c) Toxicity

Similar to penicillin.

Platelet dysfunction with bleeding diathesis.

(d) Precaution. Contains 4.7 mEq sodium per gram.

c. Aminoglycosides

(1) Pharmacokinetics

(a) CSF concentration with systemic administration is very low in normals, variable but low with inflamed meninges, and better in neonates.

(b) Excretion is by means of glomerular filtration.

(c) Half-life

Streptomycin	2–3 hours
Gentamicin	2 hours
Vancomycin	2½ hours
Tobramycin	1½–3 hours

(d) Serum drug levels achieved after a given dose may vary widely among individuals.

(2) Dosage

(a) Systemic gentamicin and tobramycin

Premature and term infants less than 1 week old: 5 mg/kg/day IV divided into two doses.

Neonates older than 1 week: 7.5 mg/kg/day IV divided into three doses.

Infants and adults: 5 mg/kg/day IV divided into three doses at 8-hour intervals.

Renal failure: 1.0–1.3 mg/kg every x hours, where x = serum creatinine × 8.

(b) Systemic kanamycin

All ages: 15 mg/kg/day divided into two doses.

Renal failure: 7 mg/kg every x hours, where x = serum creatinine × 9.

(c) Intrathecal gentamicin and tobramycin

Neonates: 1 mg every 24 hours.

Adults: 4–6 mg every 18 to 24 hours.

(3) Toxicity

(a) Vestibular disturbance is dose-related and occurs more readily in the presence of inflamed meninges. The streptomycin labyrinthine disorder occurs in four stages:

A stage of 1–2 days of headache.

An acute stage of nausea, vomiting, and vertigo lasting 1–2 weeks.

An abrupt transition to a chronic stage in which gait difficulty and imbalance are the predominant symptoms.

Finally, a compensating stage ensues, during which the patient has imbalance only with the eyes closed.

(b) Hearing dysfunction occurs less readily than vestibular dysfunction and is also dose-related. Tinnitus is often the first symptom and audiometry shows a high-tone hearing loss as the first sign, gradually progressing to involve the lower tones. Tinnitus persists as long as 2 weeks after the drug is stopped.

(c) The aminoglycosides are weak **neuromuscular blockers,** an effect that has no importance in patients with normal pulmonary function. However, it can be important in patients with myasthenia gravis, chronic obstructive pulmonary disease (COPD), acute respiratory failure, and in the immediate postoperative period when another neuromuscular blocker may still be present.

(d) Nephrotoxicity. Depressed renal function with albuminuria, glucosuria, and decreased urine output may occur as a dose-related side effect.

(e) Rare hypersensitivity reactions: rash, eosinophilia, blood dyscrasia, exfoliative dermatitis, stomatitis, fever, lymphadenopathy, and anaphylaxis.

(f) Intrathecal use is frequently associated with paresthesias of the legs and, occasionally, transverse myelitis or spinal arachnoiditis. Injection of excessive amounts of an aminoglycoside into the ventricles has produced seizures, encephalopathy, and death.

(4) Precautions

(a) Follow renal function and urinalysis at least twice weekly.

(b) Observe the patient carefully for any sign of vestibular or auditory dysfunction.

(c) Serum drug levels vary widely among individuals on a given dose of an aminoglycoside. Thus **serum drug levels,** if available, should be measured just before and ½–1 hour after a dose is given. This procedure should be followed at the initiation of therapy and at least weekly thereafter if the renal function is normal. It should be done more frequently if the renal function is abnormal.

If direct injection of the drug into the CSF is to be done, the CSF level should be checked before the second dose and before every other dose thereafter. Therapeutic serum levels are 4–6 mg/ml for gentamicin and tobramycin.

(d) If maximum doses are to be used or a prolonged course is anticipated, a baseline audiogram should be obtained before initiation of therapy and at any sign of hearing loss.

(e) Aminoglycosides should be avoided in patients with respiratory disease or neuromuscular disease that compromises respiratory function. If they must be used, respiratory function is checked before beginning therapy, after the first dose, and then as indicated. In myasthenia, depending on the severity of the respiratory involvement, respiratory function may have to be checked as often as every 4 hours. Neuromuscular blockade can be counteracted with calcium or an anticholinesterase agent (neostigmine or pyridostigmine).

d. Erythromycin

(1) Pharmacokinetics

(a) Half-life = 1½–2 hours.

(b) Erythromycin is excreted in the bile. There is no need to decrease the dose in renal failure.

(c) CSF levels are the same as with penicillin G.

(2) Dosage

(a) Neonates: 10 mg/kg IV every 12 hours.

(b) Children: 40–50 mg/kg/day IV divided into four doses.

(c) Adults: 4–8 gm/day IV divided into four doses.

(3) Toxicity

(a) Hypersensitivity reactions: fever, rash, eosinophilia, and cholestatic jaundice (with the estalate form most frequently—not seen with the parenteral form).

(b) IV use frequently causes phlebitis.

(c) High-tone hearing loss has been reported.

(4) Precautions. If used IV, infuse over ½–1 hour in 250 ml of solution.

e. Vancomycin

(1) Pharmacokinetics

(a) Half-life ≈ 6 hours.

(b) CSF levels with inflamed meninges are similar to those in patients taking penicillin.

(c) Vancomycin is excreted by the kidneys, so the dose must be adjusted in renal insufficiency.

(2) Dosage

(a) Premature infants and neonates: 6–15 mg/kg/day IV divided into four doses.

(b) Children: 40 mg/kg/day IV in divided doses every 8 to 12 hours.

(c) Adults: 1 gm IV every 8 hours.

(3) Toxicity

(a) Hypersensitivity reactions: rash, fever, and anaphylaxis.

(b) Ototoxicity with a high-tone hearing loss.

(c) Nephrotoxicity

(4) Precautions

(a) Avoid administration concurrently with an aminoglycoside, because the ototoxicity and nephrotoxicity are additive.

(b) Follow renal function at least twice weekly.

(c) When maximum doses are to be used, obtain a baseline audiogram, and repeat it at any sign of hearing loss.

f. Polymyxin B

(1) Pharmacokinetics

(a) Serum half-life > 12 hours.

(b) Excretion is by means of the kidney.

(c) CSF levels after systemic administration are negligible.

(d) There is negligible binding to serum proteins.

(2) Dosage

(a) Systemic 1.5–2.5 mg/kg/day IM in four equally divided doses at 6-hour intervals. It is not recommended for use in neonates.

(b) Intrathecal

Children under 2 years old: 2 mg daily for 3–4 days, then 2.5 mg every other day.

Children over 2 years old and adults: 5 mg daily for 3–4 days, then 5 mg every other day.

(3) Toxicity

(a) Hypersensitivity reactions are rare.

(b) Intrathecal use may produce signs of meningeal irritation with an increase in CSF cells and protein.

(c) Neuromuscular blockade can lead to respiratory failure in myasthenics and patients with borderline respiratory function. This blockade does not respond to calcium or anticholinesterase agents.

(d) Renal insufficiency occurs at doses higher than 2.5 mg/kg/day.

(4) **Precautions.** The dose must be reduced in renal failure. Renal function is monitored every other day, and respiratory function is monitored daily in patients with respiratory or neuromuscular disease. Systemic polymyxin B should be used only in the most extreme circumstances.

g. Antibiotics that penetrate into the CSF poorly and are avoided in the treatment of bacterial meningitis include **cephalosporins** and **tetracyclines**.

3. **The initial choice of antibiotics**

a. Bacteriologic identification of the infecting organism must be made, and the drug sensitivities determined. Until this information is available, the initial choice of antibiotics depends on several factors:

(1) **The Gram stain.** If a high-quality Gram stain shows an identifiable organism in abundance, the patient is treated for that organism, but, in addition, coverage for other likely infecting organisms for the age of the patient should be provided.

(2) **Identification of the organism.** Pending definite bacteriologic identification in patients without underlying immunologic disease, recent intracranial surgery, or head trauma, there is a stereotyped distribution of infecting organisms found in bacterial meningitis (according to age).

(a) **Neonatal meningitis** is considered to originate from two sources.
Infections acquired during delivery, which usually appear within the first week of life; the offending organisms are common in the female genital tract (e.g., enteric gram-negative bacilli, group B streptococci, and *Listeria monocytogenes*).
After about 1 week of age, meningitis tends to be a result of systemic sepsis from respiratory, skin, or umbilical infections, and the predominant organisms are group B streptococci, *Staphylococcus aureus,* and organisms present in hospital nurseries, such as *Pseudomonas, Proteus,* and opportunistic pathogens (such as *Flavobacterium septicum* or *Salmonella*).
The temporal division is not sharp, however, because neonates may develop delayed infections from organisms presumably acquired during delivery, and hospital-acquired organisms may infect within the first days of life. Consequently, the first 2 months of life may be considered as a unit.

(b) **Children and adolescents.** After the age of 2 months, the child loses the protection of maternal antibodies and becomes susceptible to the common organism that causes childhood meningitis (*H. influenzae* and *N. meningitidis*). Apparently the child's immune system is sufficiently developed after 2 months of age to protect him from meningitis secondary to other organisms in the environment, except for rare cases of gram-negative or *Staphylococcus* infection, which is usually associated with surgery, trauma, or systemic sepsis. The incidence of *H. influenzae* meningitis, after peaking at the age of 1 year, then drops off steadily, presumably because most children develop antibodies to the group B capsular antigen. After the age of 4 years, *H. influenzae* is rarely a cause of meningitis, leaving meningococcus as the most frequent agent for the remainder of the first two decades of life.

(c) Adults. After the age of 20 years, meningococcus becomes a rare cause of meningitis, because most adults have developed immunity to it, and pneumococcus assumes the leading role as a cause of meningitis. With its many type-specific capsular antigens and lack of cross-immunity between types, no permanent immunologic protection can develop against the pneumococcus. Virtually all other bacterial meningitis in adults occurs in the setting of some underlying predisposing disease.

(3) Predisposing factors.

(a) Head trauma. Closed head injury, with skull fractures or defects in the cribriform plate, can give bacteria access to the subarachnoid space. Usually the meningitis occurs within 2 weeks of injury, and pneumococcus is the infecting organism. With open head injuries and delayed onset of meningitis, a wide variety of organisms, including gram-negative organisms and *Staphylococcus,* may invade the CNS. Meningitis associated with CSF rhinorrhea, even long after the trauma, is penumococcal in a high percentage of patients.

(b) Parameningeal infections. Sinusitis, chronic otitis, and mastoiditis may lead to the development of meningitis, which is usually pneumococcal but is also caused by *H. influenzae* in young children and occasionally by *S. aureus.* It should be emphasized that the presence of an organism in a parameningeal focus of infection does not guarantee that organism to be the etiologic agent of the meningitis and the initial antibiotic is not chosen on that basis alone. Any organism that infects the ears or sinuses should be covered by the initial therapy; but unless there is confirmation by a strongly diagnostic CSF Gram stain, other likely organisms must be covered as well.

(c) Postneurosurgical meningitis. The organism is introduced at surgery or shortly thereafter, before healing of the incision, and most often it is a skin organism or one of the wide variety of organisms that may be acquired in the hospital environment. Consequently, broad-spectrum coverage is necessary until a definite organism can be identified. Infections of indwelling shunts or Ommaya reservoirs have a spectrum of infecting organisms that is similar to that of other neurosurgical infections.

(d) Anatomic defects. Meningomyeloceles, midline dermal sinus tracts, including pilonidal sinuses, and tumors of the head and neck that invade the skull and meninges may give organisms access to the subarachnoid space. Thus these conditions are sought in all patients with meningitis caused by unusual organisms. Conversely, in the presence of these defects and in the absence of a diagnostic Gram stain, initial antibiotic coverage must include *Staphylococcus, Streptococcus,* and enteric gram-negative organisms in addition to the common organisms for the particular age group.

(e) Evidence of systemic sepsis. The characteristic purpura or petechial skin lesions of meningococcemia may point to a diagnosis of that infection, especially if the organisms are seen in or cultured from the skin lesion. However, staphylococcal septicemia, including acute bacterial endocarditis (ABE) and, rarely, septicemia with enteric gram-negative organisms, may produce similar skin lesions.

Pneumonia may accompany meningitis and often is apparently the primary infection, with meningitis occurring as a complication of septicemia. Just as is the case with sinus and ear infections, however, the antibiotic should not be chosen purely on the basis of the respiratory pathogen.

(f) Underlying systemic illness. Splenectomy and **sickle cell anemia** predispose to pneumococcal sepsis and meningitis.

Systemic malignancy, especially hematologic malignancy, induces vulnerability to a much wider variety of organisms than the normal host, especially if the white blood count is depressed.

Cancer patients with CNS infection may be divided into several classes, each of which has its own spectrum of infecting organisms. For example, patients with malignancy and a normal white count are most often infected with *Cryptococcus,* but they may also acquire meningitis with pneumococcus or *Listeria.* When the white blood count falls below 2700, gram-negative rods become the most likely causative organisms.

Transplant recipients and other patients on **immunosuppressive therapy,** as well as patients with **renal failure,** are susceptible to a wider variety of infecting organisms than the nonimmunosuppressed host. In particular, they are susceptible to fungal infection, infection with enteric gram-negative rods, and with unusual hospital-acquired pathogens (e.g., *Pseudomonas, Mima polymorphia,* and *Serratia*). Dialysis patients are particularly likely to become infected with skin organisms, such as *Staphlococcus* and *Streptococcus.*

(g) Epidemiology. In nonhospitalized patients, knowledge of community epidemics helps determine the appropriate therapy. In hospitalized patients with malignancy, immunosuppression, or anatomic defects that predispose them to the development of meningitis with unusual organisms, initial antibiotic therapy should cover the organisms known to be present in the patient's hospital environment. Thus one should be aware of the antibiotic sensitivities of organisms being isolated in the hospital to judge therapy appropriately. It is stressed that one should err on the side of too broad a spectrum of antibiotic coverage if there is any doubt about the infecting organism, particularly in patients with inadequate host defenses and in hospital-acquired infections.

b. Recommendations for initial antibiotic therapy in various clinical situations (see Table 8-2 for summary)

(1) Neonatal meningitis (in children less than 2 months old)

(a) Ampicillin 50–100 mg/kg/day IV divided into two doses **plus**

Gentamicin 5.0 mg/kg/day IV or IM divided into two doses in premature infants and in term infants in the first week of life, 7.5 mg/kg/day IV or IM divided into three doses in neonates after the first week of life, **or**

Kanamycin 15 mg/kg/day IV divided into two doses if kanamycin-resistant organisms are very uncommon in the hospital nursery.

(b) Alternative

Chloramphenicol (succinate derivative) 25–50 mg/kg/day in four divided doses **plus**

Gentamicin or kanamycin in the same doses as listed previously.

Table 8-2. Initial Therapy of Bacterial Meningitis

Clinical Situation	Drug of Choice	Alternative
Neonatal	Ampicillin and gentamicin	Chloramphenicol and gentamicin
Infants and children	Ampicillin and chloramphenicol	Erythromycin and chloramphenicol
Adults	Ampicillin or penicillin G	Erythromycin and chloramphenicol
Neurosurgical infection	Oxacillin and gentamicin	Erythromycin and gentamicin or erythromycin and chloramphenicol
Basilar skull fracture or CSF leak	Ampicillin or penicillin G	Erythromycin and chloramphenicol
Immunosuppression or malignancy	Ampicillin and gentamicin	Erythromycin and gentamicin or erythromycin and chloramphenicol

   (2) Infants and children (over 2 months old)

      (a) Ampicillin   300–400 mg/kg/day IV in four or six divided doses **and**

         Chloramphenicol   50–100 mg/kg/day IV in four divided doses.

      (b) Alternative

         Chloramphenicol   50–100 mg/kg/day IV divided into four doses **and**

         Erythromycin   25–50 mg/kg/day in four divided doses.

   (3) Adults

      (a) Ampicillin   12–14 gm/day IV divided into four or six doses, **or**

         Penicillin G 24×10^6 units/day IV divided into 12 doses.

      (b) Alternative

         Chloramphenicol   4 gm/day IV divided into four doses **and**

         Erythromycin   4 gm/day IV divided into four doses.

   (4) Patients with basilar skull fractures or CSF leaks. Same as in **(3)**.

   (5) Postneurosurgical infections in all ages

      (a) Oxacillin   200 mg/kg/day IV in infants and children (other than neonates; see section **2.b.(3)**) and 10–12 gm/day IV in adults divided into four doses (or **nafcillin** 200 mg/kg/day IV in infants and children divided into four doses) **and**

         Gentamicin   5.0 mg/kg/day IM or IV divided into two doses in premature infants; 7.5 mg/kg/day IM or IV divided into three doses in neonates; and 5 mg/kg/day IV divided into three doses in children and adults with normal renal function.

      (b) Alternative

         Erythromycin   20 mg/kg/day IV divided into two doses in neonates; 40–50 mg/kg/day IV divided into four doses in children; 4–8 gm/day IV divided into four doses in adults **and**

Gentamicin (same doses as in **(5)(a)**) **or**

Erythromycin (same doses as in **(5)(b)**) **and**

Chloramphenicol (same doses as in **(2)** and **(3)**).

(6) Meningitis with underlying immunosuppression or malignancy

(a) Ampicillin (same doses as in **(1)**, **(2)**, and **(3)**) **and**

Gentamicin (same doses as in **(5)(a)**).

(b) Alternative

Erythromycin and gentamicin or

Erythromycin and chloramphenicol

c. Antibiotic therapy of bacterial meningitis of known etiology

(1) As soon as the identification of the infecting organism has been made and its antibiotic sensitivity is known, the broad-spectrum coverage is changed to the optimum antibiotic available for it (Table 8-3). This antibiotic is continued for the remainder of the course.

(2) With some gram-negative organisms routine sensitivity testing may rate the organism sensitive to more than one antibiotic. However, the degree of sensitivity, as measured by the respective minimum inhibitory concentrations (MIC) levels, may differ considerably. The MIC should therefore be determined, when appropriate, and used to guide therapy.

(3) *H. influenzae* presents a special problem in antibiotic choice. Until recently, virtually all isolates of *H. influenzae* from spinal fluid were sensitive to ampicillin. Within the past 3 years, however, an increasing percentage of isolates in the United States have been resistant to ampicillin by virtue of their ability to produce an enzyme, β-lactamase, which renders the ampicillin molecule inactive. As a consequence, hospitals in which ampicillin-resistant *H. influenzae* has been recovered from spinal fluid use chloramphenicol as the first-line drug for *H. influenzae* meningitis, changing to ampicillin if sensitivity to that drug can be demonstrated clearly. A direct assay of β-lactamase activity of the isolate is a more reliable indication of ampicillin sensitivity than is the more standard disc inhibition method. There have been only rare reports of *H. influenzae* isolates that are resistant to chloramphenicol, but this may become an increasing problem in the future.

(4) Refer to sec **I.C.2** for appropriate guidelines in the use of the antibiotic chosen.

D. Special problems in the management of bacterial meningitis

1. The use of intrathecal antibiotics

a. Rationale. Because of the relatively low CSF drug concentrations obtained with most antibiotics, there have been many attempts to treat CNS infections with direct subarachnoid injections of antibiotics. This procedure is used to expose the organisms in the meninges and CSF to higher concentrations of antibiotics than can be achieved with systemic administration alone. However, there are several problems with this approach.

(1) Many drugs are toxic to the CNS when they come in contact with the surface of the brain or spinal cord in high concentrations. For example, penicillin and its derivatives may cause seizures and encephalopathy. Also, many drugs, when injected into the lumbar subarachnoid space, have been reported to cause paresthesias, radiculopathies, or trans-

Table 8-3. Antibiotic Therapy of Bacterial Meningitis of Known Etiology

Organism	Drug of Choice	Alternatives	Optional Intrathecal Drug
GRAM-POSITIVE ORGANISMS			
S. pneumoniae (pneumococcus)	Penicillin G	Chloramphenicol Erythromycin	
Streptococcus, groups A and B	Penicillin G	Erythromycin	Gentamicin
Streptococcus, group D (Enterococcus)	Penicillin G and gentamicin	Vancomycin	
Staphylococcus	Oxacillin or methicillin	Vancomycin	Bacitracin
Listeria monocytogenes	Penicillin G or ampicillin	Erythromycin	
GRAM-NEGATIVE ORGANISMS			
Meningococcus	Penicillin G	Chloramphenicol	
H. influenzae	Ampicillin[a] or chloramphenicol	Chloramphenicol	
Pseudomonas aeruginosa	Carbinicillin and gentamicin (or tobramycin)	Polymixin B both IM and IT	Gentamicin or tobramycin
Enteric gram-negative organisms (E. Coli, Proteus species, Klebsiella species)	Chloramphenicol (or ampicillin, if sensitivities are known)	Gentamicin IV and IT	Gentamicin

[a]Ampicillin is recommended for *H. influenzae* only when the organism is known to be sensitive to the drug.

verse myelitis; and there have been reports of arachnoiditis following repeated intrathecal administration of drugs.

(2) Drugs do not diffuse freely throughout the CSF. When administered into the lumbar space, they reach negligible concentration in the ventricles and relatively low concentrations in the basilar cisterns.

(3) Patients with CNS infections may have blocks in CSF flow at various levels, denying the drug access to some parts of the subarachnoid space.

b. Methods. Because of the problems just listed, this type of therapy is reserved for those patients in whom systemic therapy is not recommended, since systemic therapy alone will not be curative. In these patients the organism involved requires drug levels that are higher than can be attained in the CSF by systemic administration. Of the bacteria, enteric gram-negative rods and *Staphylococcus* are the organisms that most often require the use of intrathecal (IT) drugs.

Enough experience has been obtained to state that the aminoglycoside antibiotics, gentamicin and tobramycin, as well as the polypeptide antibiotic Bacitracin, can be injected safely into the subarachnoid space in humans. However, both may produce paresthesias in the extremities if injected intracisternally or into the lumbar space, and one would expect that the aminoglycosides in high concentration may produce eighth cranial nerve damage. Nevertheless, these drugs can be used safely for a brief course of intrathecal therapy in reasonable doses.

(1) Techniques of administration

(a) Intralumbar. A lumbar puncture is performed in the usual manner, and 5–10 ml of CSF is removed for analysis, including drug-level measurement, cell count, protein, sugar, and culture. The drug to be administered is dissolved in 5 or 10 ml of sterile saline **without bacteriostatic preservative,** and it is injected through the lumbar puncture needle slowly.

(b) Intracisternal. Drugs may be injected into the basilar cistern by those skilled in the technique of cisternal puncture. The advantage over lumbar injection is that higher levels of antibiotic may be achieved at the base of the brain and over the convexities.

This technique is essentially the same as intralumbar injection, but the drug is injected over 1 minute to minimize the time the needle remains in the cistern and in danger of damaging the medulla. It is not recommended for the repeated administration of drugs and should only be undertaken by those with considerable experience with the technique of cisternal puncture.

(c) Intraventricularly. An indwelling cathether that connects one lateral ventricle with a small silicone rubber reservoir **(Ommaya reservoir),** placed beneath the scalp, may be implanted surgically. Then the reservoir can be repeatedly punctured percutaneously and becomes "self-sealing," thereby giving ready access to the intraventricular space, either for the sampling of CSF or the injection of drugs. Very high drug levels may be achieved in the ventricular CSF, and adequate levels are reached in the cisternal and lumbar CSF. With aminoglycosides, a 5-mg dose injected intraventricularly may yield therapeutic drug levels (4–6 μg/ml) throughout the CSF for as long as 24 hours after injection.

The disadvantages of this method of administration are that the patient is subjected to a neurosurgical procedure with its possible complications (although usually it can be done under local anesthesia), and the devices can become plugged, disconnected, or infected during use.

Drug administration using the reservoirs requires meticulous aseptic technique. The scalp over the reservoir must be kept closely shaved. The physician must wear a gown and mask, cover the patient's head and surrounding area with a sterile drape, and then change his gloves. With each dose, the overlying scalp is washed thoroughly with soap and water, then with iodine three times, and then with alcohol three times. Then the reservoir is punctured with a 21- or 23-gauge scalp vein needle, and 5–10 ml of CSF is withdrawn for analysis. The antibiotic, dissolved in 10 ml of normal saline **without bacteriostatic preservative** is slowly injected over 10 minutes and the needle is removed. The reservoir may then be slowly pumped to empty all its contents into the ventricle.

c. Precautions to be taken with intrathecal antibiotic administration

(1) Measure the CSF drug level with each dose to ensure that antibiotic is not accumulating excessively in the CSF.

(2) Follow the CSF protein and cell count for signs of a CSF block (greatly elevated protein) or chemical meningitis (increasing CSF white cell count, with polymorphonuclear leukocytes predominating and increasing protein).

(3) Culture the CSF with each injection. An increasing cell count may indicate iatrogenic CNS infection as well as chemical meningitis.

(4) Be aware of the possibility of blockages of CSF flow, denying the antibiotic access to regions of the subarachnoid space that may harbor "loculated infections." If this is at issue, a radioactively labeled colloid may be injected intraventricularly to determine the patency of CSF pathways by radiologic methods.

d. Indications for intrathecal therapy. Definite indications for the use of intrathecal antibiotic administration have not been defined, but there is no question that it should be limited to certain rare situations.

(1) Gram-negative meningitis

(a) If the bacteria are sensitive to chloramphenicol, this drug should be used because it gives high drug concentrations in the CSF with IV administration.

(b) If the organism is resistant to chloramphenicol, or if the patient fails to respond to chloramphenicol or relapses after a course of that drug, then gentamicin or tobramycin, depending on the organism's sensitivity, is used both systemically and intrathecally.

(c) As long as the patient is not moribund, the drug is administered into the lumbar space in a dose of 5 mg every 18 to 24 hours in adults and 1–2 mg every 24 hours in infants and children until the CSF is sterile.

(d) If the patient is moribund, or if he fails to respond to the above therapy or relapses after a full 3-week course of this therapy, then an Ommaya reservoir is installed and intraventricular gentamicin or tobramycin are used along with systemic administration of the drug.

(e) In neonates, higher levels of CSF gentamicin are achieved with systemic therapy alone than in adults. Therefore intrathecal gentamicin is not used routinely in treating chloramphenicol-resistant organisms. Rather, it is reserved for moribund neonates and those who fail to respond to systemic therapy alone.

(2) Staphylococcal meningitis. Bacitracin in doses of 5000 to 10,000 units may be injected into the subarachnoid space in the treatment of meningitis due to penicillinase-producing *Staphylococcus aureus*. However, this therapy is only clearly indicated in moribund patients and those failing to respond to systemic administration of oxacillin or nafcillin in high doses. Intralumbar administration should be tried first, except in those patients with known blocks in CSF flow that would prevent lumbar CSF from reaching the infecting organisms. The technique of administration is the same as that for the amino-glycosides.

(3) Enterococcal *(Streptococcus* group D) meningitis. This is a rare disease, at times occurring in neonates or as a complication of surgery or of bacterial endocarditis. Although sensitive to ampicillin in vitro, this organism often requires combined therapy with penicillin and an aminoglycoside to cure serious infections. Consequently, the combination of penicillin G and gentamicin is administered systemically. Intrathecal gentamicin may be added, if necessary, according to indications similar to those listed under staphylococcal infections.

e. Steroids. The only clear indication for use of steroids in the therapy of bacterial meningitis is in the treatment of symptomatic, elevated intracranial pressure. There are no conclusive data that show steroids to be of benefit in minimizing the damage caused by the inflammatory response to the bacterial infection.

f. Treatment of meningococcus contacts

(1) Patients with meningococcal disease are infectious and can spread the organism to others by means of the respiratory route until they have been on therapy for 24 hours. About 3 of 1000 family members of patients with index cases will develop meningococcal disease secondarily. Although most adults are protected by their own antibodies and will not develop meningococcal disease, many will develop an asymptomatic carrier state and will be able to expose other susceptible people to the organism. Therefore it is recommended that the following groups of people be treated with antibiotics when an index case is diagnosed.

(a) Family and household members.

(b) Others in intimate contact for prolonged periods with an index case. This does not include acquaintances or school classmates.

(c) Hospital staff members who have been directly breathed on by the patient. There is no need to treat any hospital personnel who have merely been in the room with the patient.

(2) The current recommendations for prophylactic therapy are:

(a) Rifampin   600 mg PO every 12 hours for four doses in adults; 10 mg/kg every 12 hours for four doses in children between the ages of 1 and 12 years, 5 mg/kg every 12 hours for four doses in children less than 1 year old, **or,**

(b) Minocycline   200 mg PO, then 100 mg PO every 12 hours for five doses (not to be used in children).

Both these drugs have significant side effects (primarily dizziness and gastrointestinal upset), so only those at real risk should be treated. It is crucial that all contacts be treated **simultaneously** and that they be treated as soon as possible after the index case is diagnosed. Sulfonamides may only be used in the prophylaxis of people who have had contact with patients in epidemics caused by strains of meningococcus known to be sulfonamide-sensitive.

(3) Meningococcal type A and type C polysaccharide vaccines are now available and are effective in adults and in children over 2 years of age. Their use should be considered in (a) household contacts of meningococcal disease if prophylactic therapy can be begun very early after diagnosis of the index case, and (b) in immunosuppressed children over 2 years old.

These vaccines should be used in addition to antibiotic prophylaxis. In epidemics of meningococcal disease, the Center for Disease Control (CDC) should be consulted concerning the use of these vaccines.

g. Shunt infections. Infections of shunts that are implanted for the treatment of hydrocephalus make up a special category of postneurosurgical infections. These infections are usually acquired at surgery, except for ventriculoureteral (V-U) shunts, rarely used now, which can become infected in a retrograde manner from infections of the urinary tract. Consequently, the spectrum of organisms in infections of ventriculoatrial (V-A) or ventriculoperitoneal (V-P) shunts is the same as that of other neurosurgical infections. *Staphylococcus, Streptococcus,* and anaerobes are the organisms in the vast majority of infections, with gram-negative enteric bacteria being unusual but significant pathogens. Meningococcus and pneumococcus are rare causes of shunt infections. With ventriculoureteral and lumboureteral (L-U) shunts, however, the most common organisms isolated are gram-negative enteric bacteria, followed in order of importance by *Staphylococcus.* Practically, however, the initial antibiotic coverage in the absence of a diagnostic Gram stain does not differ with either type of shunt from that for other postneurosurgical infections already discussed.

It should be borne in mind that the CSF obtained by lumbar puncture grows out the infecting organism in only about three-quarters of shunt infections. Thus the blood, surgical wound (if it is fresh), urine, and fluid obtained from a direct puncture of the shunt-valve reservoir, in addition to the lumbar CSF, are cultured. Peritonitis may occur with ventriculoperitoneal shunt infections, and the ascitic fluid may yield the organism. The treatment of a shunt infection is:

(1) Surgical removal of the shunt, and

(2) Appropriate systemic antibiotic coverage.

Usually, once the shunt is removed, the infection responds to systemic antibiotics, and there is no need for intrathecal therapy. When constant ventricular drainage is required after shunt removal, however, antibiotics can be instilled through the drainage cannula with little added morbidity.

E. Complications of bacterial meningitis

1. Increased intracranial pressure. Increased intracranial pressure is common in bacterial meningitis. It can occur through one of two mechanisms: hydrocephalus or brain swelling. The latter may be a diffuse process due to toxic effects of the infection or it may be focal, secondary to cortical venous thrombophlebitis and venous obstruction, or arteritis, with brain ischemia and infarction. The most common situation is diffuse brain swelling. However, the therapy is the same regardless of the cause.

The pressure generally returns rapidly to normal as the infection responds to therapy. If the patient is afebrile, awake, and alert, without hemispheric signs, it can safely be assumed that the increased CSF pressure has resolved.

a. If the patient is doing well clinically, avoid repeat lumbar punctures.

b. **Fluid balance.** Care must be taken to avoid overhydrating the patient. In adults, with adequate perfusion, 1500 ml of half-normal saline per day is sufficient, including the volume of fluid in which the antibiotics are administered (in children, 1000 ml/sq m antibiotics in half-normal saline). Avoid administering large amounts of free water. When the patient can regulate his or her own fluid intake, he or she should still be limited to less than 2000 ml total intake per day (oral plus IV) until the CSF pressure is no longer elevated.

c. **Steroids.** Steroids are administered in high doses initially and then rapidly tapered once the infection is under control. One program consists of dexamethasone (Decadron) 10 mg IV for the first dose, then 4 mg IV every 4 hours until the infection is under control. Then the dose is tapered to 0 over 5–10 days, assuming the total course is less than 3 weeks. If high doses are given for longer than 2 weeks, more gradual tapering is necessary to avoid hypothalamic-pituitary-adrenal insufficiency. The usual precautions necessary with high-dose steroid administration (i.e., the monitoring of blood sugars and stool guaiacs and concern for masked infection) are followed. It is generally believed that steroids only begin to exert an effect after 12–16 hours.

d. **Hyperosmolar agents.** When using hyperosmolar agents, the physician must guarantee a patent urinary system, and in comatose patients a Foley catheter is required. Furthermore, both mannitol and glycerol use are associated with hyperosmolar, hyperglycemic, nonketotic coma in diabetics (as is steroid use), so blood sugars and serum electrolytes should be followed at least every other day in patients on chronic use.

(1) **Mannitol.** 1.0–1.5 gm/kg may be given for acute, increased intracranial pressure with danger of transtentorial herniation, and the dose may be repeated twice at 4-hour intervals before the steroids take effect. Some data show that after mannitol is given, a "rebound" increase in intracranial pressure occurs, but with meningitis this effect can be minimized by using steroids and by beginning to bring the infection under control.

(2) **Glycerol.** Glycerol may be given PO or by means of a nasogastric tube in a 20% solution flavored with lemon (Osmoglyn) or in an unflavored 50% solution. The dose is 3 gm/kg/day divided into at least six doses. It is not generally available for IV use. Acutely, it has no clear advantage over mannitol, and there are no good data showing that the chronic administration of glycerol has any lasting effect on intracranial pressure. It should be tried, however, in those cases of bacterial meningitis, particularly gram-negative meningitis, that respond slowly to treatment and in which the CSF pressure may remain elevated for several days after the initiation of antibiotics, in spite of the administration of high-dose steroids.

2. Seizures

a. Seizures are a frequent manifestation of meningitis, especially in infants and children. They may occur through various etiologies:

(1) Bacterial encephalitis.

(2) Cortical vein thrombosis with venous infarction.

(3) Subdural effusions or empyemas.

(4) Infectious vasculitis.

(5) Occult brain abscess.

(6) Epilepsy exacerbated by fever in young children.

(7) Metabolic abnormalities, including hyponatremia from the syndrome of inappropriate ADH secretion (SIADH).

b. As a rule, seizures associated with meningitis resolve when the infection clears without leading to chronic epilepsy and carry no poor prognostic implications. (The treatment of seizures is described in Chapter 6.) Unless there are other indications, the occurrence of a self-limited seizure in the setting of acute bacterial meningitis (even a focal seizure) requires no further evaluation beyond a check of the serum electrolytes and assurance that cardiorespiratory function is adequate.

3. Hydrocephalus

a. Communicating hydrocephalus may complicate bacterial meningitis due to obstruction of CSF flow by thickened and fibrotic meninges. Usually the site of obstruction is at the base of the brain, leading to communicating hydrocephalus. This syndrome may occur early or late in the course of the infection and should be suspected if the patient's mental status fails to return to normal as the infection clears.

This condition is not a medical emergency, and the treatment is to cure the infection and then place a V-P or V-A shunt if necessary. It may resolve spontaneously without shunting, so the same considerations apply in deciding whether and when a shunt should be implanted as with other cases of communicating hydrocephalus (Chap. 3).

b. Noncommunicating hydrocephalus rarely occurs as a complication of meningitis due to partial or complete obstruction of CSF flow at the aqueduct of Sylvius or at the fourth ventricular outflow. **Total obstruction** of ventricular outflow is rare and difficult to recognize in acute bacterial meningitis, because its primary sign is coma, and it can be confused with the coma due to the infection itself. However, total obstruction of ventricular outflow is an emergency and will rapidly lead to death unless it is corrected. The presence of papilledema, coma, bilateral Babinski sign, and paralysis of upward gaze should suggest the diagnosis, which can be confirmed by CT scan or ventriculography. Since this syndrome generally occurs early or when the CSF is still infected, the acute treatment is constant ventricular drainage rather than shunting. After the CSF is sterile, a V-P or V-A shunt may be performed. Most surgeons prefer to use a V-P shunt soon after a CNS infection.

Partial obstruction at the aqueduct of the fourth ventricular outflow may present a picture similar to communicating hydrocephalus and is not an emergency. However, it requires careful observation for signs of total obstruction.

4. Subdural effusion. Infants less than 1 year of age are subject to the accumulation of sterile collections of fluid in the subdural space as a complication of bacterial meningitis (most often *H. influenzae*).

a. Clinical description. The signs are nonspecific: vomiting, irritability, fullness of the fontanelle, or increasing head circumference.

b. Diagnosis. The diagnosis is made through transillumination, and it is confirmed by tapping the subdural space percutaneously through the patent fontanelle.

c. Treatment is aimed at maintaining normal intracranial pressure and preventing head enlargement. Repeated percutaneous aspiration of the fluid is usually adequate, and the fluid ceases to reaccumulate after the infection is treated. Subdural taps are not indicated if there are no signs or symptoms of increased intracranial pressure and no focal neurologic deficits. The membrane that surrounds the effusion may have to be excised surgically in rare cases if the fluid continues to reaccumulate after repeated taps.

5. **Subdural empyema** is a rare complication of meningitis.

   a. **Clinical description.** Subdural empyema is suggested by the development of papilledema, persistently increased intracranial pressure, persistent fever, focal signs, or seizures.

   b. The **diagnosis** can be made most reliably by arteriography. There is too little experience with CT scanning in this relatively rare condition to know whether the test is sensitive and reliable, but one would expect it to be useful. The EEG and technetium brain scan are of little value in the diagnosis of this condition, and lumbar puncture is dangerous.

   c. Treatment is immediate surgical drainage; appropriate stains and cultures are performed at surgery and appropriate antibiotic therapy is continued for at least 1 week postoperatively.

6. **Persistent fever** during the treatment of bacterial meningitis suggests one of several conditions: an occult focus of infection that requires surgical drainage or prolonged antibiotic therapy (e.g., osteomyelitis, a parameningeal focus, an occult abscess either in the brain or elsewhere, or subdural effusion), drug fever, or inadequate antibiotic therapy.

7. **Persistent neurologic deficit**

   a. A focal neurologic deficit may indicate the destruction of brain tissue by encephalitis, arterial or venous infarction, or the presence of a mass lesion, such as a subdural effusion or empyema.

   b. Cranial nerve palsies may occur but usually resolve. Hearing deficits are the most frequent, persistent cranial nerve abnormalities.

   c. The treatment of subdural effusions and empyemas has already been discussed.

   d. Bacterial encephalitis (the direct invasion of the brain parenchyma by bacteria) is treated with systemic antibiotics. There are no data showing that steroids used to diminish the inflammatory response have an effect on the permanent deficits that may result.

   e. Venous thrombosis occurs as a result of cortical vein thrombophlebitis. Again, the only known treatment is antibiotics to prevent progression of the process. Anticoagulation is of no known benefit, and it is strongly contraindicated in the presence of CNS infections.

8. **Medical complications**

   a. Bacterial meningitis may lead to the syndrome of inappropriate ADH with hyponatremia and possible seizures.

   b. Systemic sepsis may lead to disseminated intravascular coagulation (DIC) or the development of metastatic abscesses.

   c. Antibiotics used in high doses, as is necessary for meningitis, subject the patient to their associated risks.

   d. The complications of steroids and hyperosmolar agents have been discussed.

II. TUBERCULOUS INFECTION OF THE CNS

A. Making the diagnosis

1. **Tuberculous meningitis.** The diagnosis of tuberculous meningitis must, of necessity, be made before culture results become available, because it re-

quires at least 4 weeks for the organisms to grow in vitro. The diagnosis is suggested by the clinical symptoms (fever, headache, lethargy, vomiting, and cranial nerve palsies are common), is supported by evidence of active pulmonary disease (usually miliary and present in only about one-third of cases) or by a positive PPD (present in about 50% of cases), and is confirmed by observing acid-fast organisms in the CSF. Nuchal rigidity is not often seen early in the disease. The CSF formula is most often lymphocytic, with a low sugar, but, occasionally, it is purulent early in the disease. The protein is always elevated, frequently leading to the formation of a clot, known as a **pellicle**, on standing. The CSF chloride merely reflects the serum chloride and is not useful in making the diagnosis.

The diagnostic yield of the CSF may be augmented in various ways:

a. The probability of growing the organism is directly related to the quantity of CSF cultured. Consequently, if possible, 10–15 ml of CSF are removed for culture with each diagnostic lumbar puncture.

b. Concentration of the organisms will aid in microscopic identification by the AFB smear.

    (1) The pellicle can be smeared and is an excellent source of the organism.

    (2) The CSF is centrifuged and the sediment is smeared if no pellicle forms.

    (3) Several drops of the sediment can be placed on the slide sequentially and allowed to dry in the same area.

    (4) The CSF can be examined by fluorescent-antibody staining techniques.

c. Repeated CSF examinations may show a characteristic pattern of falling sugar, rising protein, and rising or stable cell count.

2. Tuberculoma. Tuberculosis may also infect the brain parenchyma, producing encephalitis or a focal granuloma, known as a **tuberculoma,** with or without meningeal involvement. In the absence of meningeal involvement or evidence of systemic or pulmonary tuberculosis, the diagnosis may be extremely difficult, being indistinguishable from brain abscess, a brain tumor, or even viral encephalitis. Often the diagnosis is made by surgical biopsy. *Mycobacterium tuberculosis* may invade blood vessels and cause a CNS vasculitis with an associated brain infarction.

B. Therapy

1. Antibiotics

a. The first-line drug is isoniazid (INH). It is relatively nontoxic, known to be effective, and penetrates the meninges well. The dose in adults is 10–15 mg/kg/day and in children is 20 mg/kg/day. It can be given PO in a single daily dose. All patients over 6 years of age on INH should receive pyridoxine 50 mg PO daily to prevent pyridoxine-deficiency syndromes, which have been reported with INH use, that include neuropathy, encephalopathy, seizures, and anemia.

b. All cases of meningeal infection with tuberculosis are treated with at least two drugs. Many experts would use triple-drug therapy, at least in the first 2–3 months. The following are the first-line drugs that may be combined with INH:

    (1) Streptomycin. 20 mg/kg/day (maximum, 1 gm/day) IM in a single injection daily. It can only be used safely for the initial 2–3 months of therapy.

    (2) Rifampin. 600 mg/day PO in adults. The safety of this drug has not been demonstrated in children. Nevertheless, it is used in children at a dose of 10–20 mg/kg/day PO, and the drug is indicated when the organism is resistant to conventional pediatric therapy.

(3) **Ethambutol.** 25 mg/kg/day PO for the first 2 months of therapy, then 15 mg/kg/day PO for the duration of therapy.

c. In **severe infections** with a depressed mental status, with evidence of miliary disease, or with parenchymal brain involvement, three drugs should always be used.

d. After culture and sensitivity results are available, the regimen may require modification.

e. The necessary duration of therapy is not known. Most experts accept the concept of "two-phase" chemotherapy, with an initial phase of 2–3 months of intensive therapy while there are a large number of organisms present, followed by a prolonged course of less-intensive therapy, adding up to a total course of about 2 years. Furthermore, because of the eighth cranial nerve toxicity of streptomycin, it is risky to continue therapy at full dose (1 gm/day maximum) beyond 12 weeks. One effective therapeutic program is:

(1) **For the first 8–12 weeks:**

(a) **INH** 10–15 mg/kg/day in adults, 20 mg/kg/day in children **and**

(b) **Streptomycin** 20 mg/kg/day IM (maximum dose 1 gm/day) **and**

(c) **Ethambutol** 25/mg/kg/day PO, **or**

Rifampin 600 mg/day PO.

(2) Then, assuming the patient is doing well and the antibiotic sensitivity results are compatible, the following regimen should be continued for the remainder of the 2-year course:

(a) **INH** 10 mg/kg/day PO **and**

(b) **Ethambutol** 15 mg/kg/day PO, **or**

Rifampin 400 mg/day.

(3) Other regimens may also be used, such as **INH plus rifampin** with the addition of **ethambutol** for the first 2–3 months.

(4) **Second-line drugs** are included in the regimen if drug sensitivity of the patient or drug resistance of the organism preclude the use of the less toxic first-line drugs. These drugs should always be used in combination with either INH or rifampin.

(a) **Pyrazinamide** achieves high levels in the CSF, but it is relatively toxic, especially to the liver. The adult dose is 20–35 mg/kg/day PO divided into three or four doses, with a maximum daily dose of 3 gm/day.

(b) **Cycloserine** levels in the CSF are approximately equal to those in plasma. The adult dose is 250–500 mg PO BID.

(c) **Ethionamide** penetrates well into the CSF, but it commonly causes gastrointestinal, hepatic, and CNS toxicity. The adult dose is gradually increased from 500 mg to 1 gm PO daily in two to four divided doses taken with meals.

2. **Steroids.** Some have advocated the use of systemic, or even intrathecal, steroids in tuberculous meningitis. The hope is to inhibit the inflammatory response and hence attempt to prevent some of the complications of tuberculous infection, which, pathologically, often seems to result as much from exuberant granuloma formation as it does from direct destruction by the bacteria.

    a. Indications for the use of steroids in addition to antituberculous chemotherapy are:

      (1) Elevated intracranial pressure due to brain swelling.

      (2) Patients with a neurologic deficit, either from intraparenchymal disease or cranial nerve involvement.

      Tuberculous meningitis typically has an associated arteritis of the vessels at the base of the brain. Hence it can cause infarction with focal neurologic deficit in the absence of parenchymal infection. This situation is also an indication for the use of steroids.

      (3) Patients with a normal mental status and no neurologic deficit probably would **not** benefit from steroid therapy.

      (4) The **dose** of steroids for increased intracranial pressure is the same as for increased pressure of other types: dexamethasone 10 mg IV as a first dose, then 4–6 mg IV every 6 hours (the same dose is used in children). Mannitol may also be used in acute situations. Prednisone, 60 or 80 mg/day, or its equivalent, is usually chosen as an antiinflammatory agent. The high dose is generally maintained for 2–3 weeks and is then slowly tapered over about 1 month.

3. Contacts of the patient should be treated prophylactically according to the American Thoracic Society recommendations (*Am. Rev. Resp. Dis.* 110:371, 1974).

4. Tuberculomas should not be treated surgically in the acute stage of the disease because of the possibility of inducing a fatal tuberculous meningitis. Thus the disease is treated initially with antituberculous therapy and steroids. After 2–3 months of chemotherapy, the lesion can be resected if it causes intractable seizures or threatens a vital structure, such as the optic chiasm.

5. Follow-up and complications

    a. Repeat lumbar punctures are performed at 1 month, 6 months, and 2 years after beginning therapy if the patient is clinically stable. Obviously, the appearance of a new neurologic sign or symptom should prompt a lumbar puncture or other diagnostic tests that may be indicated.

    b. The major **late neurologic complication** of meningitis is hydrocephalus, and these patients are seen at least every 6 months for several years after diagnosis to screen for this development. Treatment is the same as for hydrocephalus of any other cause and depends on the site and degree of the block (see Chap. 3).

    c. Relapses may occur and are the main indication for repeat lumbar punctures. The main reasons for relapse are failure of the patient to take the medicine and the development of drug resistance (which is rare with multiple-drug therapy). At the first indication of a relapse, the patient is hospitalized, the antibiotic sensitivity of the organism is rechecked, and, pending those results, appropriate changes in the drug regimen are made. These changes may be merely the administration of the drugs under supervision or substitution or addition of alternative drugs.

6. Toxicity of antituberculous chemotherapy

    a. Isoniazid

      (1) Hepatic. About 10% of patients on INH develop elevated serum glutamic-oxaloacetic transaminase (SGOT) levels. Usually, the SGOT returns to normal even if INH is continued.

      True INH hepatitis occurs in only 1% of cases. It can occur months after beginning therapy, and it can produce jaundice, permanent liver damage, and even death. The risk of developing INH hepatitis increases with age, is not dose-dependent, and may occur principally in rapid acetylators of INH.

(2) Neurologic. Pyridoxine-deficiency syndromes, including neuropathy, anemia, encephalopathy, and seizures may occur if pyridoxine supplementation is not provided. This does not occur in children under the age of 6 years.

(3) Psychiatric. Euphoria, mania, and frank psychosis may occur and generally do not represent pyridoxine deficiency.

(4) Optic atrophy is rare.

(5) Hypersensitivity reactions are rare.

(6) Precautions

(a) Always provide pyridoxine supplementation at a dose at least one-tenth the INH dose for patients over 6 years of age.

(b) Patients should be questioned monthly concerning symptoms of liver dysfunction. Also, liver function tests should be done periodically.

(c) INH may precipitate phenytoin toxicity by interfering with that drug's metabolism.

b. Streptomycin

(1) Eighth cranial nerve damage (vestibular and hearing disturbances) limits the maximum dose of streptomycin that can be used. Doses of 1 gm/day or less are reliably tolerated for 2–3 months. Also, if it is administered to pregnant women, it may cause eighth cranial nerve dysfunction in the fetuses.

(2) Renal. As with all aminoglycosides, dose-related renal impairment may occur, but in the absence of preexisting renal disease, doses of streptomycin higher than 1 gm/day are required.

(3) Hypersensitivity reactions are unusual.

(4) Precautions

(a) Renal function is checked prior to use and the dose is adjusted accordingly.

(b) The patient should be questioned about and observed for symptoms and signs of labyrinthine dysfunction at monthly intervals.

c. Ethambutal

(1) Visual toxicity with optic nerve dysfunction can occur at doses higher than 15 mg/kg/day. However, this problem usually reverses if the drug is withdrawn promptly. The most sensitive indicators of visual toxicity are tests of color vision and visual acuity.

(2) Precautions. Patients should be questioned monthly about visual symptoms.

d. Rifampin

(1) Hepatic. Liver dysfunction may occur and may progress to jaundice.

(2) Hypersensitivity reactions and cutaneous reactions occur.

(3) Precautions. Rifampin is given daily and not on every-other-day or twice-weekly schedule, because the latter regimens and erratic use are associated with an increased risk of serious toxicity. Patients should be advised that their urine will be an orange color.

e. **Pyrazinamide**

(1) Hepatocellular toxicity necessitates the performance of baseline liver function tests before starting the drug and weekly thereafter.

(2) The drug may precipitate attacks of gout and may exacerbate diabetes mellitus.

(3) **Hypersensitivity reactions** and gastrointestinal upset are relatively frequent.

f. **Cycloserine**

(1) CNS toxicity usually appears early during administration of the drug and is reversible. Major motor seizures may occur, so the drug should not be used in epileptics.

(2) 65% of each dose is excreted in the urine, so the dose must be adjusted in renal insufficiency.

g. **Ethionamide**

(1) Gastrointestinal upset is frequent and mild, and reversible CNS toxicity may occur.

(2) Hepatocellular damage occurs in about 5% of patients taking the drug. Liver function is checked before starting the drug and every 2–4 weeks thereafter.

III. BRAIN ABSCESS

A. **Making the diagnosis**

1. **Clinical presentation.** Brain abscess generally occurs as the subacute progression of focal neurologic signs, headache, and depressed mental status. Seizures may or may not occur and systemic signs of infection are absent in about 50% of patients (i.e., peripheral white blood count, erythrocyte sedimentation rate, and body temperature are normal).

2. There may be evidence for a contiguous or systemic **source** of infection.

3. **Differential diagnosis** on admittance may include brain tumor, viral encephalitis, chronic subdural hematoma, or chronic meningitis. Signs of meningeal irritation are usually absent or mild, but the abscess may rupture into the ventricular system, producing acute bacterial ventriculitis and meningitis.

4. The definitive diagnosis is usually made only at surgery, although a characteristic CT scan in the appropriate clinical setting may be diagnostic.

B. **Localizing the lesion.** Many studies have attempted to document the relative usefulness of various techniques in the localization of brain abscesses. The techniques, with the exception of the CT scan, cannot be diagnostic but only localize and confirm the presence of a mass lesion. In order of their usefulness, the following studies may be done.

1. **A technetium brain scan** is noninvasive and highly reliable in localizing the lesion. Although not specific for brain abscesses, it is extremely useful along with other information in making the diagnosis. Also, it is the simplest method of following results of therapy radiologically.

2. **CT scanning.** There are less data concerning CT scanning than there are with radionuclide scanning, but it appears that CT scanning is highly reliable in localizing lesions. Furthermore, when the typical "donut" lesion with con-

trast enhancement (i.e., a peripheral ring around a low-density center) is present, the CT scan can be virtually specific for brain abscess in the usual clinical context. Rarely, cystic tumors or infarcts with rims of neovascularization can give the same appearance, but the absorption values of their centers are generally higher than those of abscess. The CT scan can also distinguish between an unencapsulated area of brain infection (cerebritis) and an encapsulated abscess.

3. **Ventriculography** is reliable in localizing solitary brain abscesses, localizing about 75% of cases in most series. If radionuclide or CT scanning is available, however, there is little indication for ventriculography, which is a high-risk procedure and conveys no specific diagnostic information beyond confirming the presence of a mass lesion. A pneumoencephalogram (PEG) is dangerous in the setting of a brain abscess and should be avoided.

4. **Arteriography** is relatively poor in localizing brain abscess.

5. **EEG.** Although EEG was once the only test available to localize a brain abscess, it has since been far overshadowed by other, more reliable, tests.

6. **Lumbar puncture** is hazardous when a brain abscess is present, and it should not be done when an abscess or any other intracranial mass lesion is a significant consideration. The CSF rarely discloses the organism responsible for the abscess, and the CSF formula is only of help in ruling out bacterial meningitis. In most cases, the clinical setting is such that an abscess is not confused with bacterial meningitis, but this is not invariably true. Thus, as was discussed in the section on bacterial meningitis, it is at times necessary to take the calculated risk and proceed with lumbar puncture to rule out meningitis.

7. **Skull x-rays.** This procedure is of no value in localizing the abscess. However, all suspected brain abscesses should have complete skull x-rays early in their course to search for a source of parameningeal infection. Adequate views of the mastoids and sinuses are essential, since brain abscess due to sinusitis usually occurs adjacent to the infected sinus, frequently the frontal lobe. Otitic brain abscess frequently occurs in the temporal tip or cerebellar hemisphere.

C. **Pathophysiology.** The current concept of the pathology of brain abscess involves a two-stage process.

1. Initially the infection is established as a cerebritis, with a diffuse and poorly marginated area of infection of the brain parenchyma and associated edema and destruction of brain tissue. During this stage, the infection is radiologically indistinguishable from brain edema of any cause. The ^{99}Tc brain scan should show an area of increased uptake of radionuclide; the CT scan should show a low-density area that would enhance diffusely with IV contrast material; and the arteriogram and ventriculogram may show a mass effect. At this stage, the infection is, in principle, curable with antibiotic therapy alone and is not amenable to surgical therapy.

2. Over a period of days the center of the infection turns into semiliquid pus and necrotic brain tissue. Once this stage is reached, the infection is not curable by medical therapy alone. Gradually the pus becomes encapsulated by gliotic tissue and a free abscess forms.

D. **Treatment**

1. **Surgery.** The traditional treatment of brain abscess is immediate drainage of the abscess cavity, either by needle aspiration or by total excision of the abscess, including the capsule.

   a. Most medical centers now prefer total excision whenever an abscess is accessible surgically, although there are no hard data that demonstrate this method to be superior to aspiration. Aspiration generally has to be repeated one or more times to effect a cure.

   b. As long as the patient is not endangered by increased intracranial pressure, and the abscess has not ruptured into the ventricular system, surgery may be postponed many hours to avoid operating under less than optimum conditions.

2. Medical therapy

   a. Antibiotics. The patient is started on appropriate antibiotics preoperatively. The choice of antibiotic is discussed in **D.4.** At operation, the pus from the abscess should be Gram stained and cultured for aerobic and anaerobic bacteria and for fungi. The results of these studies guide postoperative antibiotic choice.

   Antibiotics are continued for at least 2–3 weeks postoperatively, and the entire course is given parenterally and in "meningeal doses."

   b. Antiedema therapy. Patients in immediate danger of herniation are treated with mannitol 1.0–1.5 gm/kg IV over 20–30 minutes. It is common practice to treat all patients with brain abscess with high-dose steroids in an attempt to minimize brain edema. Generally dexamethasone 16–24 mg/day is given in four to six divided doses preoperatively and for several days postoperatively. If the patient is then stable, the dexamethasone dose is tapered over 1–2 weeks. There is no evidence that steroids either lead to spread of the local infection of brain abscess or that they hinder definitive therapy of the lesion.

3. Cerebritis. There are reported cases of cures of focal bacterial cerebritis with antibiotic and antiedema therapy alone, without surgical intervention. The essential factor seems to be whether or not there is a pocket of frank pus present. If so, the evidence indicates that surgical drainage is necessary.

   a. There are no strict criteria known with which to make the distinction between cerebritis and early abscess, but the following factors favor cerebritis.

   (1) Symptoms appearing early in the course of the illness.

   (2) A CT scan showing a region of diffuse low density with heterogeneous contrast enhancement and without a "donut effect," which is indicative of a central avascular area.

   b. If the patient is not severely ill, has no evidence of increased intracranial pressure, and has radiologic findings consistent with cerebritis without abscess formation, a **trial** of antibiotic and steroid therapy may be undertaken. The patient is monitored carefully and serial radiologic studies are done to follow the evolution of the focal lesion. If evidence of abscess formation appears, immediate surgery is undertaken.

4. Initial selection of antibiotics

   a. The most common sources of brain abscess are:

   (1) Direct spread of infection from a contiguous source.

   (a) Otitis

   (b) Paranasal sinus infection

   (c) Meningitis (rare)

   (d) Orbital cellulitis

   (2) Hematogenous spread.

   (a) Congenital heart disease with a right-to-left shunt or systemic A-V fistula (over the age of 2 years).

      (b) Pulmonary infection.

      (c) Bacteremia from extracranial infections other than pulmonary infections or from procedures.

    (3) Traumatic

      (a) Penetrating head trauma

      (b) Intracranial surgery

  b. Any possible source of the abscess is cultured and a Gram stain is done. As with meningitis, one cannot assume that the abscess is infected with the same organism that is obtained from the presumed source of infection. Moreover, many brain abscesses contain multiple organisms, particularly anaerobes. As a result, the organism, or organisms, recovered from a brain abscess **cannot be predicted from the clinical symptoms** with the degree of precision that is possible with meningitis.

  c. It is not known whether the ability of an antibiotic to penetrate into the CSF is as important in the therapy of brain abscess as it is in the therapy of meningitis. One might expect, however, that in the stage of cerebritis there are organisms in areas of the brain with relatively intact blood-brain barriers; hence drugs that penetrate these barriers are preferred.

  d. For the majority of brain abscesses, the **initial coverage** is broad spectrum. One regimen is **penicillin and chloramphenicol** in the same doses that are administered for meningitis. Situations in which this regimen would not be appropriate include the following:

    (1) The Gram stain or clinical situation suggests that *S. aureus* is a possible organism, in which case **oracillin** is used rather than penicillin.

    (2) The patient is allergic to penicillin, in which case **erythromycin** may be substituted for penicillin if *S. aureus* is not suspected, or **vancomycin,** if it is.

    (3) Traumatic and postsurgical abscesses require as broad a spectrum as feasible, in which case **oxacillin** and **gentamicin** are usually chosen.

    (4) If the patient has a known ear or lung infection with *Pseudomonas,* **carbenicillin** plus **gentamicin** (or **tobramycin,** depending on the sensitivity of the organism) is used.

IV. SUBDURAL EMPYEMA

  A. Making the diagnosis. In adults, subdural empyemas occur most commonly in association with ear or sinus infection, but they may also occur after head trauma or intracranial surgery and in association with meningitis or bacteremia. In children subdural empyema occurs most frequently as a complication of meningitis.

    1. Arteriography is the most reliable means of diagnosing and localizing any subdural fluid collection.

    2. CT scan experience is lacking thus far, but one would expect it to be a highly reliable and noninvasive technique for localizing subdural empyemas. However, until scanning techniques improve, it will probably prove to be somewhat less reliable than arteriography.

    3. In infants the diagnosis can be made by **transillumination** of the skull and **subdural tap.**

    4. Radionuclide brain scanning and **EEG** are of little use.

5. **Ventriculography** may be useful, but arteriography is more reliable and less invasive.

6. **Lumbar puncture** and **pneumoencephalography** are potentially hazardous and are contraindicated when a subdural empyema is suspected.

B. **Treatment**

1. **Surgery. Immediate** surgical drainage is indicated, followed by a course of high-dose antibiotics determined by the results of the Gram stains and cultures performed at surgery.

2. **Antibiotics.** The patient receives one preoperative dose of an antibiotic. The appropriate drug or drugs are chosen according to the clinical situation, obeying the same rules as in choosing antibiotics for a brain abscess.

3. The customary **duration** of postoperative antibiotics is 3 weeks, unless another focus, such as osteomyelitis, is present, which dictates a longer course.

4. **Increased intracranial pressure** may be treated the same way as it is in brain abscess, using mannitol initially and steroids if more than a few hours of therapy are necessary.

V. SPINAL EPIDURAL ABSCESS

A. **Making the diagnosis.** The presence of a spinal epidural abscess is suggested by the onset of severe back pain with local tenderness, followed within a few days by root symptoms and then later by cord compression. In acute cases the patient is febrile and has an elevated peripheral white count. However, the disease may run a chronic course, and the patient may be afebrile with a normal white count on admittance.

1. The most common infecting organisms isolated at the Massachusetts General Hospital in patients with spinal epidural abscess are:

a. *Staphylococcus aureus.*

b. *Staphylococcus pyogenes.*

c. *Streptococcus* species other than *Streptococcus pneumoniae.*

d. *Escherichia coli.*

e. *Pseudomonas aeruginosa.*

f. *Streptococcus pneumoniae.*

g. Mixed anaerobic infections.

2. The important diagnostic tests are:

a. **X-rays of the spine,** with emphasis on the area of maximum pain and tenderness, should be done in all these patients. Often an area of vertebral osteomyelitis is discovered.

b. **A CSF sample** is obtained at myelography in all patients, because there may be an associated meningitis. If the lumbar area is felt to be involved, the sample is obtained by means of a cisternal or lateral cervical puncture to avoid the possibility of introducing organisms into the subarachnoid space with the lumbar puncture needle. When the area of involvement is thoracic, as is often the case, the lumbar puncture is performed by introducing the needle in small increments. After each increment, the stylet is removed and an attempt is made to aspirate pus for Gram stain and culture. If pus is obtained, as much should be aspirated as possible and the needle is withdrawn. The CSF sample should then be obtained by means of cisternal or lateral cervical puncture.

    c. Myelography. As already mentioned, the CSF sample is obtained while the patient is on the myelography table. As long as appropriate precautions have been taken to ensure that the needle has not pierced the abscess itself, myelography should be continued to define the exact extent of the abscess.

    d. Cultures. As in other CNS infections, blood, urine, and any clinically apparent focus of infection are cultured before beginning antibiotics. The most usual associated infection is vertebral osteomyelitis, but a search is made for skin and dental infections as well.

B. Therapy

    1. Surgery. The infection is drained as soon after diagnosis as possible, because an acute spinal epidural abscess can lead to paraplegia within hours. Acute abscesses contain semiliquid pus that can be drained easily. Chronic abscesses are composed of granulation tissue, which can be removed surgically. In either case, appropriate cultures and stains for aerobic and anaerobic bacteria as well as fungi should be performed at the time of surgery. Also, the area should be liberally irrigated with a nonabsorbable antibiotic, such as Bacitracin, after the infection is removed.

    2. Antibiotics. A single dose of an antibiotic may be given preoperatively. The postoperative antibiotic therapy is determined by the results of the stains and cultures done at the time of surgery. The preoperative antibiotic can be **oxacillin** 2 gm IV (40 mg/kg in pediatric patients) or **vancomycin** (in penicillin-allergic patients) 1 gm IV in adults (20 mg/kg in children) unless there is a reason to suspect a gram-negative infection, in which case a dose of **gentamicin** 1 mg/kg IV or IM is given as well. It is notable that anaerobic infections are much less common in spinal epidural abscess than in brain abscess. The antibiotics are continued for 3–4 weeks unless there is evidence of vertebral osteomyelitis, in which case a 6–8 week course is indicated.

    3. Steroids. Although there are no good data supporting the use of steroids in spinal epidural abscess, high-dose steroids may be used in an attempt to minimize spinal cord edema. The doses are the same as for treatment of brain swelling (i.e., dexamethasone (Decadron) 10 mg IV given preoperatively, followed by 4 mg IV, IM, or PO postoperatively). This dose is continued for 7–10 days postoperatively and is then tapered over 10–14 days.

VI. NEUROSYPHILIS

A. Making the diagnosis. The chief goal of the detection and treatment of early syphilis is to prevent disability from tertiary disease, including CNS disease. Neurologic symptoms never appear earlier than the secondary stage, although treponemes presumably reach the CNS at the time of inoculation. Therefore, the main effort in syphilis treatment is devoted to identifying and treating patients in the primary and early secondary stages, before major damage can occur.

    1. In **primary syphilitic chancres,** in **secondary skin lesions,** and, very rarely, in CSF or fluid from the anterior chamber of the eye, treponemes can be identified by **dark-field examination,** giving hard evidence of active infection. Dark-field examination, to be productive, must be done by a person with experience in the technique. If active neurosyphilis is suspected and the facilities are available, fresh CSF is examined for treponemes.

    2. Since *Trepenoma pallidum* cannot be routinely cultured, when the dark-field examination does not yield a diagnosis, one must rely on **serologic tests** to make the diagnosis.

        a. Serologic test for syphilis (STS, nontreponemal tests). The VDRL, Hinton, rapid reagin, Kolmer, and Kahn tests all depend on detecting, in the patient's serum or CSF, antibodies to lipoidal substances in the treponemal cell wall or lipoidal substances resulting from the treponeme-host interaction. These are the most useful tests available.

(1) These tests are inexpensive and can be used in mass screening programs.

(2) They are less sensitive than the treponemal tests in detecting early evidence of infection, but after they become positive, they are the earliest of the serologic tests to revert to negative after treatment. Thus when the titer is obtained, the effectiveness of therapy or the possibility of reinfection can be determined.

(3) In late neurosyphilis, the serum STS may be negative in as many as one-third of cases, so a negative serum STS does not rule out neurosyphilis. The CSF STS may be positive despite a negative peripheral blood serology, but even a negative CSF STS does not absolutely rule out the diagnosis of neurosyphilis.

(4) Biologic false-positive STS tests are common and are associated with old age and rheumatic and inflammatory diseases (e.g., systemic lupus erythematosus and bacterial endocarditis). Therefore a positive STS alone does not confirm the diagnosis of syphilis, but it should lead to the performance of a more specific treponemal test.

b. Treponemal tests

(1) FTA-abs (fluorescent treponemal antibody-absorbed). This test depends on the presence of antibodies that are specific for *T. pallidum.*

(a) It is the most sensitive serologic test routinely available, being the first one to turn positive after infection and the last to revert to negative after therapy. The FTA-abs may remain positive for the remainder of the patient's life, even with adequate therapy, so its titer is not a good test to follow in judging the adequacy of therapy or possible reinfection.

(b) The FTA-abs is much more expensive than the STS, so it should only be done when specifically indicated and not as a routine screening procedure.

(c) A positive FTA-abs at a titer greater than 1:2 rules out a biologic false-positive STS.

(d) 5–10% of patients with late neurosyphilis have a negative FTA-abs, so even this test may not completely rule out neurosyphilis.

(e) There is no need to do a CSF FTA-abs for diagnosis, because all reported cases with a positive CSF FTA-abs have had a positive serum FTA-abs.

(2) TPI (*T. pallidum* inhibition). This test is less sensitive than a FTA-abs and is technically more difficult to perform. It has little usefulness.

B. Asymptomatic neurosyphilis is defined as an abnormal spinal fluid in the absence of neurologic symptoms but in the presence of serologic evidence of syphilis. It can occur as early as the primary stage in rare instances, but its progression to symptomatic neurosyphilis is 100% preventable with adequate therapy.

1. Diagnosis

a. A lumbar puncture is performed in all patients with syphilis beyond the secondary stage (latent syphilis or tertiary syphilis), even in the absence of neurologic signs and symptoms. Moreover, all patients treated for primary or secondary syphilis receive a lumbar puncture if they are possible treatment failures (STS does not become negative or reach a fixed low titer within 2 years after therapy).

b. The fluid is analyzed for cells, protein, colloidal gold curve, and STS. It is necessary to check the CSF STS to make the diagnosis of neurosyphilis, but neither it nor the CSF protein measure the activity of the disease. The cell count is the best indicator of disease activity.

c. It is generally accepted that in primary and secondary syphilis, although asymptomatic, neurosyphilis may rarely occur. A lumbar puncture is not necessary because the therapy would not be affected by the results.

2. Treatment

a. Penicillin, in a total dose of 6–9 million units, is the drug of choice, and it is probably 100% effective in preventing progression to symptomatic disease. There are several possible programs:

(1) Procaine penicillin G, aqueous, 600,000 units IM every day or every other day for 15 doses, **or**

(2) Benzathine penicillin G, 2.4 million units IM weekly for four doses.

b. Alternative therapy for penicillin-allergic patients

(1) Tetracycline, 500 mg PO QID for 20 days, **or**

(2) Erythromycin, 500 mg PO QID for 20 days.

3. Follow-up examination

a. The patient is seen and examined approximately every 3 months for the first year, and the serum STS is checked. If the patient is doing well, yearly examinations are then sufficient. In 12–24 months, the STS should revert to negative or achieve a low stable titer. Lumbar puncture is repeated 1 year after treatment.

b. Indications for retreatment

(1) Failure of the CSF cell count to revert to normal within 6 months.

(2) The CSF protein shows a marked decline by 1 year. If it does not, active disease is not necessarily present, but most syphilologists would re-treat. Some would also re-treat if the CSF STS titer does not decrease by more than one dilution by the end of the first year.

C. Symptomatic neurosyphilis

1. Diagnosis

a. When *T. pallidum* invades the CNS, several types of disease may result:

(1) Meningeal and vascular

(a) Cerebral meningeal: diffuse or focal (gumma)

(b) Cerebral vascular

(c) Spinal meningeal and vascular

(2) Parenchymatous

(a) Tabes dorsalis

(b) General paresis

(c) Optic atrophy

b. The diagnosis must often be based on clinical grounds, because in late neurosyphilis both the peripheral and CSF serology, including the FTA-abs may be negative. The spinal fluid must be abnormal, with white cells and elevated protein, to make the diagnosis. Occasionally, *T. pallidum* can be visualized in the CSF by dark-field examination.

2. Antibiotic therapy

    a. What constitutes adequate therapy of neurosyphilis is not known, since progression may occur despite massive doses of antibiotics.

    b. The United States Public Health Service recommendation is the same as for the treatment of asymptomatic neurosyphilis: 6–9 million units of penicillin. However, there are many reported cases of relapses after this therapy.

    c. There are no clear data that doses of penicillin higher than those recommended by the PHS are in any way superior. In fact, the prognosis of the disease is probably related to its duration rather than to the doses of penicillin used. Nevertheless, for patients with long-standing neurosyphilis, especially parenchymatous disease, and for those who fail to respond to 6–9 million units of penicillin, it is reasonable to attempt to re-treat with a course of high-dose penicillin.

        (1) The patient is hospitalized for the entire course of therapy.

        (2) Aqueous penicillin G 12–24 million units/day IV is given in six divided doses for 10 days.

        (3) In **penicillin-sensitive** patients, alternative regimens include:

            (a) Tetracycline 2–3 gm per day PO in four divided doses for 30 days, **or**

            (b) Erythromycin 500 mg PO QID for 30 days.

        (4) For those patients who fail to respond on the above therapy, a last trial of therapy may be attempted with **chloramphenicol** 1 gm IV every 6 hours for 6 weeks, with bone marrow function followed carefully and the dose adjusted accordingly (see **I.C.2** for guidelines on the use of chloramphenicol).

3. Steroids have no proved effect in the treatment of late neurosyphilis. Prednisone 40 mg daily or its equivalent may decrease the CSF cell count, but there is no evidence that it affects the outcome of therapy or the long-term disability. Steroids are clearly indicated for syphilitic uveitis and syphilitic involvement of the inner ear with a hearing deficit and labyrinthine dysfunction. In these diseases, it is customary to administer prednisone 80 mg every other day.

4. Follow-up

    a. The patient is seen clinically for follow-up every 3 months for the first year. At each visit, the serum STS is checked, and a lumbar puncture is performed every 6 months. If the patient is stable after 1 year, with a normal CSF cell count and a falling or fixed low value of the CSF protein, then yearly return visits are sufficient with a final lumbar puncture 2 years after treatment.

    b. As in asymptomatic neurosyphilis, if the therapy is effective, the CSF cell count is normal within 6 months after treatment. The CSF protein may be elevated for a longer time and may never return to normal, but it should level off at a fixed low level.

    c. The STS may be positive for the life of the patient in both the serum and the CSF. Paradoxically, in patients with a negative CSF STS before therapy, the test may become positive after therapy. In either case, the CSF STS titer is of little help in following the patient, the cell count and clinical course being the essential data on which therapy is based.

5. Complications of neurosyphilis

    a. Communicating hydrocephalus due to blockage of CSF flow at the base of the brain may follow neurosyphilis. Hydrocephalus should always enter the differential diagnosis of general paresis which progresses despite antibiotic therapy. The treatment is a shunt.

b. **Lightning pains** complicating tabes dorsalis have a poor prognosis. Phenytoin (Dilantin) and carbamazepine (Tegretol) may be tried, but they are often of no benefit.

c. Charcot joints

d. Perforating ulcers

e. Gummas

f. Spinal pachymeningitis

D. Congenital neurosyphilis

1. The diagnosis of congenital syphilis is often difficult to make, since the neonate's serum STS, FTA-abs, and even the CSF STS may be positive because of passively transferred maternal antibody in the absence of infection in the child.

   a. The **newborn's IgM FTA-abs** can be tested, and the total IgM in the cord blood can be measured to aid in the diagnosis. Serial titers help in this differential.

   b. **A lumbar puncture** is performed in all neonates at risk of congenital syphilis. Cells in the CSF without another cause must be considered diagnostic of congenital neurosyphilis in the appropriate setting.

2. Congenital syphilis in the neonate with normal CSF is treated with one injection of 50,000 units/kg of **benzathine penicillin G** IM or **aqueous penicillin G** 100,000 units IM every day for 10 days.

3. Congenital syphilis in the presence of an abnormal CSF is treated with one of two regimens:

   a. **Aqueous penicillin G** 25,000 units/kg IM or IV every 12 hours for 10 days, or

   b. **Aqueous penicillin G** 50,000 units/kg IM daily for 10 days.

4. Late forms of congenital neurosyphilis are treated exactly the same as acquired neurosyphilis.

E. Jarisch-Herxheimer reaction

1. The Jarisch-Herxheimer reaction is a febrile response that is believed to be caused by a release of large amounts of treponemal products into the circulation within the first 24 hours of therapy. It is characterized by fever, chills, myalgia, headache, tachycardia, tachypnea, elevated white cell count, and decreased blood pressure. During the reaction, the rash of secondary syphilis, if present, may worsen. It is a frequent occurrence on initiation of antisyphilitic therapy, usually beginning about 2 hours after the first dose of antibiotics, peaking at about 7 hours, and resolving in 24 hours.

2. The standard therapy is hydration and antipyretic therapy. It is important that the Jarisch-Herxheimer reaction not be confused with an allergic reaction to penicillin. Some physicians administer a dose of steroids with the initiation of therapy for secondary or tertiary syphilis in an attempt to abort this reaction.

VII. LEPTOSPIROSIS. *Leptospira interrogans* in man may cause several types of CNS disease: aseptic meningitis, encephalitis, myelitis, and optic neuritis. The CSF profile is typically lymphocytic, with a normal sugar. The CSF protein may be over 100 mg/100 ml on admittance.

A. The diagnosis can be made by culturing the organism from blood, urine, or CSF. Dark-field examination of the urine or CSF by an expert may demonstrate *Leptospira*. There are several serologic tests available. The usual criterion for diagnosis is a fourfold or greater rise in titer between the acute and convalescent sera.

B. If the diagnosis is made within the first 5 days of the illness, antibiotics may be of help. **Penicillin G**, 2.4 million units daily, is the drug of choice. The alternative drug for penicillin-allergic patients has not been defined for CNS disease, but **erythromycin** or **chloramphenicol** are reasonable alternatives.

VIII. FUNGAL INFECTIONS OF THE CNS

A. **Description.** The usual clinical picture is that of chronic meningitis, but intraparenchymal infections may occur with symptoms that resemble bacterial brain abscess.

The exuberant inflammatory response elicited by fungi may lead to obstruction of CSF pathways and hydrocephalus. The vast majority of cases of fungal meningitis in this country are caused by *Cryptococcus neoformans* and *Coccidioides immitis*. *Candida albicans, Aspergillus, Histoplasma capsulatum*, and blastomycetes are rare CNS pathogens, and *Phycomycetes* (mucormycosis) produces a characteristic rhinocerebral infection that can be associated with fungal meningitis. There have been rare case reports of fungal meningitis with other fungi. *Nocardia* and actinomycetes, although not strictly fungi, can infect the CNS and behave clinically like fungal pathogens. Each of these organisms has its distinctive features, but the basic approach to their therapy is similar (Table 8-4).

B. **Amphotericin use**

1. **Clinical usefulness.** Amphotericin B is an effective agent, both in vitro and in vivo, against virtually all known fungi, although resistance to the drug has been reported. Since its introduction in the late 1950s, the prognosis of cryptococcal meningitis has changed from 100% mortality within months to an expectation of recovery in all patients but those with the most advanced infections and those with an underlying fatal illness. However, there are many serious problems with its use:

    a. Almost universal **toxicity** from the drug accompanies its use, ranging from discomforting febrile reactions to renal shutdown. **Side effects of amphotericin B** are as follows:

        (1) **Dose-related effects**

            (a) **Short-term system effects**

                Fever, chills.
                Nausea, vomiting.
                Anorexia, malaise, headache.
                Hypotension.

            (b) **Renal toxicity**

                Impaired glomerular function.
                    Decreased glomerular filtration rate, increased BUN, and increased serum creatinine, with decreased creatinine clearance.

                May progress to oliguric renal failure.

                Impaired tubular function.
                    Distal renal tubular acidosis.
                    Hypokalemia that may be severe.
                    Decreased serum uric acid.

            (c) **Anemia secondary to bone marrow suppression**

Table 8-4. Antifungal Therapy

Organism	Primary Therapy	Optional Adjunctive Therapy	Comments
Cryptococcus	Amphotericin 0.5 mg/kg/day IV 5-Fluorocytosine (5-FC) 150 mg/kg/day PO	Subarachnoid amphotericin B	Each isolate should be tested for 5-FC sensitivity
Coccidioides	Amphotericin B 1.5 mg/kg/day IV Amphotericin B 0.5 mg IT 2 doses/week	Intraventricular amphotericin B	Not sensitive to 5-FC
Candida	Amphotericin B 1.5 mg/kg/day IV	5-FC 150 mg/kg/day PO Subarachnoid amphotericin B	Each isolate should be tested for 5-FC sensitivity
Aspergillus	Amphotericin B 1.5 mg/kg/day IV 5-FC may be tried	5-FC 150 mg/kg/day PO Subarachnoid amphotericin B	Each isolate should be tested for 5-FC sensitivity
Phycomycetes	Amphotericin B 1.5 mg/kg/day IV	Subarachnoid amphotericin B	Not sensitive to 5-FC
Histoplasma	Amphotericin B 1.5 mg/kg/day IV	Subarachnoid amphotericin B	Not sensitive to 5-FC
Blastomyces[a]	Amphotericin B 1.5 mg/kg/day IV	Subarachnoid amphotericin B	Not sensitive to 5-FC

[a]Hydroxystilbamidine, although useful in pulmonary blastomycosis, is not recommended as a first-line drug for CNS blastomycosis.

(d) Local toxicity

Phlebitis with IV administration.

Intralumbar injection: paresthesias, nerve palsies, back pain, paraplegia, chemical meningitis, arachnoiditis, and CSF blocks.

Intracisternal: hydrocephalus.

Intraventricular: ventriculitis, encephalopathy, seizures, and death.

(2) Idiosyncratic effects

(a) Shock.

(b) Thrombocytopenia.

(c) Acute liver failure.

(c) Seizures.

(e) Cardiac arrest, ventricular fibrillation.

Clinically, the most important toxic effects are **renal.** About one-half of patients receiving a total of 4 gm and 85% of those receiving 5 gm of amphotericin B are left with permanent renal insufficiency of clinical significance. Usually the dose of amphotericin administered to a given patient is limited by renal toxicity, often at a dose of 0.5–0.7 mg/kg/day. The other major renal effect in patients taking the drug is hypokalemia, which requires close monitoring of serum potassium and oral potassium replacement as necessary. It is recommended that amphotericin B be used according to a strict protocol (see the guidelines for the use of amphotericin B, sec **VIII.I**).

b. **Prolonged courses of therapy** at potentially toxic doses are necessary to treat fungal meningitis. However, relapse can occur even when the drug is continued until the patient is clinically well and the CSF is normal.

c. **The drug levels** in the CSF associated with IV use are extremely low, possibly accounting for the relapse rate. Injection of the drug directly into the subarachnoid space has been done extensively, in a manner that is analogous to that of using intrathecal or intraventricular amino-glycosides in the treatment of gram-negative meningitis. The problems are similar in the two cases.

(1) **Intralumbar injections** do not deliver high concentrations of drug to the basilar cisterns, the main site of most fungal infections, and virtually no drug enters the ventricles. Furthermore, subarachnoid blocks to CSF flow are frequent in fungal meningitis, complicating the problem of distribution of drug throughout the subarachnoid space.

(2) Amphotericin B has produced a large number of **irritative side effects** when injected into the subarachnoid space. Intrathecal injection frequently gives temporary paresthesias, but progressive arachnoiditis, spinal cord blocks, and transverse myelitis have occurred as well. A single intraventricular injection of 1 mg has produced encephalopathy and death within hours. Repeated intraventricular injection carries with it all the potential complications of Ommaya reservoirs.

d. In spite of adequate fungal killing and eventual cure, the inflammatory reaction set up by the fungus may produce blocks to CSF flow, hydrocephalus, and cranial nerve palsies. There are cases in which the meninges over the convexities have become so thickened they have behaved like bilateral subdural hematomas, causing herniation and death.

2. Systemic use. In spite of all these problems, amphotericin B is the first-line drug in essentially all fungal infections of the CNS. Its detailed use is described in the guidelines for the use of amphotericin B, sec **VIII.I.** Basically, a low dose is given initially and built up to the maximum tolerated daily dose, or to a maximum of 1.5 mg/kg/day (this dose will only be tolerated occasionally). During chronic administration, the renal function is followed closely, and the dose is decreased if the serum creatinine begins to rise above 3.0. In the absence of hard data on the necessary dose of amphotericin, various modifications of this approach have been suggested in an attempt to minimize the toxicity and discomfort associated with the daily administration of amphotericin B at high doses.

  a. Administration of twice the daily dose on an alternate-day basis. The advantage of this program is that fewer total injections are given, so phlebitis is less of a problem, and on the days during which the patient does not receive the drug he is free of fever, anorexia, and other debilitating effects of the drug, creating a better overall medical status.

  b. Determination of the minimal inhibitory concentration (MIC) of the patient's serum against the fungus isolated, and adjustment of the daily dose of amphotericin B to achieve a serum level of amphotericin B that is equal to twice the MIC. This generally results, for *Cryptococcus*, in a dose of 0.5–1.0 mg/kg/day. There are no data, however, that show serum levels of amphotericin correlate with clinical effectiveness.

3. Subarachnoid use

  a. Indications for subarachnoid amphotericin B administration. If a patient fails to respond to systemic therapy or if he has an overwhelming infection, the prognosis is poor. In these cases, the administration of amphotericin into the subarachnoid space has a possibility of being lifesaving.

    (1) When the patient fails to respond to systemic therapy or relapses after a full course of systemic therapy.

    (2) When the patient is moribund at the initiation of therapy.

    (3) When the patient is severely immunosuppressed.

    (4) In coccicioidomycosis with meningeal involvement, most experts would proceed immediately to subarachnoid therapy.

  b. Routes of subarachnoid injection

    (1) Intraventricular. If subarachnoid therapy is used, intraventricular injection of amphotericin B by means of an Ommaya reservoir and indwelling intraventricular cannula comprise the most reliable route of therapy. This is the preferred route at most institutions.

    (2) Intracisternal injections of amphotericin B are used routinely at some centers, but this approach is not recommended unless the injections are done by a person very experienced in the technique.

    (3) Intralumbar. A technique worthy of consideration is to inject the drug (suspended in a solution heavier than CSF, such as 10% dextrose in water) into the lumbar space and then place the patient in the Trendelenburg position for a period of time so the drug can flow by gravity to the basilar cisterns. However, there is no wide experience with this technique.

  c. The techniques of subarachnoid injection of amphotericin B are given in sec **VIII.I.** The patency of CSF pathways from the site of injection to the base of the brain must be demonstrated before initiation of subarachnoid therapy and repeatedly throughout the course of therapy if there is any indication of a block to CSF flow.

C. **Fluorocytosine** (5-FC) is active against *Cryptococcus, Candida, Aspergillus, Torulopsis,* and chlorblastomycosis. However, not all strains of these fungi are sensitive to the drug, and resistance may develop during therapy. Therefore 5-FC sensitivity must be documented in each case in which the drug is used. Since there is less experience with 5-FC than with amphotericin B, its role in the therapy of life-threatening fungal infections is less well-defined. Its **advantages** over amphotericin B are that it can be given PO and it is less toxic. Its **disadvantages** are that it has not been demonstrated to be effective when used alone against life-threatening infections and that organisms may become resistant to it when it is used alone. The following uses can be recommended at this time.

1. In cryptococcal disease, 5-FC and amphotericin B are synergistic in their action, and combination therapy suppresses the appearance of 5-FC resistant organisms. Consequently, it is reasonable to initiate therapy with the combination of amphotericin B and 5-FC and to use amphotericin B at less than the maximum dose (0.5 mg/kg/day). If the patient is moribund at the initiation of therapy, fails to respond to this regimen, or relapses after the therapy has been completed, amphotericin B can be increased to its maximum tolerated dose, in combination with 5-FC, and the addition of subarachnoid therapy can be considered.

2. There is insufficient experience with fungal disease other than cryptococcosis to know whether the combination of 5-FC plus amphotericin B, at a dose of 0.5 mg/kg/day, is as effective as amphotericin B at a maximum dose in treating organisms that are sensitive to 5-FC. In unusually severe infections with sensitive organisms and in moribund patients, 5-FC should certainly be added to full-dose amphotericin B, given both systemically and by a subarachnoid route.

3. After the patient has received a course of amphotericin B or amphotericin B plus 5-FC, 5-FC may be given alone to prolong the course of therapy.

D. **Duration of therapy.** The duration of therapy necessary to cure fungal infections of the CNS is unknown. In many cases the infection is probably never cured in the sense that every organism is not eliminated, and viable organisms remain in the patient for life. There are many cases of cryptococcal meningitis in which the india ink stain remains positive for months after therapy is stopped, but the patient remains clinically well.

1. If the patient responds clinically to the initial therapy, that regimen should be continued:

   a. For at least 6 weeks.

   b. For 1 month after the last positive CSF culture.

   c. Until there is no evidence of active CNS infection:

      (1) A stable or improving neurologic examination; or

      (2) A normal or only mildly elevated, stable CFS cell count.

   d. Until there is no evidence of active systemic infection.

   e. Until amphotericin B toxicity occurs, precluding its further use systemically.

2. **The need for prolonging therapy**

   a. An elevated CSF protein or a positive CSF india ink preparation in cryptococcal disease are not in themselves indications to continue therapy.

b. In cryptococcal disease, help may be obtained from measurements of CSF or serum cryptococcal antigen. Failure of the antigen titer to fall by more than two dilutions during therapy carries a poor prognosis in terms of relapse and should lead to a prolongation of the therapy.

c. Coccidioidal antigens may also be measured in the CSF, but their relation to prognosis has not been as clearly evaluated as it has for cryptococcal antigens.

d. One may give oral 5-FC alone after the course of combination therapy or after amphotericin B alone has been completed. At this point, there is presumably a small number of viable organisms present, so 5-FC resistance is not expected to develop.

e. Some experts recommend the administration of subarachnoid amphotericin B weekly for life in coccidioidomycosis.

f. The subarachnoid injection of amphotericin B may be continued either alone or in combination with oral 5-FC after systemic amphotericin B is stopped because of toxicity.

E. **Use of steroids**

1. **Elevated CSF pressure.** In fungal meningitis, as in other infections of the CNS, high-dose steroids are used for the treatment of elevated CSF pressure due to brain swelling or focal infection of brain parenchyma. Hydrocephalus is ruled out in all such cases, because steroids are of no benefit if this condition is the cause of the elevated intracranial pressure.

2. Pathologically, fungal meningitis, especially coccidioidomycosis, is associated with an impressive granulomatous response at the base of the brain and in the ependyma of the ventricles. This inflammatory response frequently produces blockage of CSF flow with spinal block or hydrocephalus. Some have recommended the use of steroids systemically or by means of subarachnoid injection to inhibit this response.

3. As mentioned under the guidelines for the use of amphotericin B, dexamethasone may be injected into the subarachnoid space along with amphotericin B in an attempt to minimize the local irritative effects of amphotericin B.

F. **Hydrocephalus.** As already mentioned, hydrocephalus is a frequent complication of fungal meningitis. The treatment is either a V-A or V-P shunt if hydrocephalus occurs late, after the CSF is sterile. If the CSF is still infected, either constant ventricular drainage must be used or, if the CSF block is outside the ventricular system and the hydrocephalus is temporarily being tolerated well, definitive treatment is deferred until the CSF can be sterilized.

G. **Intraparenchymal fungal infections of the CNS.** Fungi can invade the parenchyma of the brain and cause an abscess or granuloma formation. Clinically, they have the appearance of a brain abscess in either case. This process may occur with or without an associated meningitis. *Aspergillus* is the organism that most typically causes focal intraparenchymal disease, but any fungus that infects the CNS may cause intraparenchymal infection, including *Cryptococcus, Candida,* and phycomycosis. The prognosis for intraparenchymal disease is worse than that for meningeal involvement alone. The diagnostic approach and treatment is similar to that of bacterial brain abscess, with surgical excision of solitary lesions being indicated. If the etiologic agent is known or strongly suspected preoperatively, antifungal therapy in the maximum tolerated doses should be begun 48 hours preoperatively. There may be no choice but to attempt to treat multiple lesions medically, in which case the dose of amphotericin B is pushed to its absolute maximum, and 5-FC is added if the organism is sensitive.

H. **Actinomycetes and *Nocardia*** are acid-fast organisms with properties that are intermediate between those of bacteria and fungi. When they infect the CNS, it is usually by causing a disease similar to brain abscess. Spinal cord abscess and meningitis may also occur, and actinomycetes may cause an intracranial epidural abscess from contiguous cranial osteomyelitis. Unlike the fungi, however, these organisms respond to antibacterial drugs. Single abscesses may require surgical excision. The drugs of choice are:

1. **Actinomycetes**

   a. **Penicillin G.** 24 million units/day in adults and 200,000 units/kg/day in children in 12 divided doses for 4–6 weeks.

   b. **Erythromycin.** 4 gm/day IV in adults, and 50 mg/kg/day IV in children in four divided doses.

2. *Nocardia*

   a. **Triple sulfa** 75 mg/kg/day in four divided doses.

   b. **Cycloserine** 15 mg/kg/day PO in four divided doses in combination with sulfa for severe disease, moribund patients, multiple intracranial abscess, or failure to respond to sulfa alone.

   c. **Trimethoprim-sulfamethoxazole** (Bactrim, Septra) is a promising, but unproved, therapy.

   d. **Minocycline** is the alternative drug in patients who are allergic to sulfa drugs.

I. **Guidelines for the use of amphotericin B**

1. **Intravenous administration**

   a. **Premedication of the patient**

      (1) Aspirin 60 mg/year of age to a maximum of 600 mg PO or PR or acetaminophen, 60 mg/year of age to maximum of 600 mg PO or PR for fever.

      (2) An antihistamine or phenothiazine as an antiemetic.

         (a) Promethazine HCl (Phenergan) 25–50 mg PO, PR, or IM.

         (b) Prochlorperazine (Compazine) 10 mg PO or IM or 25 mg PR. Prochlorperazine is avoided in infants and small children.

      (3) **Steroids.** The mechanism of steroids in minimizing the side effects of amphotericin B is not known. Hydrocortisone may be given in a dose of 25–50 mg IV before beginning the infusion of amphotericin B or it may be added to the infusion mixture.

      (4) Since one site of renal toxicity of amphotericin B is in the distal tubule of the kidney, the point in the nephron at which the concentration of the drug in the urine would be expected to be the highest, a high urine flow is maintained during the administration of the drug. Adequate hydration should also protect against the hypotension that may occur in some patients during the infusion. Some physicians recommend maintenance of an alkaline urine during therapy by adding 44 mEq of $NaHCO_3$ to each liter of IV fluid or by giving the patient oral sodium citrate solutions.

   b. **Preparation of the solution**

      (1) Each dose is mixed immediately before use. The commercial preparation contains amphotericin B 50 mg per vial.

      (2) 10 ml of sterile water for injection **without bacteriostatic preservative** is added to the dry powder, and the vial is shaken until the

suspension becomes clear. This yields a suspension of amphotericin 5 mg/ml.

(3) The appropriate amount of suspension is then withdrawn from the vial and is added to a bottle of 1000 ml 5% D/W, again **without bacteriostatic preservative,** to be infused into the patient.

(4) Electrolyte solutions, acidic solutions, and solutions with preservatives may not be used, because they may cause precipitation of the antibiotic.

(5) If the patient is oliguric and a smaller volume must be used, the final concentration of amphotericin B should in no circumstance exceed 0.1 mg/ml.

(6) The possible advantages of using a large volume to maintain rapid urine flow have been mentioned.

(7) Heparin 25 mg added to the IV bottle may help to prevent phlebitis at the IV site.

(8) Another maneuver that has been claimed to lessen the incidence of phlebitis is to interrupt the infusion once or twice each hour to run 50 ml 5% D/W into the vein.

c. The infusion mixture is administered through a "scalp vein" needle, if possible, over 4–6 hours. The rate of infusion may be varied according to the severity of the side effects encountered. In some patients, the side effects will be severe, with high fever, chills, nausea, and vomiting, even with slow infusion rates. Rarely is there any alternative but to persist with the infusion. Generally, the side effects tend to diminish after the first few doses but will recur in their initial severity if the course of treatment is interrupted for longer than 1–2 weeks. Since amphotericin B is administered as a colloidal suspension, no filter should be in the IV line.

d. **Initial doses.** When beginning treatment with amphotericin B, it is prudent to start with a very small dose. Then gradually build up to the planned therapeutic dose over 5–10 days to avoid precipitation of any side effects that are so severe as to threaten the life of the patient. It is recommended that the first dose be 1 mg. Then each succeeding dose may be doubled until 16 mg/day is reached, and thereafter the dose can be increased by increments of 10 mg/day each day until the therapeutic dose is attained. If the therapy is interrupted for more than 10 days, it is necessary to repeat this gradual buildup of the dose. If alternate-day doses are planned for the complete course of therapy, administer the initial doses on a daily basis until the full therapeutic dose is attained. Unfortunately, in many cases of CNS fungal infection, it may not be possible to increase the dose slowly. In that case, a 1-mg test dose is given on the first day. If it is tolerated, a therapeutically significant dose (0.2 mg/kg) of antibiotic can be given on the first day of therapy, and then it can be increased by increments of 0.2 mg/kg each day.

e. **Monitoring of drug toxicity.** Renal and bone marrow function are closely observed during therapy. The following tests are performed before initiating therapy and at least twice each week while systemic amphotericin B is being administered.

(1) CBC

(2) Peripheral blood smear or platelet count or both

(3) Reticulocyte count

(4) BUN or creatinine

(5) Serum electrolytes

(6) Bilirubin

(7) SGOT

(8) Alkaline phosphatase

(9) Urinalysis

f. The maximum dose is 1.5 mg/kg/day IV, or 2.0 gm/kg, given on an alternate-day basis. The dose does not have to be adjusted in renal failure.

2. Intrathecal administration

a. Preparation of solution. Mix amphotericin B 50 mg in 200 ml 5% D/W **without preservative** to give a final concentration of 0.25 mg/ml. The solution must be made up immediately before each dose, as possible. Dexamethasone, to give a total dose of 0.5 mg with each dose of amphotericin B, may be added to this suspension as indicated.

b. Premedicate the patient with an antiemetic, and perform a lumbar puncture in the usual manner. With each dose, CSF is removed and the cell count, protein, sugar, and culture are checked to monitor the progress of the therapy. Fungal antigen titers, if available, are checked weekly.

c. The first dose should be 0.025 mg (0.10 ml of the solution as prepared in step 1). A dose is given every other day and is increased slowly by 0.025-mg increments with each dose until a maximum dose of 0.50 mg (2.0 ml) is achieved on the seventh day. At that point, the frequency of administration is decreased to two times per week.

d. Ommaya reservoirs. Inject the dose of drug in a small volume into the reservoir, and then express it into the ventricle gradually over 3–6 hours to duplicate, as much as possible, a slow infusion.

e. Subarachnoid therapy of fungal meningitis is complicated by the frequent development of blocks to CSF flow, which is caused by either the inflammatory response to the fungus or amphotericin B itself. A block may occur in the cervical region, preventing drug injected into the lumbar space from ascending beyond the foramen magnum; or a block may occur at the base of the brain, producing a communicating hydrocephalus, and deny access to the surfaces of the hemispheres. CSF flow may be evaluated by injecting a radioactively labeled colloid and following its movement with repeated imaging of the neuraxis (cisternography). This study is performed before initiating subarachnoid therapy with amphotericin B, and the patency of the CSF pathway is checked at any indication of a developing block (very high CSF protein, hydrocephalus, rising CSF pressure, or mental deterioration).

J. Guidelines for the use of 5-FC. 5-FC is well absorbed when taken PO, and CSF concentration reaches 80–100% that of serum.

1. Dose

a. 100–150 mg/kg/day in four divided doses at 6-hour intervals.

b. In renal failure, the frequency of doses must be reduced as follows:

Cl_{cr}	Interval between doses of 25–40 mg/kg
100	6
40–25	12
25–12	24
12	48

2. The sensitivity of the organism being treated must be checked at the initiation of therapy and at least monthly thereafter.

3. Toxicity

a. Gastrointestinal upset, with anorexia, nausea, vomiting, and diarrhea, is the most frequent untoward effect.

b. Elevation of SGOT and alkaline phosphastase may occur, possibly in association with hepatic necroses. Liver function should, therefore, be checked weekly during therapy.

c. Anemia, leukopenia, or thrombocytopenia may occur. These reactions are dose-dependent and occur primarily in azotemic patients. Because of the renal toxicity of amphotericin B, the combination of 5-FC and amphotericin B is especially likely to lead to bone marrow dysfunction. Blood counts are checked at least twice weekly in all patients during therapy with 5-FC.

IX. VIRAL MENINGITIS

A. Description. Viruses often infect the subarachnoid space and leptomeninges, with little or no parenchymal involvement of the CNS. The clinical syndrome produced is that of an acute febrile illness, with headache, meningismus, and often vomiting. The neurologic signs are sparse. There may be lethargy, irritability, mild drowsiness, isolated transient cranial nerve dysfunction, or minor reflex changes. Seizures, aside from febrile convulsions, or any severe and persistent neurologic deficit implies an encephalitis component to the illness. Also, there may be associated findings of systemic viral infection, and these may help to identify the etiologic agent.

The total duration of the illness is 10–14 days, and the course is benign, without significant sequelae in over 90% of cases. There is no relation between the identity of the etiologic agent and the severity of the infection. About 10% of cases require prolonged convalescence, and rare cases have a permanent residual deficit, usually spasticity or intellectual changes. Death from aseptic meningitis is exceedingly rare. A careful history may reveal evidence of concurrent viral illness in family members or other contacts of the patient.

B. Etiology. The most common single cause is mumps, but the enteroviruses, primarily coxsackie B and ECHO, comprise the most common viral group that infects the meninges. Next in order of frequency are lymphocytic choriomeningitis (LCM), herpes simplex, and arthropod-borne viruses. Leptospirosis is an unusual cause of the syndrome in the United States, and *Mycoplasma* is a very rare cause. All other agents account for less than 1% of cases of aseptic meningitis in the United States.

C. Diagnosis. The most important clinical problem in aseptic meningitis is to verify that the CSF is indeed aseptic; i.e., no bacterial, mycobacterial, or fungal agent is causing the infection. (*Leptospira* and mycoplasmas, although bacteria, are included in the causes of aseptic meningitis, since they do not grow on the usual culture media, and they cause a benign neurologic disease that is indistinguishable from viral illness.) The CSF profile is lymphocytic, with normal glucose, but very early in the course the CSF may have a purulent profile. A repeat lumbar puncture 8–24 hours after the first will show a shift to lymphocytic predominance in these cases. Identification of the specific infecting organism is useful in confirming the diagnosis and for epidemiologic purposes, but it has no therapeutic importance.

D. Treatment consists of supportive measures. There is no known specific therapy.

E. Complications

1. Hydrocephalus. In spite of the generally benign cause of aseptic meningitis, there are reported cases of noncommunicating hydrocephalus, due to aqueductal stenosis, that occur following mumps meningitis. Mumps and possibly other viruses cause an ependymitis throughout the ventricular system. The resultant chronic scarring leads to aqueductal stenosis as a late complication of the original infection, in which case shunting is required.

2. **Residual neurologic deficits** occur rarely.

X. VIRAL ENCEPHALITIS

A. Description. Viral encephalitis, like aseptic meningitis, is usually an acute febrile illness. It is often associated with meningismus and a lymphocytic normal glucose profile in the CSF. However, there is also evidence of parenchymal involvement of the CNS, with seizures or focal neurologic signs. Depressed mental status is the rule and coma may occur. Rarely, the CSF may contain no, or only a few, white blood cells. The disease is more prolonged than aseptic meningitis, lasting 2 weeks to several months. There is significant mortality during the acute illness (about 10% for all cases of clinically recognized viral encephalitis), and there is a high incidence of permanent disabling sequelae.

B. Etiology. The most frequent etiologic agents identified in this disease are mumps, lymphocytic choreomeningitis (LCM), herpes simplex, and arboviruses. Enteroviruses, in contrast with aseptic meningitis, are unusual causes of encephalitis. The prognosis depends on the etiologic agent.

1. Herpes simplex has been reported to have a 10–40% mortality with a corresponding high incidence of sequelae. Herpes characteristically produces destructive lesions of the inferior frontal and anterior temporal lobes, so dementia, personality disorders, memory loss, and aphasia are frequent sequelae of herpes encephalitis.

2. The arboviruses have a variable prognosis.

   a. Eastern equine encephalitis is the most severe, with a 70–90% incidence of death or disabling sequelae.

   b. The mortality from western equine encephalitis and St. Louis encephalitis is less than 10%, and the disease is usually benign, although it may be severe in younger children.

   c. California and Venezuelan equine encephalitis generally cause benign infections; death and disability are unusual.

3. Encephalitis caused by mumps or LCM virus is benign except in rare instances.

4. Neonatal viral encephalitis may occur and has a poor prognosis. Neonatal encephalitis due to herpes type 2 is usually a fulminant, generalized, and rapidly fatal disease.

C. Treatment. Therapy for viral encephalitis is limited to therapy for cerebral edema and general supportive measures.

1. **Edema.** In viral encephalitis the CSF pressure may be very high, and focal areas of infection with edema or hemorrhage may act as a mass lesion. Herniation may occur. Osmotic agents may be used in acute situations, and high-dose steroids may be used over the longer run. There is experimental evidence that steroids can potentiate the spread of herpes in nervous tissue, so steroids should not be used in viral encephalitis without definite indications.

2. **Seizures** resulting from viral encephalitis may be extremely difficult to control, but their treatment is identical to that of seizures of other etiologies (Chap. 6).

3. **Complications** of coma must be prevented, if possible, but treated as they occur.

4. **Experimental chemotherapy** of herpes simplex encephalitis with adenine

arabinoside (Ara-A) is currently being employed at several centers as part of a controlled study.

D. Prognosis. An overall prognosis can be stated for encephalitis due to each of the common agents, but in any individual case there are no known rules to guide the physician in arriving at a prognosis. It is not uncommon for patients, at some point in the course of their illness, to be comatose, yet to make a full recovery. Some cases have been astounding in the degree of recovery achieved after a severe illness. Therefore this is a disease in which aggressive supportive care is indicated, even though the patient, at a given point in the disease, may be severely affected.

XI. RABIES

A. Description. Rabies is a form of viral encephalitis. It is characterized by its mode of transmission to humans by means of animal bites and by severe brainstem encephalitis, with resultant high mortality. The usual incubation period in man is 3–60 days for bites on the extremities, but periods as long as 6 months have been reported. Bites on the face and neck can have an incubation period as short as 2 weeks.

The clinical disease usually begins with personality change and a period of excitement. Then focal neurologic signs, especially those referable to the brainstem, develop. The characteristic hydrophobia is caused by dysphagia and probably hyperirritability of the respiratory tract and pharynx. Death results from respiratory failure or cardiac arrhythmia; the latter is associated with myocarditis in some cases. In rare cases, the clinical syndrome may begin with ascending paralysis of the Guillain-Barré type. The disease is fatal during the acute stage in over 95% of cases, but with intensive respiratory support and nursing care, complete recovery has been reported.

B. Postexposure prophylaxis

1. **Local wound therapy.** All animal bites that break the skin are debrided and scrubbed with generous quantities of soap and water as soon after the bite as possible. The wound is then rinsed with ethyl alcohol and washed with a quaternary ammonium antiseptic in high concentration (1% Zephiran or 1% Cetavlon). Before coming to the hospital, patients may be instructed to wash the wound at home and flush it with alcohol (in any form available; 86 or higher proof whiskey can be used, if necessary). The wound is not sutured primarily. Local anesthesia may be used if the extensive cleansing measures are painful.

2. **Active immunization.** Formerly, a nervous tissue–derived vaccine was used in the prevention of rabies, but postimmunization encephalomyelitis was a frequent and dreaded complication. Presently, duck embryo vaccine (DEV) is available and carries a much lower risk of allergic encephalitis. It is therefore the preferred agent.

   The usual course of therapy consists of 14 daily subcutaneous injections of 1 ml of the vaccine in adults (0.5 ml in children under 3 years of age). Booster doses of 1 ml are then given 10 and 20 days following completion of the initial series. Mild local and systemic reactions to duck embryo vaccine are frequent, but systemic anaphylaxis is rare. In severe exposures, some would extend the initial course of injections to 21 days.

3. **Passive immunization.** Horse antirabies antiserum is administered in a total dose of 40 units/kg as soon after exposure as possible. Half the antiserum is given IM and half is used to infiltrate the area of the wound. The injection of horse serum is accompanied by a risk of allergic reactions, including anaphylaxis and serum sickness.

4. Patients receiving the combination of active and passive immunization and those receiving steroids may fail to develop adequate serum antibody responses to duck embryo vaccine. Moreover, about 10% of patients receiving

duck embryo vaccine alone do not develop protective titers of antirabies antibodies. Therefore **serum antirabies antibody titers** are measured in all patients receiving postexposure prophylaxis 30–40 days after the initiation of therapy.

5. **When to treat.** The major clinical problem in dealing with rabies is deciding who should be treated with these measures when the bite is from an animal that is not definitely rabid. Several types of observations are important in making this decision (Table 8-5).

   a. **The severity of the wound.** If the skin is not broken, immunotherapy is not necessary. Deep puncture wounds and wounds around the face and neck pose the greatest risk, while lacerations and abrasions of the extremities are of intermediate concern.

   b. **Geography.** Many areas of the country have had no reported cases of rabies in many years. Thus the physician should consult local health authorities to be advised on the prevalence of rabies in his or her area.

   c. **The species of animal.** Most reported rabies in mammals of the United States is from skunks, foxes, and raccoons. Domestic animals are a minor source of infection in this country. Bats pose a special problem in that they can harbor rabies virus in their saliva for many months without developing the disease. Furthermore, rabies may be transmitted in caves from bats to humans by means of aerosol contamination.

   d. **Status of the animal at the time of the attack and circumstances of the attack.** A wild animal that bites a human in an unprovoked attack must be assumed to be rabid if it is a member of a species known to carry rabies in that area. If the animal can be recovered, immunization may be deferred so the animal's brain can be examined pathologically and immunologically if the exposure is not severe. Domestic animals can be assumed to be nonrabid unless they exhibit clear signs of rabies or a recent "personality change," but they should be impounded and observed for 7–10 days for the development of signs of rabies. The vaccination status of the animal and whether the bite was at all provoked are also important considerations.

C. **Preexposure prophylaxis.** Persons who are constantly exposed to animals (e.g., veterinarians, animal handlers, and spelunkers) should receive preexposure immunization with duck embryo vaccine in 1-ml subcutaneous doses. Only three doses are given; the first two are administered 1 month apart, followed by a booster dose at 7 months. The presence of serum antirabies antibody should be documented and a further dose of vaccine is administered if necessary. Individuals who have had a course of rabies immunization, and who have had serum antirabies antibody documented, require only one to five inoculations of vaccine if postexposure immunization is required at a later time.

XII. **POLIOMYELITIS.** A special form of viral infection of the CNS is caused by enteroviruses, with a special predilection to damage of the anterior horn cells of the spinal cord. The clinical picture is one of an acute febrile illness with lower motor neuron paralysis. Fortunately, immunization has made this a rare disease, although cases continue to be reported sporadically, either secondary to poliovirus in unimmunized individuals or as atypical cases secondary to other enteroviruses. The treatment is purely supportive.

XIII. **"SLOW VIRUSES" AND PROGRESSIVE MULTIFOCAL LEUKOENCEPHALOPATHY**

A. **Creutzfeldt-Jakob disease and kuru** are transmissible diseases, but the agent has not been characterized. Creutzfeldt-Jakob disease is seen in this country. It is a subacutely progressive dementia, usually beginning in middle age and progressing relentlessly to coma and death. Ataxia and myoclonus are striking fea-

Table 8-5. WHO Recommendation for Postexposure Treatment of Rabies

Nature of Exposure	Status of Biting Animal (Whether Vaccinated or Not)		Recommended Treatment
	At Time of Exposure	During Observation Period of 10 Days	
I. No lesions; indirect contact	Rabid	—	None
II. Licks:			
(1) Unabraded skin	Rabid	—	None
(2) Abraded skin; scratches and unabraded or abraded mucosa	(a) Healthy	Clinical signs of rabies or proved rabid (laboratory)	Start vaccine at signs of rabies in the biting animal
	(b) Signs suggestive of rabies	Healthy	Start vaccine immediately; stop treatment if animal is normal on the fifth day after exposure
	(c) Rabid, escaped, killed, or unknown	—	Start vaccine immediately
III. Bites	(a) Healthy	Clinical signs of rabies or proved rabid (laboratory)	Start vaccine at first signs of rabies in the biting animal
	(b) Signs suggestive of rabies	Healthy	Start vaccine immediately; stop treatment if animal is normal on the fifth day after exposure
	(c) Rabid, escaped, killed, or unknown	—	Start vaccine immediately
	(d) Wild (wolf, fox, bat, etc.)	—	Serum immediately, followed by a course of vaccine

Severity of exposure	Status of biting animal at time of exposure	Status during observation period	Recommended treatment
(2) Severe exposure (multiple; or face, head, finger, or neck bites)	(a) Healthy	Clinical signs of rabies or proved rabid (laboratory)	Serum immediately; start vaccine at first sign of rabies in the biting animal
	(b) Signs suggestive of rabies	Healthy	Serum immediately, followed by vaccine; vaccine may be stopped if animal is normal on the fifth day after exposure
	(c) Rabid, escaped, killed, or unknown		Serum immediately, followed by vaccine
	(d) Wild (wolf, jackal, pariah dog, fox, bat, etc.)		

tures clinically. The CSF is normal but the EEG is distinctive. There is no known specific therapy (see Chap. 3).

B. **Subacute sclerosing panencephalitis** (SSPE) is a syndrome that occurs in childhood, is almost always the result of measles infection, but is rarely caused by rubella. The first symptoms are personality change and intellectual deterioration, followed by the development of myoclonus seizures, ataxia, and visual impairment. There are reports of spontaneous remissions, but often only after permanent damage has occurred to the brain. Usually, the disease progresses to death in a matter of months or a few years. The CSF may contain a few lymphocytes, but, most importantly, it contains an elevated gamma globulin and elevated titers of measles antibodies. There is no known specific therapy.

C. **Progressive multifocal leukoencephalopathy** (PML) can be caused by either the SV40-PML virus or the JC virus, both of which are papovaviruses. The disease begins with subacutely progressing multifocal white-matter deficits, with normal CSF, generally causing death within months, although occasionally it stabilizes spontaneously. There is a dramatic correlation with disorders of immunity, especially Hodgkin's disease and other lymphomas. There is no known specific therapy.

XIV. TOXOPLASMOSIS

A. **Description.** *Toxoplasma gondii* is an intracellular parasite that infects man and animals. It usually infects totally asymptomatically, but it can cause several varieties of disease.

1. **Congenital toxoplasmosis** classically causes a specific syndrome of choreoretinitis, retardation, and intracranial calcifications, often associated with microcephaly, hepatosplenomegaly with jaundice, and rash or purpura. Any of the components of the syndrome may be missing in any given case.

2. **Acquired toxoplasmosis** usually occurs in a host with defective cellular immunity and may occur as a CNS disease with encephalitis, meningitis, or an intracerebral mass lesion. Myositis has been reported. Diagnosis requires identification of the organisms in a tissue biopsy (either brain, meninges, or lymph node) and has seldom been made with the patient alive.

B. **Treatment.** Prompt treatment of the acquired disease may result in a cure, but the congenital disease is only treated in an attempt to prevent progression of the disease; the CNS damage that is present at birth is irreversible. There is a high spontaneous remission rate of acquired toxoplasmosis, but active CNS disease with an abnormal CSF is indication for treatment. The recommended therapy is:

1. **Sulfadiazine.** 100 mg/kg/day in combination with **pyrimethamine** 1 mg/kg/day, both given in divided doses.

2. **Folinic acid** (Leukovorin). 1 mg/day may be given to counteract the bone marrow depressant effects of pyrimethamine. Trimethoprim, a folate antagonist similar to pyrimethamine, cannot be used in place of pyrimethamine, because it has no activity against toxoplasmosis.

XV. AMEBIC MENINGOENCEPHALITIS. *Naegleria,* a free-living ameba commonly present in warm, fresh water, can cause an acute meningoencephalitis with purulent CSF and hemorrhagic brain lesions. The organisms can be identified as mobile, large organisms on a wet preparation of fresh CSF. In one reported case, amphotericin B was of possible benefit, but there is no known generally effective therapy. All forms of antibiotic therapy, including metronidozole (Flagyl), sulfamethoxazole and trimethoprim (Bactrim), and assorted antibacterial agents, have been tried in vain. The disease is universally fatal.

XVI. HERPES ZOSTER (shingles) is caused by reactivation of latent varicella-zoster virus. Although the infection may be generalized, the brunt of the clinical syndrome

is due to the predilection of the virus for the dorsal root ganglia and cranial nerve ganglia. The virus migrates both antegrade and retrograde in the axons to reach the skin and dorsal horn of the spinal cord, respectively. The virus can be recovered from the vesicles that appear on the skin. Most cases (about 50%) involve the thoracic dermatomes, with pains and parasthesias often preceding the vesicular eruption. Some cases involve the lumbo-sacral and cervical dermatomes while a small number (about 15%) affect cranial nerve ganglia, most often the gasserian and geniculate. When the geniculate ganglion is involved, there is an ipsilateral lower motor neuron–type facial palsy and vesicles are seen in the external auditory canal or on the tympanic membrane (the Ramsay-Hunt syndrome).

There is no specific treatment for the viral infection. Patients with symptomatic herpes zoster infection have an increased incidence of immune deficiency states, particularly lymphomas, and these should be sought using a careful physical examination and complete blood count in every such patient. Steroids should be avoided in the acute period and should be decreased or stopped if their use preceded the infection. Treatment of pain may be difficult, especially if the pain and parasthesias persist long after the vesicles have disappeared (postherpetic neuralgia). Guidelines for the treatment of chronic pain outlined in Chapter 9 apply here. Use of narcotics should be avoided if possible. Carbamazepine or imipramine may be of particular value in these patients.

SELECTED READINGS

General
Hoeprich, P. D. (ed.) *Infectious Diseases.* Hagerstown, Md.: Harper and Row, 1972.
Petito, F., and Plum, F. The lumbar puncture. *N. Engl. J. Med.* 290:225, 1974.
Thompson, R. A., and Green, J. R. (eds.) Infectious diseases of the central nervous system, in *Advances in Neurology,* Vol. 16. New York: Raven, 1974.

Bacterial Meningitis
Carpenter, R. R., and Petersdorf, R. G. The clinical spectrum of bacterial meningitis. *Am. J. Med.* 33:262, 1962.
Hyslop, M. E., Jr., and Swartz, M. N. Bacterial meningitis, *Postgrad. Med.* 58:120, 1975.
Kaiser, A. B., and McGee, Z. A. Aminoglycoside therapy of gram-negative bacillary meningitis. *N. Engl. J. Med.* 293:1215, 1975.
Overall, J. G., Jr. Neonatal bacterial meningitis. *J. Pediatr.* 76:449, 1970.
Schoenbaum, S. C., et al. Infections of cerebrospinal fluid shunts: Epidemiology, clinical manifestations and therapy. *J. Infect. Dis.* 131:543, 1975.
Swartz, M. N., and Didge, P. R. Bacterial meningitis—A review of selected aspects. *N. Engl. J. Med.* 272:725, 779, 842, 898, 954, 1003, 1965.

Tuberculous Meningitis
American Thoracic Society Preventive therapy of tuberculous infection. *Am. Rev. Respir. Dis.* 110:371, 1974.
Escobar, J. A., et al. Mortality from tuberculous meningitis reduced by steroid therapy. *Pediatrics* 56:1050, 1975.
Johnson, R. F., and Wildrick, K. H. State of the art review: The impact of chemotherapy on the care of patients with tuberculosis. *Am. Rev. Respir. Dis.* 109:636, 1974.
O'Toole, R. D., et al. Dexamethasone in tuberculous meningitis. *Ann. Intern. Med.* 70:39, 1969.

Brain Abscess
Brewer, N. S., et al. Brain abscess: A review of recent experience. *Ann. Intern. Med.* 82:571, 1975.
Crocker, E. T., et al. Technetium brain scanning in the diagnosis and management of cerebral abscess. *Am. J. Med.* 56:192, 1974.
Heineman, H. S., and Braude, A. I. Anaerobic infection of the brain. *Am. J. Med.* 35:682, 1963.
Heineman, H. S., et al. Intracranial suppurative disease: Early presumptive diagnosis and successful treatment without surgery. *J.A.M.A.* 218:1542, 1971.

Subdural Empyema
Coonrod, J. D., and Dans, P. E.   Subdural empyema. *Am. J. Med.* 53:85, 1972.
Kaufman, D. M., et al.   Subdural empyema: Analysis of 17 recent cases and review of the literature. *Medicine* 54:485, 1975.

Spinal Epidural Abscess
Baker, A. S., et al.   Spinal epidural abscess. *N. Engl. J. Med.* 293:463, 1975.

Neurosyphilis
Center for Disease Control.   Syphilis recommended treatment schedules, 1976. *Ann. Intern. Med.* 85:94, 1976.
Sparling, P. F.   Diagnosis and treatment of syphilis, *N. Engl. J. Med.* 284:642, 1971.
Hooshmand, H., et al.   Neurosyphilis: A Study of 241 patients. *J.A.M.A.* 219:726, 1972.
Wilner, E., and Brody, J. A.   Prognosis of general paresis after treatment. *Lancet* 2:1370, 1968.
Yoder, F. W.   Penicillin treatment of neurosyphilis. *J.A.M.A.* 232:270, 1975.

Fungal Diseases
Alazraki, N. P., et al.   Use of a hyperbaric solution for administration of intrathecal amphotericin B. *N. Engl. J. Med.* 290:641, 1974.
Bennett, J. E.   Chemotherapy of systemic mycoses. *N. Engl. J. Med.* 290:30, 1974.
Block, J. T.   Cerebral candidiasis: Case report of brain abscess secondary to *Candida albicans,* and review of the literature. *J. Neurol. Neurosurg. Psychiatry* 33:864, 1970.
Burgess, J. L., and Birchall, R.   Nephrotoxicity of amphotericin B, with emphasis on changes in tubular function. *Am. J. Med.* 53:77, 1972.
Chernik, N. L., et al.   Central nervous system infections in patients with cancer. *Medicine* 52:563, 1973.
Diamond, R. D., and Bennett, J. E.   Prognostic factors in cryptococcal meningitis. *Ann. Intern. Med.* 80:176, 1974.
Lewis, J. L., and Rabinorich, S.   The wide spectrum of cryptococcal infections. *Am. J. Med.* 53:315, 1972.
Littman, M. L., et al.   Coccidioidomycosis and its treatment with amphotericin B. *Am. J. Med.* 39:568, 1958.
Ratchesan, R. S., and Ommaya, A. K.   Experience with the subcutaneous cerebrospinal fluid reservoir. *N. Engl. J. Med.* 279:1025, 1968.
Rieschbrech, R. E., et al.   Subarachnoid distribution of drugs after lumbar injection. *N. Engl. J. Med.* 267:1273, 1962.

Rabies
Christie, A. B.   *Infectious Diseases—Epidemiology and Clinical Practice.* New York: Livingstone, 1974. Pp. 816–841.
Corey, L., et al.   Serum neutralizing antibody after rabies postexposure prophylaxis. *Ann. Intern. Med.* 85:170, 1976.
Plotkin, S. A., and Clark, H. F.   Prevention of rabies in man. *J. Infect. Dis.* 123:227, 1971.

Toxoplasmosis
Feldman, H. A.   Toxoplasmosis. *N. Engl. J. Med.* 279:1370, 1431, 1968.
Ruskin, J., and Remington, J. S.   Toxoplasmosis in the compromised host. *Ann. Intern. Med.* 84:193, 1976.

Amebic Meningoencephalitis
Duma, R. J., et al.   Primary amoebic meningoencephalitis. *N. Engl. J. Med.* 281:1316, 1969.

Herpes Zoster
Weller, T. H.   Varicella-herpes Zoster Virus. In F. L. Horsfall and I. Tamm (Eds.) *Viral and Rickettsial Diseases of Man.* Philadelphia: Lippincott, 1965. Pp. 915–925.

9
Neuropsychiatric Disorders

I. DEPRESSION

A. Depression is encountered in neurologic practice primarily under the following circumstances:

1. **Depression as a reaction to neurologic disability.** Reactive depressions (grief reactions) complicate many neurologic illnesses, especially when there is a significant loss of neurologic function. Some patients become depressed early in the course of neurologic illness as a result of fear of future disability. Others become depressed only as their disability increases.

2. **Depression manifested as neurologic complaints.** A variety of somatic complaints, including dizziness, headache, backache, memory loss, facial pain, and diffuse weakness, may reflect an underlying depressive illness, while simulating a neurologic disorder. These somatic complaints may remit with treatment of the depression.

3. **Depression as a reflection of CNS dysfunction.** Both anatomic lesions and metabolic derangements within the brain can produce symptoms that closely mimic depression.

B. The manifestations of depression. The behavior of the depressed patient is a combination of altered affect (mood) and disordered somatic (vegetative) function. Common manifestations of depression are as follows:

Affective	Somatic
Sadness	Fatigue
Tearfulness	Weakness
Despair	Anorexia
Pessimism	Insomnia
Anhedonia (loss of pleasure)	Headache
Suicidal ideation	Dizziness
Loss of mirth	Constipation
Sense of worthlessness	Loss of libido

Patients who exhibit both affective and somatic signs pose no difficulty in diagnosis. However, when somatic complaints overshadow alterations in mood, depression can be easily confused with neurologic disease.

C. Classification and treatment of the depressive syndromes. Numerous schemes for classifying depressive illnesses have been proposed, testifying to the fact that no one is completely satisfactory. One system is shown in Figure 9-1.

1. **Reactive depressions** (grief reactions) are often appropriate responses to serious losses. Patients with neurologic disease may face loss of bladder and bowel control, sexual dysfunction, progressive paralysis, intellectual decline, and impending loss of life. Grief reactions can be effectively managed by supportive psychotherapy aimed at permitting the patient to grieve over his losses, while emphasizing the hopeful aspects of the illness. Thus therapy, whether it is specific or symptomatic, is essential to foster a positive attitude in the patient. The correction of any misconceptions the patient may have about the nature of his or her illness is also helpful. Antidepressant medications are generally of limited benefit.

2. **Primary (endogenous) depressions** occur without relation to other illnesses (either medical or psychiatric) and are out of proportion to life events (losses).

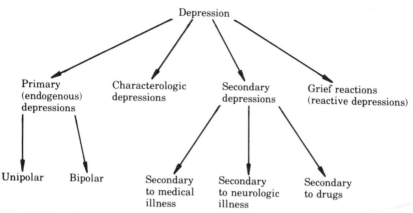

Fig. 9-1. Classification of depressive illnesses.

Primary depressions may be either unipolar (depressive episodes only) or bipolar (manic and depressive episodes).

a. Tricyclic antidepressants

(1) In uncomplicated **primary depressions,** the drug of first choice is one of the tricyclic antidepressants. In cases of severe depression or when suicidal ideation is prominent, immediate psychiatric referral is indicated.

(2) The tricyclic antidepressants have three major actions: antidepressant, sedative, and anticholinergic. The antidepressant action of these drugs appears to be related to their ability to block the reuptake of norepinephrine and serotonin at the neural synapse.

(3) Six tricyclic antidepressants are currently available in the United States (Table 9-1). Their effectiveness is similar, although protriptyline is considered to be less sedating than the others, and doxepin is alleged to have greater antianxiety properties.

(4) To **minimize side effects,** it is best to begin therapy at low dosages, usually imipramine or amitriptyline 25–50 mg at bedtime. Several days later an additional 25–50 mg can be added in the morning, and the dose can then be gradually increased to 150 mg daily. Some patients require higher dosages for relief of depression (up to 300 mg daily). Also, changing the administration to a **single bedtime dose** increases patient compliance and helps to correct sleep disturbances. The tricyclics often take 3–4 weeks to become fully effective.

(5) **Side effects** are numerous and are occasionally troublesome to the patient. Drowsiness, fatigue, and excessive sedation usually diminish as tolerance to the drug increases. However, some patients develop psychosis, hallucinations, and severe anxiety, which necessitates the discontinuance of medication.

Cardiovascular side effects (hypotension and tachycardia) occur in some patients, and these drugs are not prescribed immediately after a myocardial infarction or in the presence of severe coronary artery disease. Also, a variety of anticholinergic side effects may occur, including dry mouth, urinary retention, aggravation of glaucoma, and

Table 9-1. Tricyclic Antidepressants

Drug	Maximum Total Daily Dosage (mg)
Imipramine (Tofranil)	150–300
Amitriptyline (Elavil)	150–300
Doxepin (Sinequan)	150–300
Desipramine (Norpramin)	150–200
Nortriptyline (Aventyl)	75–100
Protriptyline (Vivactil)	40– 60

constipation; and sweating, tremor, and weight gain are common, while seizures are rare.

(6) Drug overdosage is a serious danger in depressed suicidal patients. Fatal overdoses are unlikely when these patients are limited to a week's supply of a tricyclic antidepressant at a time (about 1000 mg), but doses as little as 2500 mg may cause death.

Patients who are still alert after an overdose may be treated with emetics, and obtunded or comatose patients should receive endotracheal intubation before undergoing gastric lavage. Also, cardiac monitoring is desirable in most of these patients.

Massive overdoses may produce seizures, hypotension, and cardiac arrhythmias. CNS depression and cardiac toxicity may be reversed rapidly by IV administration of physostigmine 1–2 mg, repeated as necessary, and seizures can be treated with conventional anticonvulsants. Hemodialysis and peritoneal dialysis are not of benefit.

b. **Major tranquilizers.** When primary depression is complicated by **psychosis** (delusions, paranoia) or **agitation,** therapy is usually initiated with a major tranquilizer (either a phenothiazine or a butyrophenone). Tricyclic antidepressants can be added later, if necessary.

c. **Monoamine oxidase inhibitors** are less effective than the tricyclic antidepressants, and their use is associated with more serious side effects.

d. **Stimulant drugs** (amphetamines, methylphenidate) are not ordinarily used in the treatment of primary depression. However, patients who develop depressive symptoms while taking sedating anticonvulsant medications (primidone, phenobarbital) may improve on small doses of dextroamphetamine (5–15 mg each morning).

e. **Lithium carbonate.** Patients with **bipolar depressions** should be under the care of a psychiatrist. Lithium prophylaxis is often of benefit.

3. **Characterologic depressions** are lifelong illnesses marked by unremitting unhappiness. These patients may become quite vocal in expressing their complaints and their dissatisfaction with the medical profession's inability to do anything to help them. However, they generally defy satisfactory management.

Hypochondriacal and characterologically depressed patients respond poorly to antidepressant medications. Not only do their depressions persist unabated, but drug side effects often lead to new complaints.

4. **Secondary depression.** Finally, depression may be a secondary manifestation of medical illness (myxedema, Cushing's disease, hyperparathyroidism, or viral illness), neurologic disease (stroke, brain tumor, multiple sclerosis, or

parkinsonism), or drug therapy (reserpine, α-methyldopa, propranolol, barbiturates, or benzodiazepine tranquilizers).

II. HYSTERIA

A. **Definition.** There is some unfortunate confusion over the use of the word **hysteria.** It is used variously to describe:

1. A chronic personality disorder (the hysterical personality);

2. The psychogenic involuntary loss of neurologic function (conversion reaction); and

3. A nonclinical state of emotional instability (e.g., a hysterical outburst).

The current *Diagnostic and Statistical Manual of Mental Disorders (DSM-II)* has added to this confusion by listing both hysterical personality disorder and hysterical neurosis as acceptable diagnoses. **Hysterical neurosis** is meant to encompass the phenomena of conversion and dissociative reactions, while the **hysterical personality** is defined as a disorder of character marked by narcissism, frigidity, self-dramatization, exhibitionism, manipulativeness, seductiveness, and overreactivity. To avoid this confusion we suggest that the term **hysteria** be used only to describe conversion and dissociative reactions, such as:

1. Paralyses: e.g., hemiparesis, quadraparesis, paraparesis, and monoparesis.

2. Anesthesias.

3. Movement disorders: e.g., chorea, tremor, and ataxia.

4. Gait disorders: e.g., astasia-abasia.

5. Dysphagia (globus hystericus) and dysphonia.

6. Urinary retention.

7. Pain.

8. Seizures.

9. Visual loss, anosmia, and deafness.

10. Amnesia.

11. Fugue states and coma.

12. Somnambulism.

13. Multiple personality states.

Tentative plans for *DSM-III* include the abandonment of the diagnosis of hysterical personality in favor of the more descriptive diagnoses, **histrionic personality** and **narcissistic personality.**

B. **Epidemiology.** Conversion reactions can occur in both sexes and at all ages, although they are most common in young women with the diagnosis of hysterical personality. Furthermore, hysteria appears to be more common in less sophisticated and often less well-educated individuals. Thus the neurologist may be faced with the problem of conversion symptoms that complicate known neurologic deficits. Under these circumstances, special care must be taken to separate conversion symptoms from those that are attributable to the underlying neurologic disease.

C. **Diagnosis.** The absence of an organic etiology for the symptoms is necessary, but not sufficient, for the diagnosis of a conversion reaction. This diagnosis is not made by exclusion but, rather, rests on positive evidence. The following findings support a diagnosis of conversion reaction:

1. A history of **previous conversion reactions,** unexplained illnesses, or multiple surgical procedures for doubtful indications.

2. A history of **psychosomatic symptoms,** including hyperventilation, headaches, dizziness, vomiting, and ill-defined abdominal pains.

3. A history of **psychoneurosis,** including depression, phobia, anxiety, or obsessiveness.

4. The presence of **la belle indifférence** (emotional impassivity in the face of neurologic disability). Care must be taken not to confuse emotional impassivity due to hysteria with stoicism in the face of organic disease.

5. Demonstration that the neurologic deficit can be modified by **suggestion** is useful in confirming the diagnosis of hysteria.

6. Finally, the presence of **inconsistencies** in the neurologic examination lends support to a diagnosis of hysteria.

   a. Patients with **paralysis** due to hysteria rarely manifest alterations of tone or reflexes. Muscle bulk is usually well preserved, even when the paralysis has been long-standing, and Babinski signs are rare except in medically sophisticated patients. The paralysis often occurs in nonanatomic patterns. "Giving-way weakness" (the obvious relaxation of muscular effort by the patient) often characterizes hysterical paralysis, although some patients with organic paralysis also exhibit this phenomenon as a means of emphasizing the seriousness of their problem to the physician.

   b. As with paralysis, **hysterical anesthesias** are often nonanatomic in their distribution. Extremely sharp borders to the areas of sensory loss as well as dense stocking-glove anesthesias are common. In cases of hysterical hemianesthesia, it is often useful to test vibratory sensation on both sides of the forehead. Patients with hysteria perceive diminished vibration on the anesthetic side, while patients with organic hemianesthesias usually perceive vibration equally on both sides due to bone conduction. Again, the physician must be wary of patients with true anesthesias who embellish their deficits by reporting a more severe anesthesia than exists.

   c. **Astasia-abasia** is a hysterical gait disorder that is characterized by a wild staggering gait despite the absence of paralysis, ataxia, or sensory loss. Falls tend to be either abortive or into the arms of a nearby physician or nurse.

   d. The wild flailing activity of patients with **hysterical seizures** rarely imitates the tonic-clonic activity of those with true seizures. Urinary incontinency and tongue-biting rarely occur. In cases of **hysterical coma,** awareness can often be demonstrated by gently dropping the patient's hand over the face—the hand rarely falls downward onto the unprotected face.

   e. On testing visual fields, many patients with hysterical symptoms exhibit **constricted (tubular) fields.** Yet these same patients rarely complain spontaneously of visual loss and do not behave as if their fields were severely constricted. The explanation for this common phenomenon is uncertain, but its elicitation can be a helpful confirmation of the diagnosis of hysteria.

D. Nature of the conversion reaction

1. Patients with conversion reactions are not malingering—their deficits seem real to them.

2. The sophistication with which the conversion reaction simulates neurologic disease partially reflects the medical sophistication of the patient. Thus

patients with some knowledge of neurology may have more elaborate conversion symptoms.

3. Conversion reactions have psychiatric significance as both **defenses** and **symbols.** These reactions serve to substitute physical symptoms for unacceptable emotional conflicts, and they may also serve as icons (body symbols), acting as nonverbal forms of communication. For example, the paraplegia that besets a woman soon after she threatens to leave her husband defends her against the anger she feels toward him, while symbolizing her inability to leave him.

E. Management of conversion reactions

1. There is no standard therapy for conversion hysteria. The patience and ingenuity of the physician are tested in each case.

2. Nothing is gained by threatening or scolding the patient. Accusing the patient of malingering will only destroy the patient's trust in the physician.

3. Reassurance, persuasion, and suggestion are the mainstays of short-term management. Many patients improve quickly with a simple and convincing reassurance that the symptoms will disappear in so many hours or so many days. Placebos, administered convincingly and coupled with appropriate suggestions, are often helpful.

4. The patient should not be allowed to lose face. Allowing the patient a vehicle by which his or her symptoms can gradually improve is often useful (e.g., physical therapy).

5. Long-term psychotherapy to direct attention away from somatic concerns and toward underlying emotional conflicts is indicated in appropriately motivated and psychologically equipped individuals.

III. PAIN

A. Guidelines for the management of pain

1. The first priority is to establish the cause of the pain. Pain must be treated cautiously when the cause is unknown.

2. Pain is not always synonymous with somatic disease. Many medical patients experience pain in the absence of any obvious somatic disorder. Therefore when no etiology for the pain is present initially, careful follow-up is necessary. The diagnosis of psychogenic pain must not be made lightly, and once made, it must remain open to revision in case an organic cause for the pain becomes apparent.

3. When available, specific therapy rather than analgesia is used to relieve the pain (e.g., lumbar puncture for the headache of pseudotumor cerebri and carbamazepine for the pain of trigeminal neuralgia).

4. In the absence of specific therapy, analgesic drugs may be administered to relieve the pain. Mild superficial pain may be relieved by nonnarcotic analgesics, while deep (visceral) or severe pain generally requires treatment with narcotics. The dosage of these drugs should be gradually increased until either pain relief or drug toxicity occurs.

5. If a narcotic is used, therapy is initiated with drugs that have a low abuse potential (e.g., pentazocine and codeine) rather than the highly addicting narcotics (e.g., morphine, oxycodone, and meperidine). On the other hand, fear of producing drug addiction should not discourage the physician from prescribing dosages that are adequate for pain relief.

6. Administration of narcotics as needed (PRN) places the unnecessary psychological burden of having to ask for medication on some patients, especially those with recurrent or persistent severe pain.

7. Prolonged use of narcotics produces both tolerance (diminishing analgesic effect from given doses of narcotic) and dependency (psychic and physical).

8. Anxiety commonly accompanies acute pain and is usually related to fear of an underlying disease, future disability, or recurrent pain. Although reassurance and antianxiety drugs are often indicated, they are not substitutes for adequate analgesia.

9. When analgesic medications in adequate dosages fail to relieve the pain, the possibility that the pain is psychogenic in origin should be considered. On the other hand, somatic (organic) pain that is unrelieved by analgesic drugs may necessitate use of an ancillary technique for pain control.

10. Ancillary techniques of pain control that rely on the neurosurgical or neurolytic interruption of pain pathways are often successful initially, but recurrence of the pain over a period of months to years is common. This exasperating tendency for pain to circumvent destructive lesions in the nervous system is unexplained. Thus neurosurgical techniques for pain control are best applied to patients with limited life expectancies (usually patients with malignant disease).

    The long-term results of neurosurgery to control pain due to nonmalignant causes (e.g., postherpetic neuralgia, phantom limb pain) have not been satisfactory. A notable exception to this rule has been the excellent long-term relief of trigeminal neuralgia achieved by electrocoagulation of the gasserian ganglion.

B. **Antipyretic analgesics.** Most of the nonnarcotic analgesics possess antipyretic properties. These agents alleviate pain primarily by peripheral mechanisms, and CNS side effects are uncommon.

1. **Aspirin**
   a. **Actions.** Antipyretic, antiinflammatory, and analgesic.

   b. **Metabolism.** Conjugation in the liver, followed by renal excretion. Renal excretion is greatly enhanced by alkalinization of the urine.

   c. **Adverse reactions** include gastric irritation and hemorrhage as well as allergy (uncommon).

   d. **Toxicity** (overdose) is manifested by salicylism (tinnitus, vertigo, and hearing loss), stupor, hyperthermia, metabolic acidosis, hyperventilation, and bleeding diathesis (inhibition of both plasma- and platelet-clotting mechanisms).

   e. **Dosage** is usually 600 mg every 4 hours.

2. **Acetaminophen (Tylenol)**
   a. **Actions.** Antipyretic, analgesic.

   b. **Metabolism.** Conjugation in the liver.

   c. **Side effects** are uncommon.

   d. **Overdosage** occasionally produces hepatotoxicity.

   e. **Dosage** is usually 600 mg every 4 hours. Analgesic potency is approximately equal to that of aspirin (Table 9-2).

3. **Indomethacin (Indocin), phenylbutazone (Butazolidin), and oxyphenbutazone (Tandearil)** are potent antipyretic, antiinflammatory agents that are never used solely for their analgesic properties. Adverse gastrointestinal reactions can occur with these drugs.

C. **Narcotic analgesics**
   1. **Action.** The narcotic analgesics relieve pain by means of an unknown central action within the nervous system. The relief of pain occurs in the absence of

Table 9-2. Relative Potencies of the Commonly Used Oral Analgesics and Narcotics

Drug	Approximate Equivalent Analgesic Dose (mg)
Aspirin	600
Acetaminophen	600
Propoxyphene (Darvon)	65
Meperidine (Demerol)	50
Codeine	30
Pentazocine (Talwin)	30
Oxycodone (Percodan)	4
Hydromorphone (Dilaudid)	1
Levorphanol (Levo-Dromoran)	0.5

obtundation of other sensory stimuli (touch, temperature, etc.), and it is out of proportion to the impairment of consciousness produced (cf. general anesthetics). The relief of pain produced by narcotics can be partially understood as a blunting of the affective component (suffering) that accompanies pain, rather than as a dulling of the painful sensations.

2. **Overdosage.** All the narcotics can produce coma and fatal respiratory depression. However, the toxic effects of these agents can be quickly reversed by the parenteral administration of the narcotic antagonist **naloxone** (Narcan). The usual dose of 0.4–1.2 mg IV may have to be repeated over 12–24 hours if overdosage involved a long-acting narcotic (e.g., methadone).

3. **Morphine** is the prototypical narcotic, and other narcotics share many properties with it. (However, important differences in potency, abuse potential, and side effects exist.)

   a. **Actions** include analgesia and sedation, although a variety of other mental changes may occur, including euphoria, dysphoria, and relief of anxiety.

   b. **Side effects**

      (1) Respiratory depression.

      (2) Decreased gastrointestinal motility and constipation.

      (3) Miosis.

      (4) Nausea and vomiting (due to direct stimulation of the chemoreceptor zone of the medulla).

      (5) Postural hypotension and peripheral vasodilatation.

   c. **Metabolism.** Conjugation in the liver, followed by renal excretion.

   d. **Contraindications** include head injury, status asthmaticus, and respiratory insufficiency.

   e. **Tolerance** and **habituation** (psychic and physical) limit the long-term usefulness of morphine.

   f. **Dosage.** Maximum pain relief is achieved by administering morphine 10–15 mg parenterally every 4 hours. Lower dosages yield lesser degrees of analgesia, while higher dosages rarely improve on pain relief. Morphine, like meperidine, pentazocine, and hydromorphone, has much less potency when it is administered PO. **Potent oral narcotics include methadone, codeine, levorphanol, and oxycodone.** Some of the unpleasant side effects of the parenteral administration of morphine (vomiting and nausea) can be greatly diminished by the simultaneous administration of promethazine or chlorpromazine 25 mg. Some authorities also believe that concomitant administration of phenothiazine potentiates the analgesic effect of narcotics, although studies to date are equivocal on this point.

4. **Hydromorphone (Dilaudid)** is a synthetic narcotic that is five times as potent as morphine (Table 9-3), and it has the same actions and dependency-producing properties. Thus it has no distinct advantages or disadvantages compared with morphine. The usual dosage is 2 mg parenterally every 4 hours. Hydromorphone is similar to morphine in that oral preparations are much less potent analgesically.

5. **Meperidine (Demerol)** is a completely synthetic narcotic with approximately one-tenth the potency of morphine. Meperidine has one-half the duration of action of morphine, and it must be administered more frequently to alleviate pain. Because meperidine (unlike morphine) has spasmolytic properties in vitro, it has been proposed as the drug of choice for biliary colic and pancreatitis. However, these spasmolytic properties have not been duplicated in vivo and may not be of clinical significance. The usual dosage is 50–150 mg parenterally every 3 hours. The oral preparation has much less analgesic potency.

6. **Codeine** is the oral narcotic of choice, because its oral potency is about equal to its parenteral potency. Also, it produces less euphoria and dependency than morphine. The usual dosage is 30–60 mg PO every 4 hours. **Oxycodone** (the narcotic ingredient of Percodan) is also highly effective orally, but its abuse potential approaches that of morphine.

7. **Levorphanol (Levo-Dromoran)** is a potent synthetic narcotic that is highly effective when administered PO. However, its abuse potential and side effects are similar to those of morphine. The usual dosage is 2 mg every 4 hours.

8. **Methadone (Dolophine)** has the longest duration of action of the commonly used narcotics. It is effective when administered PO or parenterally, and its potency is equal to that of morphine. Because of its long duration of action, it is administered PO once daily to forestall the development of narcotic withdrawal.

9. **Pentazocine (Talwin)** is an analgesic with weak narcotic antagonistic properties. Pentazocine is about one-fiftieth as potent as naloxone (Narcan) in antagonizing the action of morphine, and the administration of pentazocine to narcotic addicts can precipitate an acute withdrawal syndrome. Nonetheless, overdosage with pentazocine is reversible if the usual dosage of naloxone is given.

   The initial claim that pentazocine could not be abused has proved to be incorrect, but the liability for dependency on this drug is much smaller than that for either morphine or codeine (Table 9-3). Further, the narcotic antagonizing properties of pentazocine make abuse of this drug by known narcotic addicts extremely unlikely, and tolerance to pentazocine does not produce tolerance to other narcotic drugs. The toxic effects of pentazocine are somewhat different than those of morphine and include respiratory and CNS depression, tachycardia, and hypertension. The usual dosage of pentazocine is 30–60 mg parenterally or 50–100 mg PO, both every 4 hours.

10. **Propoxyphene (Darvon)** is a weak analgesic that has a low abuse potential. Some have attributed its wide popularity to the mild euphoria it sometimes produces rather than to its weak analgesic properties. Side effects are rarely troublesome and include constipation, drowsiness, anorexia, and nausea. Overdosage produces CNS and respiratory depression, which are reversible by the administration of naloxone (Narcan). Various combinations of prop-

Table 9-3. Abuse Potential and Relative Analgesic Potency of the Commonly Used Parenteral Narcotics

Drug	Abuse Potential	Equivalent Analgesic Dose (mg)
Codeine	Medium	130
Meperidine (Demerol)	High	100
Pentazocine (Talwin)	Low	60
Morphine	High	10
Methadone	High	10
Hydromorphone (Dilaudid)	High	2

oxyphene with caffeine, aspirin, phenacetin, and acetaminophen are currently available.

D. Other drugs useful in the management of pain

1. **Psychotropic drugs** are sometimes useful in the alleviation of intractable pain. The most effective regimen appears to be a combination of a phenothiazine tranquilizer (e.g., chlorpromazine 50–150 mg daily) and a tricyclic antidepressant (e.g., imipramine 50–150 mg daily). The mechanism by which these drugs relieve pain is uncertain, but they may be effective even in the absence of overt psychopathology.

2. **Carbamazepine** (Tegretol) or **phenytoin** (Dilantin) may alleviate a variety of brief, lancinating, neuritic pains. These drugs are often effective therapy for **trigeminal neuralgia** (Chap. 2), as well as for the brief lancinating pains associated with **multiple sclerosis** (Chap. 13) and **tabes dorsalis.** These drugs may also be of use in controlling the lancinating component of pain associated with **postherpetic neuralgia** (although the persistent burning component of the pain is not usually affected) and some of the lancinating pains that follow **spinal cord injury.**

   Phenytoin is given in a dosage of 200–400 mg/day. The dosage of carbamazepine needed to control lancinating pain ranges from 400 to 1000 mg daily in divided doses. **Adverse reactions** to carbamazepine include skin rash, ataxia, drowsiness, nausea, hepatic dysfunction, and bone marrow depression. Blood count and liver function should be monitored monthly.

3. **Baclofen (Lioresal)** is chemically related to gamma-aminobutyric acid. This drug appears to control effectively the **painful flexor and extensor spasms** that commonly accompany spinal cord disease (multiple sclerosis, spinal cord compression, or spinal cord trauma). Dosage is started at 5 mg TID and is gradually increased to a maximum of 30–80 mg daily in divided doses. **Side effects** include lightheadedness, nausea, drowsiness, dry mouth, weakness, dizziness, leg edema, and postural hypotension.

E. Thermocoagulation of the gasserian (trigeminal) ganglion, using a percutaneously inserted radiofrequency electrode, is the surgical treatment of choice for trigeminal neuralgia when drug therapy with phenytoin or carbamazepine is ineffective (Chap. 2). An intracranial approach to the trigeminal nerve is indicated for the unusual case in which thermocoagulation of the gasserian ganglion is ineffective.

F. Cordotomy

1. **Rationale.** Interruption of the spinothalamic pathways in the spinal cord.

2. **Technique.** Cordotomy may be performed by either an open or closed approach. The **open approach** involves laminectomy and direct exposure of the

spinal cord to interrupt the spinothalamic tract. The **closed approach** involves the insertion of a radiofrequency electrode percutaneously, and a thermocoagulative lesion may be produced in the anterolateral quadrant of the spinal cord.

One approach to unilateral pain is to begin with a percutaneous cordotomy at the C1–2 level contralateral to the painful side. If this measure is ineffective, it is usually necessary to proceed to an open cordotomy. If the pain is bilateral, cordotomies of both spinothalamic tracts may be necessary. Since bilateral, high cervical cordotomies run a high risk of producing sleep apnea (Ondine's curse), the second cordotomy is usually done at a high thoracic level by an open approach.

3. **Results** are excellent in patients with pain due to malignant disease; 75–80% get good relief.

4. **Complications**

   a. Pain recurrence is uncommon in patients with malignant disease, because they generally have a short life expectancy. About one-half of patients who have cordotomies for nonmalignant neuralgias have recurrence of pain within 2 years.

   b. Mortality is about 2–5%.

   c. Sleep apnea (Ondine's curse) may complicate bilateral, high cervical cordotomies.

   d. Bladder and bowel incontinence may occur after bilateral cordotomies.

   e. Transient ataxia.

   f. A disconcerting postcordotomy syndrome, characterized by painful dysesthesias, occurs in about 5% of patients.

   g. Paresis.

5. **Comment.** Cordotomy is the procedure of choice for relief of intractable pain due to malignancy that affects the trunk or limbs.

G. **Posterior rhizotomy**

   1. **Rationale.** Relief of regional pain by division of the dorsal roots that innervate the painful area.

   2. **Technique.** The segmental levels that innervate the painful area are ascertained by nerve blocks. After laminectomy, the dorsal roots at the affected levels plus one further root above and below are sectioned (rhizotomy).

   3. **Results.** Posterior rhizotomy is not effective for postherpetic neuralgia, phantom limb pain, or causalgia. When pain is well localized to the segmental distribution of a few sensory roots, the procedure is successful in about 60–70% of cases. Pain produced by localized malignancy or the entrapment of nerves by operative scars, traumatic scars, or herniated discs is most likely to respond favorably to posterior rhizotomy.

   4. **Complications** include traumatic skin ulceration due to anesthesia as well as the usual complications associated with laminectomy.

H. **Intrathecal dorsal root block**

   1. The **rationale** is similar to that of posterior rhizotomy.

   2. **Technique.** Several methods are currently used to produce dorsal root damage intrathecally. These include barbotage (the withdrawal and rapid replacement of CSF), intrathecal irrigation with hypertonic saline, and intrathecal injection of phenol in glycerol. The intrathecal injection of alcohol has been practically abandoned. Before proceeding to intrathecal destruction

of dorsal roots, the likelihood of pain relief should be ascertained by administering a short-acting spinal anesthetic.

3. **Results.** Intrathecal dorsal root blocks are usually reserved for patients with pain due to malignancy. Barbotage gives only short-term pain relief, usually of less than 3 months' duration. Relief of pain after intrathecal phenol blocks is longer lasting, often persisting for 6 months to 1 year.

4. **Complications** include urinary retention (20%), paresthesias (5%), rectal sphincter paralysis (5%), paresis (10%), and headache (10%).

5. **Comment.** Intrathecal blocks are useful in patients who cannot tolerate bilateral cordotomies, but the incidence of disabling complications is quite high.

I. Thalamotomy

1. **Rationale.** Thalamotomy is an attempt to alleviate pain by interrupting pain pathways in the thalamus proximal to their cortical projections.

2. **Technique.** Electrocoagulative lesions are produced in thalamic nuclei after the stereotactive introduction of electrodes. Lesions produced in the venteroposterior lateral nucleus produce profound sensory loss but little pain relief. However, lesions produced in the parafascicular, intralaminar, and median nuclei may relieve pain with minimal sensory loss.

3. **Results.** This procedure has been used with limited success to treat the pain of head and neck cancer, facial postherpetic neuralgia, and thalamic syndrome. While the relief of pain by thalamotomy is of immense theoretical interest, in practice it has limited use, because bilateral lesions must be produced in most patients for pain relief. Currently, few neurosurgeons use thalamotomy for pain relief.

4. **Complications** include ataxia, dementia, and personality changes. The mortality from the procedure is about 4%.

J. Dorsal column stimulation

1. **Rationale.** It has been proposed that electric stimulation of the dorsal columns could relieve pain by eliciting the closure of hypothetical "pain-gates" in the dorsal horns. However, this intriguing hypothesis has not yet received strong experimental confirmation.

2. **Technique.** After laminectomy, electrodes are placed subdurally against the posterior columns. Then the electrodes are connected by insulated wires to a subcutaneously implanted receiving coil. This coil can be activated by an externally placed battery-powered transmitter to stimulate the posterior columns.

3. **Results.** The initial enthusiasm generated by dorsal-column stimulators has waned considerably. Although the technique is undergoing extensive investigation, truly favorable results have been achieved only with phantom limb pain (see sec **N.1**).

4. **Complications** include spinal cord compression, transient paraplegia, CSF leaks, and wound infection.

K. Transcutaneous stimulation is under investigation as a possible technique for chronic-pain relief. Most systems use a portable battery-powered transmitter that delivers a low-voltage, low-frequency (10–150 Hz) current to the skin. Thus electric stimulation may be applied to both the painful area itself and the nerves innervating it.

About 15% of patients with diverse regional pains (nerve entrapment, arthritis, phantom limb pain, causalgia) experience relief of pain after 1 year. Transcutaneous nerve stimulation appears to be especially useful in the management of pain due to peripheral nerve entrapment.

L. Cingulotomy

1. **Rationale.** Pain is relieved by creating destructive lesions in the limbic system, where affective responses to pain are presumed to originate.

2. **Technique.** Electrodes are introduced into the anterior cingulate gyri under radiographic control through frontal burr holes. Electrocoagulative lesions are produced bilaterally (approximately 2–3 cm in diameter).

3. **Results.** About 25% of patients with intractable pain due to malignancy have marked or moderate relief of pain after cingulumotomy. In patients with pain due to nonmalignant causes (thalamic syndrome, phantom limb pain, postherpetic neuralgia), about 25% have marked relief of pain and 25% have moderate relief of pain 3 months after the procedure.

4. **Complications** include transient bladder and bowel incontinence, transient headache, and fever. Unwanted personality changes are unusual.

5. **Comment.** Cingulumotomy remains a radical approach to the control of intractable pain, although it is being evaluated further.

M. Hypnosis and **acupuncture** have produced disappointing results in the control of severe intractable pain. Hypnosis raises the threshold to experimental pain slightly; acupuncture does not raise it at all. Hypnosis is rarely effective against chronic organic pain and is only occasionally effective against psychogenic pain. At present, we do not recommend the routine use of either of these techniques for the control of chronic pain.

N. Special pain problems

1. **Phantom limb pain**

   a. **Description.** About 35% of amputees experience transient pain in a phantom limb, while 5–10% of amputees develop severe, chronic phantom limb pain. The pain is described variably as cramping, shooting, burning, or crushing. Phantom limb pain is more common in individuals who experienced pain in the limb prior to amputation, and the phantom pain often resembles the preamputation pain.

   b. **Etiology.** There is no satisfactory explanation for the development of phantom limb pain.

   c. **Treatment.** Care must be taken to distinguish phantom limb pain from local pain in the stump. Stump pain is effectively managed by either excision of neuromas or reamputation. However, treatment of phantom limb pain has proved to be difficult. Cordotomy (either percutaneous or open) has given the best results, but pain may recur months or years later. Recent experience with the dorsal-column stimulator has been encouraging.

2. **Causalgia**

   a. **Description.** Causalgia is a severe, superficial burning pain that may occur after incomplete nerve injury. It is estimated that causalgia occurs after about 2–5% of peripheral nerve injuries. The pain may begin immediately after injury or after an interval of several weeks, and trivial sensory stimuli (even light touch) may trigger severe paroxysms of pain.

   b. **Etiology.** It has been speculated that causalgia is produced by short circuits in the area of damaged nerve between unmyelinated postganglionic sympathetic efferent fibers and poorly myelinated afferent fibers. This hypothesis has received support from the observation that electric stimulation of sympathetic ganglia produces pain in patients with causalgia, but not in normal individuals.

   c. **Treatment.** Sympathectomy is curative in nearly all cases if it is performed soon enough after the injury. If sympathetic blockade by injection of a local anesthetic produces pain relief, permanent sympathectomy by surgery or phenol injection yields excellent results.

3. **Thalamic syndrome**

a. **Description.** In 1906, Dejerine and Roussy identified the essential features of the thalamic syndrome as mild hemiparesis, hemianesthesia, and hemiataxia, associated with "severe, persistent, paroxysmal, often intolerable pains of the hemiplegic side, not yielding to any analgesic treatment." The thalamic syndrome occurs most commonly after strokes in the distribution of the posterior cerebral artery with thalamic infarction.

b. **Treatment.** Analgesics and anticonvulsants (carbamazepine and phenytoin) may be tried, but they are rarely of benefit. An occasional patient responds to a combination of tricyclic antidepressants and phenothiazine tranquilizers.

4. **Psychogenic pain**

a. Pain is generally considered a symptom of somatic disease. The term *psychogenic pain* implies that it may also be a symptom of psychiatric disease.

b. Engel has described the many psychological meanings of pain:

(1) Pain is a warning of impending damage to the body.

(2) The announcement that one is in pain elicits comforting and caring from others.

(3) Pain is associated with punishment and may become a vehicle for the expiation of guilt.

(4) The infliction of pain on others symbolizes power and aggression.

(5) The experience of having pain may allow an individual to identify with others who are in pain.

c. **Hysteria.** Pain is one of the most common conversion reactions. The criteria for diagnosis of pain due to conversion reaction are similar to those outlined above. For example, the site of the pain often has symbolic significance. The treatment of hysterical pain disorders is not well established. However, some patients benefit from psychotherapy aimed at shifting their attention away from matters of somatic concern and toward psychic and interpersonal issues.

d. **Delusional pains** may occur in psychotic individuals and respond to specific antipsychotic medications.

e. **Depression** is probably the most common cause of psychogenic pain, which includes ill-defined complaints of backache and headache. However, these patients must be distinguished from those who become depressed because of intractable pain. Also, pain may serve to lessen the patient's degree of depression (because pain acts as expiation for the guilt that commonly accompanies severe depressions). Thus emphasis must rest on treating the depression rather than on the associated pain. The pain that accompanies depression does not usually yield to conventional analgesics, but it may improve dramatically with tricyclic antidepressant therapy. In drug-refractory cases of severe depression complicated by pain, ECT may be curative.

5. **Hypochondriasis** and **malingering** are often associated with unremitting pain. Szasz introduced the term *l'homme douloureux* ("pained man") to describe the individual who has decided to make a career of pain and suffering. The rewards for a career of pain are diverse and include money (through litigation for injuries), love and caring (which is bestowed on individuals in

pain), expiation (pain as punishment for wrongdoings), and power (over the physicians and nurses who are inadequate to relieve the pain).

Pain relief in these individuals can come only when they decide to seek a new career that is free of pain. Comprehensive psychological rehabilitation is necessary in many cases. Analgesics and neurosurgical interventions are rarely of benefit. About one-third of these patients improve after extended hospitalization in a pain rehabilitation unit that gives emphasis to psychological interventions. Psychotropic drugs are sometimes a useful adjunct to therapy.

SELECTED READINGS

Depression

Appleton, W. S., and Davis, J. M. *Practical Clinical Psychopharmacology*. New York: Medcom Press, 1973.

Burks, J. S., Walker, J. E., Rumack, B. H., and Ott, J. E. Tricyclic antidepressant poisoning: Reversal of coma, choreoathetosis, and myoclonus by physostigmine. *J.A.M.A.* 230:1405, 1974.

Frazier, S. H. Changing patterns in the management of depression. *Dis. Nerv. Syst.* 37:25, 1976.

Hollister, L. E. Clinical use of tricyclic antidepressants. *Dis. Nerv. Syst.* 37:17, 1976.

Sachar, E. J. Evaluating Depression in the Medical Patient, in J. J. Strain and S. Grossman (eds.), *Psychological Care of the Medically Ill*. New York: Appleton-Century-Crofts, 1974. Pp. 64–75.

Shader, R. I. Problems of polypharmacy in depression. *Dis. Nerv. Syst.* 37:30, 1976.

Woodruff, R. A., Jr., Goodwin, D. W., and Guze, S. B. *Psychiatric Diagnosis*. New York: Oxford University Press, 1974.

Hysteria

Lewis, W. C. Hysteria: The consultant's dilemma—Twentieth century demonology, pejorative epithet, or useful diagnosis. *Arch. Gen. Psychiatry* 30:145, 1974.

Nemiah, J. C. Hysterical Neurosis, Conversion Type, in A. M. Freedman, H. I. Kaplan, and B. J. Sadock (eds.), *Comprehensive Textbook of Psychiatry II, 2nd Ed.* Baltimore. Williams and Wilkins, 1975. Pp. 1208–1220.

Szasz, T. S. *The Myth of Mental Illness*. New York: Harper and Row, 1974.

Nature of Pain

Melzack, R. *The Puzzle of Pain*. New York: Basic Books, 1973.

Nathan, P. W. The gate-control theory of pain—A critical review. *Brain* 99:123, 1976.

Drug Treatment of Pain

Goodman, L. S., and Gilman, A. *The Pharmacologic Basis of Therapeutics*, 5th ed. New York: Macmillan, 1975.

Merskey, H., and Hester, R. A. The treatment of chronic pain with psychotropic drugs. *Postgrad. Med. J.* 48:594, 1972.

Ancillary Techniques of Pain Control

Boshes, B., and Arieff, A. J. Clinical experiences in the neurologic substrate of pain. *Med. Clin. North Am.* 52:111, 1968.

Hammington-Kiff, J. G. *Pain Relief*. London: Medical Books, 1974.

Hurt, R. W., and Ballantine, T. H., Jr. Steriotactic anterior cingulate lesions for persistent pain: A report of 68 cases. *Clin. Neurosurg.* 21:334, 1974.

Li, C. L., Ahlberg, D., Lansdale, H., Gravitz, M. A., Chen, T. C., Ting, C. Y., Bak, A. F., and Blessing, D. Acupuncture and hypnosis: Effects on induced pain. *Exp. Neurol.* 49:272, 1975.

Loeser, J. D., Black, R. G., and Christman, A. Relief of pain by transcutaneous stimulation. *J. Neurosurg.* 42:308, 1975.

Northfield, D. W. C. *The Surgery of the Central Nervous System*. Oxford: Blackwell Scientific, 1973. Pp. 575–617.

Strain, J. J.   The Problem of Pain, in J. J. Strain and S. Grossman (eds.), *Psychological Care of the Medically Ill.* New York: Appleton-Century-Crofts, 1975. Pp. 93–107.

Sweet, W. H.   Pain: Mechanisms and Treatment, in T. N. Chase (ed.), *The Clinical Neurosciences.* New York: Raven Press, 1975. Pp. 487–500.

Swerdlow, M. (ed.)   *Relief of Intractable Pain.* London: Excerpta Medica, 1974.

White, J. C.   Neurosurgical Treatment of Pain in Neuralgias of Nonmalignant Etiology, in F. D. Hart (ed.), *The Treatment of Chronic Pain.* Philadelphia: Davis, 1974. Pp. 113–156.

Phantom Limb, Causalgia, and Thalamic Syndrome

Nashold, B. S., Jr.   Central pain, its origins and treatment. *Clin. Neurosurg.* 21:311, 1974.

Nielson, K. D., Adams, J. E., and Hosobuchi, Y.   Phantom limb pain: Treatment with dorsal column stimulation. *J. Neurosurg.* 42:301, 1975.

Thompson, J. E., Patman, R. D., and Persson, A. V.   Management of posttraumatic pain syndromes (causalgia). *Am. Surg.* 41:599, 1975.

Wilkins, R. A., and Brody, I. A.   The thalamic syndrome. *Arch. Neurol.* 20:559, 1969.

Psychogenic Pain

Altman, N.   Hypochondriasis, in J. J. Strain and S. Grossman (eds.), *Psychological Care of the Medically Ill.* New York: Appleton-Century-Crofts, 1975. Pp. 76–92.

Engel, G. L.   Psychogenic pain and the pain-prone patient. *Am. J. Med.* 20:899, 1959.

Mandell, M. R.   Electroconvulsive therapy for chronic pain associated with depression. *Am. J. Psychiatry* 132:632, 1975.

Sternbach, R. A.   Psychological aspects of pain and the selection of patients. *Clin. Neurosurg.* 21:323, 1974.

Szasz, T. S.   A Psychiatric Perspective on Pain and Its Control, in F. D. Hart (ed.), *The Treatment of Chronic Pain.* Philadelphia: Davis, 1974. Pp. 37–62.

Stroke

Stroke is one of the most commonly encountered neurologic disorders, and it can almost always be distinguished clinically from other such illnesses by the suddenness with which the neurologic deficit develops. Stroke is generally divided into two categories. (1) **Ischemic strokes** include embolic and thrombotic strokes, and (2) **hemorrhagic strokes** encompass primary intraparenchymal brain hemorrhage as well as subarachnoid hemorrhage, which is usually the result of a ruptured cerebral aneurysm or an arteriovenous malformation. Successful prevention of stroke is now becoming possible with the identification of important risk factors, such as hyptertension, atrial fibrillation, hyperlipidemia, and oral contraceptives.

In this chapter, guidelines for treatment of the various types of stroke are presented. Although a general orientation to the clinical picture for each variety of stroke is provided, a detailed description is beyond the scope of this text.

I. **Ischemic strokes.** The clinician is most commonly confronted with two types of ischemic strokes: **primary thrombotic occlusion** of a vessel and occlusion of a vessel by material from a distant source **(embolism).** The most common source of embolic material is the heart (e.g., mural thrombus formation in the setting of atrial fibrillation or myocardial infarction, prosthetic valves, septic emboli in bacterial endocarditis, marantic (nonbacterial) endocarditis, Libman-Sacks endocarditis, and atrial myxoma). Another common source is the carotid artery system in the neck. Less commonly emboli may result from mural thrombus formation in the aortic arch or at the origin of the great vessels. Rare causes of ischemic stroke include cerebral vein thrombosis, polycythemia vera, meningovascular syphilis, arteritis secondary to tuberculosis, arteritis in association with collagen vascular disease, giant cell arteritis, Takayashu's arteritis, moyamoya, fibromuscular dysplasia, subclavian steal, and dissecting aortic aneurysm.

A. **Clinical description.** Although not invariable, the neurologic deficit associated with embolism characteristically begins suddenly, with a maximum deficit occurring at the onset; preceding transient ischemic attacks occur in only a small percentage of cases.

In contrast, thrombotic strokes are often preceded by transient ischemic attacks (defined as transient neurologic deficits that often last only seconds or minutes, but never longer than 24 hours). Thrombotic strokes may progress over hours or days, but the neurologic deficit changes in a step-wise fashion with a series of sudden events, the so-called stroke-in-evolution.

1. **Middle cerebral artery syndrome.** Middle cerebral artery occlusions are usually embolic. When the entire territory of the middle cerebral artery is affected, the clinical picture includes: contralateral hemiplegia and hemianesthesia; contralateral homonymous hemianopia with impairment of conjugate gaze in the direction opposite the lesion; aphasia with dominant hemispheral involvement; and apractognosia, asomatognosia, and anosognosia, with nondominant hemispheric involvement. When middle cerebral branch occlusions occur, which is often the case, incomplete syndromes result: motor or Broca's aphasia with contralateral lower-face and arm weakness from upper-division middle cerebral artery occlusion, Wernicke's aphasia with lower-division middle cerebral artery occlusion, and others.

2. **Anterior cerebral artery syndrome.** Anterior cerebral artery occlusion, also usually embolic, may **lead to** paralysis of the opposite foot and leg, with sensory loss, contralateral grasp reflex, gegenhalten rigidity, abulia, gait apraxia, perseveration, and urinary incontinence. Occlusion of the stem of the anterior cerebral artery is often inconsequential because of collateral flow

through the anterior communicating artery. However, when both anterior cerebral arteries arise from a common stem, occlusion can result in a severe deficit, involving the territories of both arteries.

3. **Carotid artery syndrome.** Disease of the carotid artery can **produce symptoms** in two ways: as vascular insufficiency secondary to stenosis or occlusion and as a source of embolic material. Even when the artery is only minimally narrowed by atheroma, ulceration of the atheromatous plaque is often a nidus for thrombus formation; thus it is a source of embolic material. Although occlusion of the carotid artery is at times asymptomatic, symptomatic occlusion most commonly produces deficits that involve all or part of the middle cerebral artery territory.

Because of variations in the origins of cerebral vessels, the territory supplied by the anterior cerebral artery, and at times the posterior cerebral artery, may be involved. When the internal carotid artery is severely narrowed and collateral flow is compromised, the most distal regions supplied by the middle cerebral, anterior cerebral, and at times the posterior cerebral arteries (the so-called border zones) may be affected. These zones represent the areas of collateralization between the three arteries. The damage in this situation typically produces weakness or paresthesias in the contralateral arm and, if it is more extensive, the face and tongue.

Carotid artery disease is responsible in approximately 50% of patients with transient unilateral loss of vision (transient monocular blindness), occurring with or without other neurologic symptoms. This may be the result of platelet emboli from atheromatous plaques in the carotid system. Occlusion of the central retinal artery or one of its branches, with total or partial permanent loss of vision, is less commonly caused by carotid artery disease. Nevertheless, there is an association, and carotid artery disease should be excluded in this case.

The presence of prominent facial pulses or low retinal artery pressure by ophthalmodynamometry usually signifies severe stenosis or occlusion of the ipsilateral internal carotid artery. The Doppler procedure, ultrasonography, and phonoangiography are useful noninvasive procedures for the diagnosis of carotid artery disease.

4. **Posterior cerebral artery syndrome.** The posterior cerebral artery may be occluded by embolus or thrombosis, **resulting in** various combinations of the following neurologic signs: contralateral homonymous hemianopia (often upper quadrantanopia), memory loss, dyslexia without dysgraphia, color anomia, mild contralateral hemiparesis, contralateral hemisensory loss, and ipsilateral third-nerve palsy, with contralateral involuntary movements, hemiplegia, or ataxia.

5. **Vertebrobasilar artery syndrome.** The basilar and vertebral arteries are usually involved with atherosclerotic narrowing and thrombosis, but they can be subject to embolism. Disease in the **branches of the basilar artery** is usually manifested by unilateral pontine or cerebellar dysfunction or both. Depending on the level of involvement, this includes combinations of ipsilateral ataxia; contralateral hemiplegia with sensory loss; ipsilateral horizontal gaze palsy, with contralateral hemiplegia (the opposite of that seen in hemispheric lesions); ipsilateral peripheral seventh-nerve lesion; internuclear ophthalmoplegia; nystagmus, vertigo, nausea, and vomiting; deafness and tinnitus; and palatal myoclonus and oscillopsia.

Occlusion or severe stenosis of the **basilar artery itself** usually **gives rise to** bilateral signs, such as quadriplegia, bilateral conjugate horizontal gaze palsies, coma, or the de-efferented ("locked-in") syndrome. These same signs may be produced by bilateral vertebral artery disease or unilateral disease when one vertebral artery is the dominant source of blood supply.

Damage to structures in the medulla results from occlusion or stenosis of the intracranial vertebral arteries. This **leads to** various symptom complexes: the most well-known is the lateral medullary syndrome, consisting of nystagmus, vertigo, nausea, vomiting, dysphagia, hoarseness, impaired sensation on the ipsilateral side of the face, ipsilateral ataxia, ipsilateral Horner's syndrome, and impairment of pain and thermal sense over the contralateral side of the body.

6. **Cerebellar infarction.** Early in the course, cerebellar infarction usually produces dizziness, nausea, vomiting, direction-changing nystagmus, and ataxia, with inability to stand or walk unaided. Over 1–3 days, there may be resultant edema of the cerebellum, manifested by signs of brainstem compression, such as conjugate gaze palsy, ipsilateral fifth-nerve dysfunction, and ipsilateral facial nerve palsy. The patient may then progress rapidly to coma and death. Patients with these clinical signs are always thoroughly evaluated and observed for several days, since the complication of brainstem compression can be remedied by surgical decompression of the posterior fossa.

7. **Lacunar infarction.** Hypertension commonly leads to a special type of vascular disease that is characterized by hyaline thickening of the small penetrating arteries of the brain. This can result in small, often cystic infarcts in the brain parenchyma, which are referred to as *lacunar infarcts*. These infarcts are often asymptomatic but may **result in** certain clinical syndromes, such as pure motor strokes, pure sensory strokes, clumsy hand–dysarthria syndrome, homolateral ataxia and crural paresis, and pure motor hemiparesis, with contralateral paralysis of lateral gaze and internuclear ophthalmoplegia. This diagnosis may be suspected when no arterial occlusions are seen on arteriography and the clinical symptoms fit one of the syndromes already discussed.

B. **Diagnostic evaluation.** A fairly accurate clinical impression can usually be formulated after the initial history-taking and physical examination. It is critically important to distinguish hemorrhage from infarction. Thus diagnostic studies should be arranged early in the course to clarify the diagnosis beyond a doubt, so an appropriate course of therapy can be planned.

1. **Lumbar puncture.** Examination of the cerebrospinal fluid (CSF) is carried out early, since most cases of intracerebral hemorrhage and all cases of subarachnoid hemorrhage produce blood in the CSF. Note that diagnostic confusion may arise when bleeding into the CSF is induced by needle insertion at lumbar puncture—the so-called traumatic tap.

Thus if four to six successive tubes of CSF are collected, traumatic taps usually result in a diminishing number of red cells per cubic millimeter in each successive tube, while true hemorrhage produces a more uniform red cell count in each tube. Moreover, when blood has been present in the CSF for approximately 6 hours or longer, the supernatant CSF will appear xanthochromic after centrifugation.

Small intraparenchymal hemorrhages that do not communicate with the subarachnoid space will not yield positive CSF early. The same is often true of hemorrhage into an area of infarction (hemorrhagic infarction), which is usually the result of an embolus. In these situations, the CSF is almost always positive by 48 hours due to seepage of blood into the ventricular system.

2. **Computed tomography (CT scan).** This is an extremely useful radiographic procedure, because it distinguishes hemorrhage from infarction easily. It demonstrates virtually all instances of supratentorial intracerebral hemorrhage, although it may fail to detect hemorrhagic infarction, and most cases of cerebellar hemorrhage will be detected. Pontine hemorrhage may or may not be demonstrated. Thus, when available, CT scan is employed in all cases in which hemorrhage is suspected.

3. **Angiography.** Once a presumptive diagnosis of ischemic infarction has been made, angiography should be carried out within 24 hours. The complications

of angiography are usually avoided if the procedure is done by an experienced person, especially when the femoral or brachial approach is used. Also, a clear understanding of the pathologic process is essential to determine a course of therapy.

Angiography may be foregone if the diagnosis of lacunar infarct is certain. Likewise, if no specific therapy (e.g., anticoagulation) is planned, then angiography is not as important.

4. **Brain scan and electroencephalogram (EEG).** The EEG is usually abnormal in cerebral infarction, with slowing over the area of infarction. Brain scan often shows increased uptake in the area of infarction, but it often does not become positive for 4–5 days or longer. Also, the diphosphonate scan seems to give positive evidence of infarction more often than does the conventional technetium scan.

Although EEG and brain scan usually give positive evidence of infarction, they add little to the diagnostic evaluation of patients with stroke. However, they are at times useful in determining whether infarction or merely transient ischemia has occurred. Also, a negative EEG may be supportive of the diagnosis of a lacunar infarct, since it is only rarely positive in this type of stroke.

When a diagnosis of embolism has been made and no source is identified, two uncommon diagnoses are **infective endocarditis** and **atrial myxoma.** Both these disorders may produce an increased sedimentation rate and fever as well as other constitutional symptoms. Serial blood cultures are indicated if there is any evidence of infective endocarditis. Echocardiography is positive in virtually all cases of left atrial myxoma and, in addition, may be useful in detecting unsuspected mitral valve disease.

C. Treatment

1. General precautions

a. Rapid lowering of blood pressure is avoided in the first 10 days unless it is critically high (persistent diastolic pressure greater than 120 mm Hg), and, of course, hypotension is reversed. The patient may be kept in the horizontal position with the feet slightly elevated for a few days, especially for stroke-in-evolution.

b. **Vomiting** is common in the early stages of some types of stroke, particularly vertebrobasilar strokes and hemorrhages. If vomiting occurs, nasogastric suction is instituted along with intravenous fluid and electrolyte maintenance; close attention must be given to the control of nasopharyngeal secretions. Patients who are dysphagic must also be maintained on intravenous fluids.

c. **Intravenous solutions** which contain excessive amounts of free water (such as 5% dextrose in water) may increase cerebral edema and are **contraindicated.**

d. **Inactivity** can itself be a problem. Antiembolic stockings, although of doubtful efficacy in preventing thrombophlebitis, are usually worn, and a footboard is placed at the foot of the bed. With prolonged inactivity, the patient is turned every 2–3 hours to prevent decubitus ulcers.

e. Within 24–48 hours of completion of the stroke, passive range-of-motion exercises are begun three to four times a day to prevent the development of **contractures.**

2. Specific therapy

a. **Anticoagulants.** The most commonly used anticoagulants for cerebrovascular disease are the coumarin agents and heparin. These drugs should not be given to irresponsible patients or to those who cannot be followed closely with clotting tests. They are contraindicated in patients with bleeding diatheses, active peptic ulcer disease, uremia, severe liver disease, or in patients who are at risk of falling frequently.

(1) Coumarin agents. Either bishydroxycoumarin (average maintenance dose, 75 mg/day) or warfarin (maintenance dose, 2–15 mg/day) may be used for oral long-term anticoagulant therapy. These agents result in decreased hepatic synthesis of the vitamin K-dependent clotting factors (i.e., prothrombin and factors VII, IX, and X).

Although prolongation of the prothrombin time may be achieved in 48 hours or so, this is merely a reflection of the short half-life of factor VII, and the patient's intrinsic clotting mechanism is still very much intact. It is usually 5 days or longer before the other factors reach their lowest levels and adequate therapeutic anticoagulation is achieved. For this reason, a loading dose at the commencement of therapy is unnecessary, and a daily maintenance dose, such as warfarin 10 mg/ day, may be started. Daily prothrombin time (protime) determinations are made, and the dosage is adjusted to maintain the protime level at 17–19 seconds (although variations from one laboratory to another may dictate a different value).

Once the protime has been controlled and the patient has been discharged from the hospital, the protime is determined no less frequently than every 2 weeks. Other drugs that may augment or antagonize the effect of the coumarin agents are always kept in mind.

(2) Heparin. When heparin therapy is indicated, two methods of administration can be used. An intravenous bolus of 5000–10,000 units may be given, followed by a **continuous infusion** by syringe pump of 1000–2000 units/hour. The alternative method calls for an initial intravenous bolus of 5000–10,000 units followed by **repeated bolus** injections of 5000–10,000 units every 4 hours.

Either the Lee-White whole-blood clotting time or the activated partial thromboplastin time (PTT) may be used to adjust the heparin dose to maintain the clotting time at approximately double the control. If the continuous-infusion method is used, the clotting tests can be performed at any time, while with the intermittent-infusion method, the tests are performed approximately 4 hours after a bolus of heparin has been given. Coagulation tests are performed at least once a day.

Watch for hemorrhagic areas on the patient's skin or microscopic hematuria, because these often indicate excessive anticoagulation and allow reversal of the anticoagulant effect before serious hemorrhage occurs.

In case of hemorrhagic side effects, the effects of heparin can be reversed in minutes by IV administration of **protamine** given in a 2 mg/ml solution (5 ml of a 1% solution is mixed with 20 ml of saline). The protamine is injected slowly IV, with no more than 50 mg given in any 10-minute period. If the protamine is needed just after a dose of heparin has been given, the amount of protamine required may be calculated by assuming that 1 mg of protamine will neutralize approximately 100 units of heparin; however, the package insert for heparin should be checked, since preparations vary. After a half-hour has elapsed since the last heparin dose, the dose of protamine is usually 1 mg/ml. If 4 hours or more have passed, no protamine is given, since an overdose of protamine may produce a hemorrhagic state. **Side effects** include hypotension, bradycardia, dyspnea, and flushing.

Coumarin effects can be reversed in 6–12 hours after the IV injection of 50 mg of vitamin K, provided the liver is functioning properly. Rapid reversal of coumarin effects can be achieved by administering fresh frozen plasma IV, starting with 15–20 ml/kg, followed by one-third the dose at 8–12-hour intervals.

(3) Antiplatelet agents. Although the effectiveness of platelet-inhibiting drugs, such as aspirin, dipyridamole (Persantine), and sulfinpyrazone (Anturane), has not yet been established in the treatment of stroke, large well-designed long-term studies are in progress. There is evidence of some effectiveness in preventing embolic complications in patients with prosthetic cardiac valves. Because the risk of hemorrhagic side effects may be smaller with these agents, they may be tried as alternative forms of therapy in patients in whom the coumarin agents and heparin are contraindicated.

In this situation, aspirin is given in a dose of 600 mg PO BID. Dipyridamole (50 mg PO TID) or sulfinpyrazone (200 mg PO TID) may be given along with aspirin, although the combinations have not been shown to be more effective than each individual agent used alone.

Although the side effects of aspirin are numerous, the major ones at this dosage are gastrointestinal, with gastric irritation and aggravation of peptic ulcer disease. Side effects with dipyridamole are uncommon but include headache, dizziness, nausea, flushing, weakness or syncope, mild gastrointestinal distress, and skin rash. Sulfinpyrazone, a uricosuric agent, can lead to urolithiasis and upper gastrointestinal disturbances, with aggravation of peptic ulcer disease, skin rash, anemia, leukopenia, agranulocytosis, and thrombocytopenia. It may augment the effect of the coumarins.

(4) Indications for anticoagulation. Anticoagulants may be beneficial in the following situations, except when a surgical lesion is present in the carotid artery, in which case surgery is the treatment of choice.

(a) Transient ischemic attacks (TIAs). Approximately one-third of patients with TIAs will go on to develop a cerebral infarct. Long-term therapy with the coumarin agents has been shown to be effective in preventing further TIAs and perhaps in lowering the incidence of subsequent cerebral infarction.

If there are no contraindications, one of the coumarin drugs is administered indefinitely according to the guidelines discussed. When no lesion is demonstrated and no source of embolism is identified, there is less certainty about what to do. Probably antiplatelet agents are the safest choice in this situation.

(b) Stroke-in-evolution. Early in the course of a thrombotic stroke-in-evolution, before maximum injury has occurred, the acute administration of heparin may prevent further damage. Maintenance warfarin or bishydroxycoumarin is started along with the heparin, and after the therapeutic coumarin effect is achieved (in 5–6 days), the heparin is discontinued and the coumarin is continued indefinitely.

(c) Completed stroke. Unfortunately, once completion of a stroke has occurred, nothing can be done to reverse the damage. When the deficit is so severe there is little hope for a reasonably normal existence, most would agree that little can be done. However, when the patient is not totally devastated, measures are directed toward preventing a recurrence of the stroke. It is well to keep in mind that most nonfatal strokes are associated with some degree of improvement, and one should not give up hope too early.

Anticoagulation may be effective in preventing a recurrent stroke, especially in the case of embolic infarction. Maintenance therapy with one of the coumarin agents can be started on admittance, and it is continued indefinitely. If there is any evidence that multiple emboli are being generated, then heparin is also probably given for 5–6 days until an adequate coumarin effect is attained.

Although hemorrhagic infarction is a complication of embolism, heparin usually does not worsen the situation if gross hemorrhage has been ruled out by the initial lumbar puncture and CT scan, if available. As previously stated, while CSF examination may be negative early in hemorrhagic infarction, it is almost always positive by 48 hours.

Patients with lacunar infarcts are not anticoagulated except when they are at the TIA stage. While the data are inconclusive with regard to anticoagulation for embolic complications of infective endocarditis, these patients probably should not be anticoagulated because of the risk of hemorrhage.

b. Surgery. Carotid endarterectomy is the most commonly performed surgical procedure for ischemic cerebrovascular disease. Also, surgery may be effective for the rare cases of symptomatic extracranial vertebral artery disease, subclavian steal, and aortic arch disease. As previously mentioned, posterior fossa decompression can be lifesaving in the case of massive cerebellar infarction and brainstem compression.

Therapeutic value has not yet been established for the newer procedures currently under evaluation, such as anastomosis of the temporal artery to the middle cerebral artery, saphenous vein bypass graft from the carotid artery to the middle cerebral artery, and anastomosis of the occipital artery to the basilar or posterior inferior cerebellar artery.

Carotid endarterectomy is probably the treatment of choice in the following situations rather than long-term anticoagulation, provided there are no serious medical contraindications to surgery.

(1) TIAs. Carotid endarterectomy is indicated for hemispheric TIAs in the carotid territory when either an ulcerated plaque or severe stenosis (defined by narrowing of the lumen to 2 mm or less) is demonstrated by angiography.

(2) Completed stroke and stroke-in-evolution. When carotid artery disease leads to massive infarction of a cerebral hemisphere, surgical results are poor. However, carotid endarterectomy is indicated when there is less than maximum damage and the potential for an acceptable recovery exists. Potential surgical lesions include ulcerated plaque, severe stenosis (2 mm or less), and acute occlusion. Although coexisting asymptomatic stenosis or occlusion of the contralateral carotid artery may be present, this does not alter the decision to operate on the symptomatic side.

The timing of the surgical procedure is a subject of controversy. Some think that sudden restoration of blood flow to an area of infarction may result in a more serious hemorrhagic infarct and will delay surgery for days to weeks. However, with a fluctuating or progressive deficit, such as a stroke-in-evolution, early revascularization may be very important; and if the blood pressure is maintained in the normal range at surgery and postoperatively, the hemorrhagic complication is usually avoided.

(3) Asymptomatic occlusion or stenosis. Old carotid occlusions usually cause no symptoms and do not require surgery. Although the natural course of asymptomatic carotid artery stenosis has not yet been determined, at the present time these patients are not usually referred for carotid endarterectomy.

(4) If the carotid artery has clearly been the source of the symptoms, the patient is not usually put on anticoagulants postoperatively.

(5) When a surgical carotid lesion is present but severe coexisting medical illness precludes an operation, anticoagulants are administered according to the guidelines in sec **I.C.2.a.**

    c. Antiedema agents. Corticosteroids have not been shown to be useful in cerebral infarction, although there is some evidence that they are effective in reducing cerebral edema in other conditions. They are withheld in cerebral infarction unless there are signs of increased intracranial pressure, such as obtundation, coma, or signs of herniation. In this situation, dexamethasone is given in an initial bolus of 10 mg IV or IM, followed by 4 mg IV or IM every 4–6 hours. Glycerol (1 gm/kg PO every 6 hours) may be substituted or used adjunctly with dexamethasone.

    d. Anticonvulsants. Some patients with cerebral infarction develop seizures, but this is usually a late complication. Anticonvulsants are usually withheld until there is evidence of a seizure disorder.

    e. Vasodilators. In spite of evidence that cerebral blood flow is increased by amyl nitrate, papaverine, isoxsuprine, acetazolamide, carbon dioxide, and other agents, these agents do not seem to alter the course of ischemic strokes favorably. Indeed, some feel that the resultant vasodilation from these agents reduces perfusion to the area of ischemia (so-called intracerebral steal).

    f. Others. While other agents have been tried in brief clinical trials in the treatment of stroke, there is little evidence that they have therapeutic value. These include low-molecular-weight dextran, clofibrate, and thrombolytic agents, such as streptokinase and urokinase.

  3. In the recovery phase, where some degree of improvement almost always occurs, **speech, occupational,** and **physical therapy** are beneficial.

II. HEMORRHAGIC STROKES. The most common varieties of hemorrhagic stroke are hypertensive intracerebral hemorrhage and subarachnoid hemorrhage secondary to ruptured saccular aneurysm or arteriovenous malformation. Other less common causes of hemorrhage are anticoagulants, bleeding diatheses, trauma, hemorrhage into a primary or metastatic brain tumor, idiopathic subarachnoid hemorrhage, and rupture of a mycotic aneurysm. Rare causes include carotid cavernous arteriovenous fistulas, hemorrhage after vasopressor drugs, hemorrhage on exertion, encephalitis, and pituitary apoplexy.

A. Hypertensive intracerebral hemorrhage

  1. Description. Hypertensive hemorrhage proceeds from the small penetrating vessels of the brain that have been damaged by hypertension. As a consequence, the hemorrhage almost always arises in the following locations in decreasing order of frequency: putamen, thalamus, pons, and cerebellum. Hemorrhage secondary to anticoagulants, bleeding diatheses, or trauma often involves other areas of the brain, such as the frontal, temporal, or occipital lobes—sites rarely involved with hypertensive hemorrhage. The onset of intracerebral hemorrhage is abrupt, and the stroke usually evolves gradually over minutes or hours without the stepwise progression seen in thrombotic strokes.

    a. Putaminal hemorrhage. When first seen, patients with putaminal hemorrhage often present a clinical picture that is almost indistinguishable from that of middle cerebral artery occlusion, with contralateral hemiplegia, hemianesthesia, homonymous hemianopsia, aphasia (if the dominant hemisphere is involved), and hemineglect, anosognosia, and the like, with nondominant hemispheral involvement. There is usually a greater alteration in the state of consciousness in patients with hemorrhage. Smaller hemorrhages produce more restricted deficits, while larger ones may produce coma and signs of herniation.

    b. Thalamic hemorrhage. Thalamic hemorrhage produces contralateral hemiparesis or hemiplegia with contralateral hemianesthesia. The sensory loss may be disproportionately greater than the motor deficit. Unusual eye signs provide a clue to the diagnosis of thalamic hemorrhage. Often there is restriction of upward gaze, at times with forced downward deviation of the eyes, and skew deviation of the eyes is common. The eyes may even be deviated conjugately away from the side of the lesion (so-called wrong-going eyes). As in putaminal hemorrhage, massive hemorrhage in the thalamus leads to coma and signs of herniation.

c. **Pontine hemorrhage.** Pontine hemorrhage usually results in early coma, pinpoint pupils that react to light, and bilateral decerebrate posturing. The eyes are often in midposition, with impaired or absent response to caloric testing. More restricted hemorrhages in the pons, although uncommon, may produce deficits that resemble those seen in pontine infarction.

d. **Cerebellar hemorrhage.** Cerebellar hemorrhage is a diagnosis not to be missed, since with proper treatment this type of hemorrhage has by far the greatest potential for complete recovery. Patients typically develop sudden dizziness and vomiting, along with marked truncal ataxia. On examination they are unable to stand or walk because of the ataxia. They are often perfectly alert early in the course. Frequently there are signs of compression of the ipsilateral pons, such as paresis of lateral conjugate gaze to the side of the lesion, ipsilateral sixth-nerve weakness, ipsilateral facial weakness, and diminished corneal reflex on the affected side. Untreated, they rapidly progress to coma and death from brainstem compression. It is critically important to make the diagnosis early, since surgical evacuation of the hematoma can result in complete recovery.

2. **Diagnosis.** General guidelines for the diagnosis of intracerebral hemorrhage are provided in sec **II.A.** Almost all cerebellar and pontine hemorrhages produce bloody spinal fluid, as do most hemorrhages in the putamen and thalamus. Some of the small hemorrhages in the putamen and thalamus may not show blood in the CSF early; however, as previously mentioned, the spinal fluid is almost always positive within 48 hours.

Lumbar puncture is performed without worry of producing herniation in most cases of intracerebral hemorrhage. Although lumbar puncture may be safe in the case of cerebellar hemorrhage, if CT scan can be performed without delay, one might forego lumbar puncture. CT scan is the procedure of choice, if available, to confirm the diagnosis of intracerebral hemorrhage and to determine the extent of damage. The pons is the only area where hemorrhage might be missed by CT scan. When CT scan is not available, angiography often shows an avascular mass in the region of hemorrhage.

3. **Treatment**

a. **General measures.** The same general measures listed in the section on ischemic stroke apply to the management of intracerebral hemorrhage, with the exception of blood-pressure control. In the patient with intracerebral hemorrhage, efforts are made to maintain the blood pressure in the normal range.

b. **Antiedema agents.** Patients with intracerebral hemorrhage may have considerable cerebral edema and, if drowsiness or evidence of herniation is present, antiedema agents, such as steroids or glycerol, are given in the doses already discussed.

Because of their transient effect, mannitol or urea has no place in the management of intracerebral hemorrhage, except when it is given just before surgery or as a last-resort effort to reverse herniation.

c. **Surgery.** Evacuation of a hematoma in the cerebellum can be lifesaving. If this diagnosis is suspected, the neurosurgeon is contacted early in the course to avoid any delay. Procedures for evacuation of clots in the putamen, thalamus, and even the pons are under investigation, although it is too early to reach any firm conclusions regarding their effectiveness.

   d. **Anticonvulsants.** Anticonvulsants are withheld until there is evidence of seizure activity.

   e. **Clotting abnormalities.** In those patients with hemorrhage secondary to clotting abnormalities or anticoagulant therapy, appropriate measures are taken to reverse the abnormality (e.g., platelets for thrombocytopenia, fresh frozen plasma and vitamin K for coumarin agents, and protamine for heparin).

B. Subarachnoid hemorrhage

1. Description

   a. **Aneurysmal rupture.** Subarachnoid hemorrhage most commonly results from rupture of a saccular aneurysm, which is a defect in the arterial wall that occurs at sites of arterial bifurcation or branching. The majority of patients who experience rupture are between the ages of 35 and 65 years. Associated conditions include polycystic kidneys and coarctation of the aorta. Other aneurysms occur along the trunk of the internal carotid, vertebral, or basilar arteries, and they are described in terms of their morphology: fusiform, globular, or diffuse. These aneurysms may cause symptoms by compressing local structures or thrombosis, but they seldom rupture. A rare cause of subarachnoid hemorrhage is rupture of a mycotic aneurysm, resulting from septic embolism. Unfortunately, aneurysms are usually asymptomatic until they rupture.

   Typically there is a sudden onset of severe headache, usually the worst headache the patient has ever experienced. The patient may or may not lose consciousness, which may herald the onset of coma, although often the patient reawakens somewhat confused. At times the loss of consciousness is sudden and unaccompanied by headache. The event often occurs during physical exertion, such as during sexual intercourse. Although patients with ruptured cerebral aneurysms usually have supportive clinical signs, their examination may be perfectly normal early, and a high index of suspicion is in order for patients with **severe** headache of **sudden** onset. On examination, signs of **meningeal irritation** are common as well as a **low-grade fever.** Subhyaloid **hemorrhages** are often seen on funduscopic examination.

   The hemorrhage may be only subarachnoid or blood may dissect into the brain parenchyma itself, resulting in **focal neurologic deficits. Infarction** early in the course may also result from compromise of blood flow or thrombosis in the arteries involved by the aneurysm. Clinical localization of the aneurysm is usually difficult, although **certain signs** may be helpful (e.g., pain behind the eye and dysfunction of cranial nerves II to VI with cavernous carotid artery aneurysms; hemiplegia, aphasia, etc., with middle cerebral artery aneurysms; third-nerve palsy with aneurysm at the juncture of the posterior communicating and internal carotid arteries; abulia or weakness of the lower limb with anterior communicating artery aneurysms; and involvement of the lower cranial nerves with basilar and vertebral artery aneurysms).

   Neurologic deficits that occur 2–3 days after the initial hemorrhage, either transient or permanent, are often caused by **vasospasm,** resulting from the presence of blood in the subarachnoid space.

   Hydrocephalus may occur as an early or late complication of subarachnoid hemorrhage, although it usually does not occur before a week or longer after the initial hemorrhage.

   b. **Vascular malformations.** Vascular malformations or angiomas are usually brought to clinical attention because of seizures or hemorrhage, although large ones may shunt enough blood to result in ischemia of the surrounding brain. Symptoms are most likely to occur in childhood or young adulthood. Since they commonly extend from the surface into the brain parenchyma, hemorrhage from these malformations is often a combination of intracerebral and subarachnoid hemorrhage. A chronic headache is a common complaint prior to hemorrhage, and the presence of a bruit over the eyeball, carotid artery, or mastoid of a young patient strongly suggests the presence of a cerebral angioma.

In any large series of patients with subarachnoid hemorrhage, a considerable number will have no demonstrable lesion. At least some of these result from rupture of so-called cryptic arteriovenous malformations, which are too small to be detected angiographically. Spinal arteriovenous malformations must be considered in young patients with subarachnoid hemorrhage and no demonstrable cerebral lesion. Also, a bruit may sometimes be heard over the spine in these patients.

2. **Diagnosis**

   a. **CSF examination.** Bloody cerebrospinal fluid on lumbar puncture examination is the sine qua non of subarachnoid hemorrhage. Traumatic tap can usually be ruled out according to the guidelines in sec **I.B.1.**

   b. **Skull x-rays** may show calcification in an arteriovenous malformation and occasionally in an aneurysm.

   c. **Angiography.** Many would perform angiography shortly after admission to clarify the picture fully. This is particularly important when diagnostic confusion exists between ruptured aneurysm or arteriovenous malformation and hypertensive intracerebral hemorrhage. However, one of the mainstays of early therapy for ruptured aneurysm is avoidance of stress, and angiography is a somewhat stressful procedure.

   If a surgically accessible lesion exists, such as an aneurysm, then a repeat angiogram is usually performed just before surgery. For this reason, postponement of angiography until a time when surgery might be contemplated is an acceptable alternative in those patients whose history strongly suggests ruptured aneurysm.

   d. If no lesions are demonstrated by cerebral angiography and no localizing neurologic signs are present, probably no further diagnostic studies are indicated for middle-aged to elderly adults. In **children** or **young adults,** spinal angiography must be strongly considered, especially if a bruit is heard over the vertebral column.

   e. Other lesions that produce subarachnoid hemorrhage and may at times present some diagnostic confusion, such as hypertensive intracerebral hemorrhage or hemorrhage into a tumor, are usually demonstrated by angiogram. The CT scan is useful in further characterizing these lesions.

3. **Treatment.** Surgery is the treatment of choice for aneurysms that are surgically accessible in suitable candidates. In the preoperative period, therapeutic efforts are directed toward prevention and treatment of the two most important complications: **recurrent hemorrhage** and **vasospasm.** Arteriovenous malformations may or may not be amenable to surgery. Since there is risk of recurrent hemorrhage from arteriovenous malformations (AVMs), although less than that for aneurysms, the preoperative measures listed as follows apply in the early period after bleeding.

   a. **Preoperative measures**

      (1) **General precautions**

         (a) **Elevation of blood pressure is avoided** if possible. If hypertension exists, antihypertensive drugs are used to maintain the blood pressure in the normal range.

(b) Sedation with phenobarbital or diazepam is instituted to prevent excitement and elevation of blood pressure.

(c) Seizures are a complication and raise the blood pressure, so prophylactic anticonvulsants are given. Phenobarbital is an effective anticonvulsant (starting dose, 30 mg PO TID) and may serve a dual purpose: sedative and anticonvulsant.

(d) To prevent straining with bowel movements, **stool softeners** are given, such as dioctyl sodium sulfosuccinate (Colace), 100 mg PO TID.

(e) The room is darkened and loud noises are avoided to prevent startling the patient.

(2) Antifibrinolytic agents. It is thought that lysis of the clot formed at the point of bleeding is partly responsible for recurrent hemorrhage from aneurysms and arteriovenous malformations. This provides some rationale for the use of antifibrinolytic agents; and, indeed, the early studies suggest considerable efficacy of these agents in preventing rebleeding.

Epsilon-aminocaproic acid (Amicar) 30–36 gm/day is given IV. This is usually prepared by mixing 30–36 gm in 1 L of dextrose 2½% and saline 0.45% or a similar solution. The mixture is infused over 24 hours with a microdrip apparatus. Alternatively, the drug may be administered PO, but if so it must be given at least every 3 hours (4 gm PO every 3 hours). The drug is continued until the time of surgery, or for 6 weeks if surgery is contraindicated. **Complications** include nausea, cramps, diarrhea, dizziness, tinnitus, conjunctival suffusion, nasal stuffiness, headache, skin rash, thrombophlebitis, and pulmonary embolus.

(3) Antiedema agents. Corticosteroids or glycerol are given if there are signs of increased intracranial pressure, as discussed previously.

(4) Antivasospasm agents. Vasospasm may be responsible for drowsiness or focal neurologic signs, but these signs do not usually occur until 2–3 days after the initial hemorrhage. The spasm is thought to result from the release of vasoactive compounds, one of the most important of which is serotonin. Although agents that deplete serotonin stores in the body are being evaluated, such as reserpine and kanamycin, their effectiveness has not been established. Intravenous **isoproterenol,** with its beta-adrenergic vasodilatory effects, is currently being evaluated. If spasm occurs, it is often necessary to raise the blood pressure to prevent infarction of brain tissue that is supplied by the constricted arteries.

The concomitant use of pressors (e.g., **dopamine** or **isoproterenol**) and vasodilators (e.g., **nitroprusside** or **nitroglycerine**) may be useful in this circumstance, but definite data regarding the efficacy of this therapy are still lacking. The risk of rebleeding is probably raised as the blood pressure is increased, but this risk must sometimes be taken to prevent severely disabling or even fatal cerebral infarction due to arterial spasm.

b. Surgery. Patients who undergo surgery for ruptured aneurysm generally fare somewhat better than those who are treated medically, because of the sharp reduction in the incidence of rebleeding with surgery. The decision to operate is made with the guidance of the neurosurgeon and depends to a certain extent on his or her preferences. However, certain generalizations can be made.

Surgery is not usually performed on patients in coma or with severe neurologic deficits because of the high mortality and low potential for recovery. The mortality is high for surgery undertaken in the first 24 hours following hemorrhage, so operation is usually delayed for a few days at least. On the other hand, a large number of recurrent hemorrhages will have occurred by 2 weeks, so surgery is not postponed indefinitely. Repeat (or initial) angiography is usually performed on the day before surgery, and if significant vasospasm is present, the operation is delayed until this has disappeared.

Various procedures have been devised for dealing with aneurysms surgically (e.g., clipping the neck of the aneurysm, wrapping it with muscle, coating it with plastic, and occluding the internal carotid artery in the neck). In those in whom surgery is contraindicated, embolization procedures are sometimes employed in an effort to induce thrombosis of the aneurysm, using such material as horse hair and iron filings. When surgery is contraindicated, the preoperative measures already listed are continued for approximately 6 weeks, after which time activity is gradually increased.

Block resection or ligation of the major arteries is done for arteriovenous malformations, although the importance of the involved vessels in supplying blood to critical areas of the brain often precludes this form of therapy. When this is the case, embolic procedures may be used, employing such material as gel foam and silastic balls. Conventional x-ray irradiation of arteriovenous malformations in an attempt to induce hyalinization and occlusion of the involved vessels has been used in the past with little success. However, radiotherapy using a proton beam has enabled more accurate focusing of the beam and has produced encouraging results.

Hydrocephalus may occur as an early or late complication of subarachnoid hemorrhage and may require a shunt procedure.

SELECTED READINGS

Ischemic Strokes
Fisher, C. M.   The use of anticoagulants in cerebral thrombosis. *Neurology* 8:311, 1958.
Fisher, C. M.   Anticoagulant therapy in cerebral thrombosis and cerebral embolism: A national cooperative study, interim report. *Neurology* 11: (Part 2) 199, 1961.
Genton, E., Gent, M., Hirsh, J., and Harker, L. A.   Platelet inhibiting drugs in the prevention of clinical thrombotic disease (First of three parts). *N. Engl. J. Med.* 293:1174, 1975.
Lehrich, J. R., Winkler, G. F., and Ojemann, R. G.   Cerebellar infarction with brain stem compression. *Arch. Neurol.* 22:490, 1970.
Millikan, C. H.   Reassessment of anticoagulant therapy in various types of occlusive cerebrovascular disease. *Stroke* 2:201, 1971.
Ojemann, R. G., Crowell, R. M., Roberson, G. H., and Fisher, C. M.   *Clin. Neurosurg.*, Vol. 22, The Congress of Neurological Surgeons, 1975.

Hemorrhagic Strokes
Browne, T. R., and Poskanzer, D. C.   Treatment of strokes. (Second of 2 parts) *N. Engl. J. Med.* 281:650, 1969.
Nibbelink, D. W., cited by Millikan, C. H.   Summary of the ninth Princeton conference on cerebral vascular disease, January 9–11, 1974. *Stroke* 5:249, 1974.
Sengupta, R. P., So, S. C., and Villarejo-Ortega, F. J.   Use of epsilon aminocaproic acid in the preoperative management of ruptured intracranial aneurysms. *J. Neurosurg.* 44:479, 1976.
Walshe, T., Hier, D.   The diagnosis of intracerebral hemorrhage. Submitted for publication.

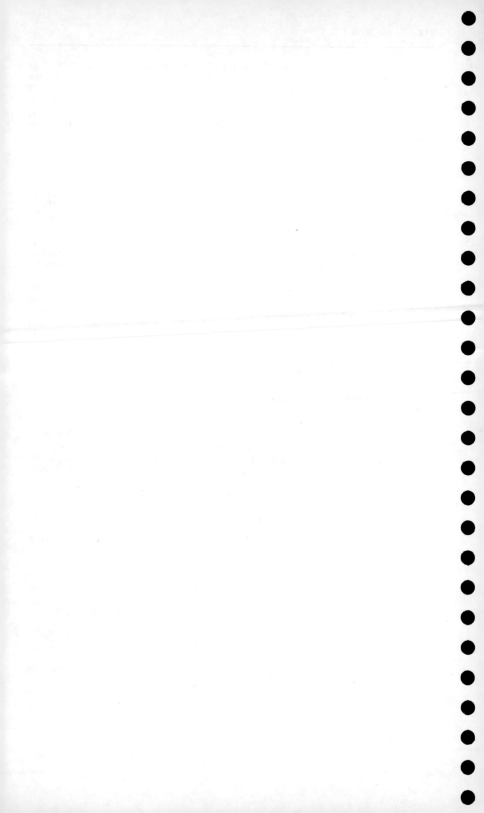

Neoplasms

I. INTRODUCTION

A. Classification. Many different histologic types of neoplasms can arise in the central nervous system. For example, there are tumors of glial cell origin (e.g., astrocytoma, glioblastoma multiforme, oligodendroglioma, and ependymoma), tumors of meningeal origin (e.g., meningioma), tumors of nerve sheath origin (e.g., schwannoma and neurofibroma), tumors of primitive bipotential cells (e.g., medulloblastoma and pineal germinoma), and metastatic tumors (e.g., from lung cancer, melanoma, and breast cancer). Figure 11-1 is a simplified classification of the most common neoplasms of the central nervous system.

B. Prevalence. Malignancy of the brain is not rare; there are approximately 8500 deaths per year in the United States due to primary brain tumors and many more due to metastases.

C. Symptoms. All tumors of the nervous system cause signs and symptoms by five main mechanisms.

1. **Direct (local) effects.** Some examples are tumors that disrupt the optic radiations, producing contralateral hemianopsia; and schwannomas of the acoustic nerve, producing ipsilateral hearing loss.

2. **Effects related to cerebral edema and increased intracranial pressure.** The edema surrounding a cerebral neoplasm increases the neurologic deficits by compressing nearby structures. Brain edema may also cause a marked increase in intracranial pressure, with headache, vomiting, papilledema, and, ultimately, fatal cerebral herniation.

3. **Indirect effects.** One example is a midline cerebellar tumor that may compress the aqueduct of Sylvius, thereby causing symptomatic internal (noncommunicating) hydrocephalus.

4. **Convulsions.** A supratentorial neoplasm may produce focal or generalized seizures.

5. **Remote effects.** Examples are the Eaton-Lambert syndrome, cerebellar degeneration, and progressive multifocal leukoencephalopathy.

The location of the tumor is usually of greater importance than the histology in evaluating the patient's symptoms.

D. Diagnosis. Both the **histology** and the **neuroanatomic** localization of the lesion(s) must be known to determine the best treatment and assess the prognosis. With relatively few exceptions, this implies obtaining a biopsy of the tumor before instituting or withholding other forms of therapy.

There are often preoperative clues to the correct diagnosis. For example, posterior fossa tumors in adults are more likely to be metastases than primary CNS neoplasms. Also, relatively slow-growing tumors (such as meningiomas, low-grade astrocytomas, oligodendrogliomas, and craniopharyngiomas) frequently show abnormal calcification on skull radiographs, whereas malignant gliomas and metastases rarely, if ever, calcify.

Numerous ancillary studies are available for the diagnosis of brain tumor. The most important ones are as follows:

1. **Skull x-rays** may show evidence of increased intracranial pressure (e.g., demineralization of the dorsum sella or floor of the sella turcica), mass effect (shift of the pineal organ from the midline), or abnormal calcifications (e.g., in a craniopharyngioma, meningioma, or oligodendroglioma). In children sep-

216

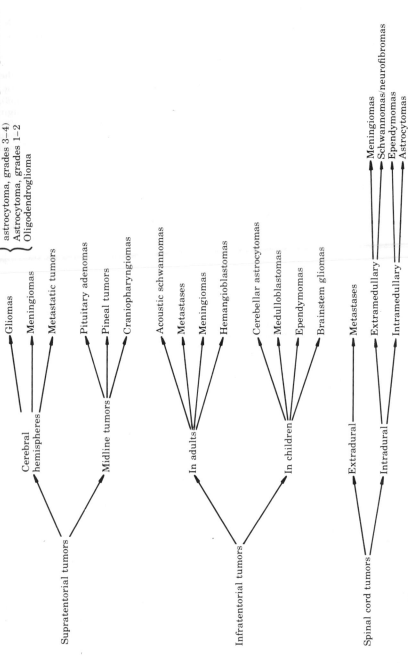

Fig. 11-1. Most frequent CNS tumors and their sites of predilection.

Supratentorial tumors

Cerebral hemispheres → Gliomas, Meningiomas, Metastatic tumors

Gliomas → { Glioblastoma multiforme (malignant glioma and astrocytoma, grades 3–4), Astrocytoma, grades 1–2, Oligodendroglioma }

Midline tumors → Pituitary adenomas, Pineal tumors, Craniopharyngiomas

Infratentorial tumors

In adults → Acoustic schwannomas, Metastases, Meningiomas, Hemangioblastomas

In children → Cerebellar astrocytomas, Medulloblastomas, Ependymomas, Brainstem gliomas

Spinal cord tumors

Extradural → Metastases

Intradural → Extramedullary → Meningiomas, Schwannomas/neurofibromas

Intramedullary → Ependymomas, Astrocytomas

aration of sutures is the most frequent sign of increased intracranial pressure.

2. **EEG** is abnormal in most patients with supratentorial tumor, often revealing focal disturbance.

3. **CT scan** reveals the presence of most supratentorial tumors and also allows detection of cerebral edema, mass effect, and associated hydrocephalus. The sensitivity of CT scanning for brain tumors is increased by obtaining scans with and without intravenous contrast material. Unfortunately, some posterior fossa tumors can escape detection on CT scan.

4. **Radionuclide brain scan** reveals most supratentorial and some posterior fossa tumors. Radionuclide scans will miss some tumors that are detectable by CT scan, and they do not reveal information about cerebral edema or ventricular size.

5. **Arteriography** shows the vascular supply of some tumors, and it provides indirect evidence for mass effect (displaced vessels).

6. **Pneumoencephalography** (PEG) outlines subarachnoid cisterns and the ventricular system (which is especially useful for the evaluation of posterior fossa, suprasellar, and third-ventricle tumors).

7. **Lumbar puncture** may reveal increased intracranial pressure or nonspecific findings, such as elevated protein. Lumbar puncture is potentially dangerous in patients with intracranial mass lesions and **should not** be part of the routine preoperative evaluation of most patients with brain tumor.

8. **CSF cytology.** Malignant cells are found in the CSF in patients with meningeal carcinomatosis and meningeal leukemia. CSF cytology is the only way to confirm either of these diagnoses, and it sometimes gives positive evidence of medulloblastoma, pineal tumors, and ependymoma.

However, there is still no substitute for histologic diagnosis, since, despite the recent advances in diagnostic techniques (see sec **I.D**), patients who are suspected of harboring an untreatable malignant glioma are still occasionally found to have a treatable meningioma or brain abscess.

II. **CORTICOSTEROIDS FOR TUMOR-RELATED BRAIN EDEMA.** Although only palliative, no drug other than the corticosteroids has had as great an impact on the preoperative and postoperative management of patients with brain tumor.

A. **Mechanism of action.** Corticosteroids can decrease cerebral edema in patients with brain tumors. As already mentioned, most brain tumors (primary or metastatic) cause edema in the surrounding brain parenchyma. If the edema is considerable or widespread, it can produce a marked increase in intracranial pressure and produce new deficits by compressing nearby structures. Thus in some patients the neurologic deficits may be more a reflection of uncontrolled cerebral edema than actual tumor destruction of the brain. The mechanism by which steroids act to reduce cerebral edema is not known.

B. **Clinical effects.** Improvement in neurologic signs (e.g., papilledema, aphasia, and hemiparesis) and symptoms (e.g., headache and lethargy) begins within 12–24 hours in a significant number of patients treated with very large doses of steroids (Table 11-1). Also, the clinical improvement may be more dramatic in patients with metastatic tumors than in those with primary brain tumors. The maximum degree of improvement is usually obtained by the fourth or fifth day, although further improvement may continue for several weeks.

C. **Choice of corticosteroid.** A variety of glucocorticoids (e.g., prednisone, methylprednisolone, hydrocortisone, and dexamethasone) have been of benefit in relieving tumor-related edema. Dexamethasone has been the most widely used steroid due to its relatively insignificant salt-retaining side effects. There is no evidence,

Table 11-1. Improvement of Neurologic Signs and Symptoms Following Steroid Treatment in Patients with Primary or Metastatic Brain Tumors

Symptom	Percent of Patients in Whom Symptoms Were Improved by Dexamethasone Therapy (4 mg every 6 hours)
Headache, vomiting, lethargy	89
Papilledema	37
Hemiparesis	70
Hemisensory deficit	56
Visual field deficit	31

Data from French and Galicich, 1962.

however, that there is a significant difference among these drugs in relieving cerebral edema when they are used in equivalent doses.

D. Initial dose. The use of steroids in brain tumor patients was derived from empirical observations, and most clinical studies have employed different dosages of steroid administration. Consequently, the information regarding optimal dosage is largely anecdotal.

However, several guidelines have been established. For example, there is a clear dose-dependency of clinical response to corticosteroids. The great majority of patients with brain tumors who respond favorably to steroids do so with dexamethasone 4–5 mg, given PO or parenterally, every 6 hours. This is a very large dose of steroid (dexamethasone 20 mg/day is roughly equivalent to prednisone 130 mg/day); but there is no advantage to starting therapy at lower doses, because the drug toxicity is similar, while the therapeutic benefit may be greatly diminished.

Most neurologists begin a course of treatment with an initial loading dose of dexamethasone 10 mg parenterally. If 5 mg every 6 hours does not produce some clinical improvement, a trial at even higher doses may be warranted. Also, administering dexamethasone in daily divided doses seems to be necessary, because some patients begin to suffer recurrent symptoms if there is a prolonged interval between doses.

Many patients do not have a favorable clinical response to dexamethasone at total doses of 20 mg/day. These patients may show improvement if the total dose is increased to 32 mg/day or even as high as 96 mg/day. These doses are well tolerated and do not increase the incidence of serious complications during short-term use.

E. Indications. Steroid therapy is indicated for brain tumor patients who have progressive, disabling neurologic signs and symptoms that can be at least partially attributed to brain edema. For example, a patient who develops intractable headaches and papilledema is a logical candidate for steroid therapy. Steroids are also extremely valuable for reducing cerebral edema in the perioperative period; and steroid therapy has been a major factor in reducing the morbidity and mortality associated with neurosurgical procedures.

F. Duration of treatment. It is difficult to give rational guidelines for the optimal length of steroid treatment. (There is currently no way to predict the duration of favorable steroid response or whether the patient will tolerate tapering dosages). Some patients will relapse before the steroid dosage has been tapered, and others will suffer a recurrence of neurologic dysfunction when the dosage is tapered below a critical level. In these patients, high dosages are reinstituted and most will improve again, although some patients will never return to their previous level of function.

A smaller group of patients remain neurologically stable while steroids are tapered to a low maintenance dosage or discontinued. These patients may continue comfortably on an ambulatory basis for weeks or even months before symptoms recur. Empirically, high-dose steroid therapy should be continued for 10 days or more before dosage reduction is contemplated.

G. **Effect of corticosteroids on prognosis.** It seems that steroid therapy alone does not dramatically alter the patient's length of survival or ultimate prognosis. In most cases the favorable response to steroids lasts for only a matter of weeks. If other potentially helpful therapies (e.g., surgery or radiotherapy) have already failed to arrest the tumor growth, the patient's death is often imminent. Thus although steroids have done much to relieve the operative mortality and diminish the postoperative morbidity, their use is strictly a palliative measure.

H. **Side effects.** The complications and side effects of steroid therapy in brain tumor patients are similar to those that occur in any other group of patients (e.g., hypothalamic-pituitary-adrenal axis suppression, carbohydrate intolerance, Cushing's syndrome, and "steroid psychosis"). However, fear of inducing iatrogenic side effects is seldom a good reason for withholding steroid therapy from patients with brain tumor.

I. **Osmotic agents for lowering intracranial pressure acutely.** Occasionally patients with brain tumor suffer a sudden dramatic increase in intracranial pressure (e.g., due to hemorrhage within the tumor), with signs of cerebral herniation and imminent death. Situations in which a very rapid reduction in intracranial pressure is needed are indications for therapy with osmotic agents, such as mannitol, glucose 50% in water, glycerol, or urea.

Rapid infusion of hypertonic solutions of mannitol quickly reduces brain water by creating an osmotic gradient between the brain and plasma. When mannitol 1 gm/kg is given over 10–15 minutes (i.e., about 250 ml of a 20% solution in an average adult), a reduction of intracranial pressure of 30–60% can be expected for 2–4 hours. It is important to administer mannitol with a filter in the IV apparatus to prevent undissolved crystals from entering the circulation. At the same time steroid therapy should be started for its longer-term antiedema effects.

A massive osmotic diuresis will follow mannitol therapy, so all patients should have a bladder catheter inserted and careful monitoring of fluid and electrolyte balance. Smaller doses of mannitol (i.e., 0.25–0.5 gm/kg) may be repeated every few hours thereafter, if needed, to control intracranial pressure.

At some point after the administration of mannitol there is often a **rebound rise** in intracranial pressure. Thus hyperosmolar therapy is useful only in the short term until more definitive therapy, such as surgery and steroids, can be instituted.

Glycerol, an oral hyperosmolar agent, may be administered (1–5 ml/kg/day in divided doses) and eliminates the need for IV lines. Serum osmolarity and blood glucose should be monitored at least daily during glycerol therapy so that the dosage may be adjusted to avert serious hyperosmolarity syndromes.

III. BRAIN TUMORS IN ADULTS

A. Glioblastoma multiforme

1. **Incidence.** The most common primary brain tumor in adults is glioblastoma multiforme, which is also known as malignant glioma and astrocytoma, grades 3–4.

   There are approximately 5000 new cases of this disorder each year in the United States. The age of peak incidence is between 45 and 55 years, and males are more frequently afflicted than females by a ratio of 3:2. The tumor may arise in any portion of the cerebral hemispheres, the frontal and temporal lobes being the most frequent sites. The cerebellum, brainstem, and spinal cord are rare sites for glioblastoma multiforme.

2. **Prognosis.** Glioblastoma multiforme is a rapidly growing anaplastic tumor, with a uniformly fatal prognosis. Although these tumors are highly invasive within the CNS, they do not metastasize outside the nervous system. Several years ago a review of the medical literature (encompassing over 2000 cases) revealed the median survival of patients having these tumors to be approximately 5½ months. At the end of 1 year only 20% of patients were alive and fewer than 10% survived 2 years.

Unfortunately, the best modes of therapy currently available have not dramatically altered this dismal prognosis.

3. **Surgical therapy.** The surgical treatment of choice is open craniotomy followed by extensive resection. It is the most reliable method for obtaining adequate histologic sampling and results in "internal decompression" of the swollen brain. (Many neurosurgeons contend that internal decompression results in fewer cases of postoperative mortality than biopsy alone.) A limited biopsy is indicated only in those cases where extensive resection is not possible, such as a tumor of the basal ganglia.

Following internal decompression, patients may have significant temporary amelioration of their symptoms. Their overall survival time is not greatly lengthened, but aggressive surgical intervention probably prolongs the patient's useful period of survival.

Although glioblastomas often appear relatively well circumscribed on gross examination, the tumor invariably shows extensive microscopic infiltration into other regions. Infiltration into adjacent lobes or across cerebral commissures to the opposite hemisphere occurs commonly. Therefore, although the neurosurgeon may optimistically report "gross total removal of the tumor," the tumor will always recur, usually within months. Thus surgery cannot cure glioblastoma multiforme.

4. **Radiation therapy**

   a. **Dosage and fields.** Glioblastoma multiforme is not a "radiosensitive" tumor. However, the functional tolerance of the brain to radiation is relatively high, so a dose of 6000 rads (supervoltage) can be given with relative safety to the whole brain over a period of 6 weeks at five fractions per week. At even slightly higher doses there is a considerable risk of radiation-induced brain damage that outweighs any further therapeutic advantage.

   These tumors are widely invasive, and their full extent is never known with certainty. Therefore radiotherapy must be delivered to the whole brain (e.g., 5000–6000 rads over 5 or 6 weeks). Some radiotherapists advocate an additional "boost" of 1000–2000 rads to the primary tumor site in 1–2 weeks after the initial course of radiotherapy.

   b. **Complications of radiation therapy.** The complications of modern cranial irradiation are seldom significant and the incidence of radiation-induced brain damage is small if standard doses are used. Also, radiation, as described, does not increase cerebral edema significantly. Consequently, corticosteroids need not be administered to all patients during radiotherapy as prophylaxis against radiation-induced edema.

   All patients suffer loss of hair as a result of therapy, although in many instances the hair regrows over the next few months. Perhaps the greatest morbidity most patients suffer as a result of cranial irradiation is the extra 5 or 6 weeks during which they must either remain in the hospital or return each day for treatment. In view of the poor prognosis of glioblastoma, this is a considerable period.

   c. **Value of radiotherapy.** Many neurologists and neurosurgeons have been reluctant to refer their patients with glioblastoma for radiation therapy, because they question whether the treatments are of any real benefit.

However, recent clinical data from several sources have confirmed the value of cranial irradiation in glioblastoma multiforme.

The Brain Tumor Study Group prospectively evaluated several modes of therapy in over 160 patients with glioblastoma multiforme (Table 11-2). The median survival following surgery alone was only 17 weeks, whereas surgery followed by radiotherapy more than doubled the median survival to 38 weeks (a statistically significant difference). Although this difference is not impressive in the total life span of a human being, radiotherapy also results in considerable improvement in the quality of survival. Thus although cranial irradiation does not cure glioblastoma multiforme, it does ameliorate symptoms and lengthen short-term survival. These modest benefits justify the continued routine use of postoperative cranial irradiation in glioblastoma multiforme.

5. Chemotherapy

a. **Early drug trials.** The failure of surgery and radiation therapy to alter the grim prognosis dramatically has led to clinical trials of antineoplastic agents in glioblastoma multiforme. Over the past 20 years numerous chemotherapeutic agents, including nitrogen mustard, cyclophosphamide, 5-fluorouracil, methotrexate, vincristine, and mithramycin, have been employed against this type of tumor.

Although initial reports were enthusiastic for all these drugs, the studies were uncontrolled, and the data were often subjective and anecdotal. There is no objective evidence that any of these drugs exert clinically useful antineoplastic effects against glioblastoma multiforme. Various modes of administration (e.g., intravenous, intrathecal, intracavitary, and intracarotid infusion) have been tried and have failed.

b. **Lipid-soluble drugs—the nitrosoureas.** The blood-brain barrier is deficient in brain tumors. Thus small lipid-soluble molecules that can cross the normal blood-brain barrier may have the best chance of attaining sufficient concentration for chemotherapeutic effectiveness in **all** areas of the tumor.

A new group of antineoplastic agents, the nitrosoureas, have pharmacologic properties that enable them to cross the blood-brain barrier. Two nitrosourea compounds, BCNU (Carmustine) and CCNU (Lomustine) have undergone extensive clinical trials in glioblastoma multiforme (Table 11-2).

The Brain Tumor Study Group found that postoperative BCNU (80

Table 11-2. Treatment of Glioblastoma Multiforme[a]

Therapy		Median Survival (Weeks)	18-Month Survival (%)
Group I	Surgery alone	17	0
Group II	Surgery plus BCNU[b]	25	5
Group III	Surgery plus radiation therapy[c]	38	5
Group IV	Surgery plus radiation therapy plus BCNU[b]	41	23

[a]Preliminary data of the Brain Tumor Study Group.
[b]BCNU = 80 mg/sq m × 3 days every 2 months.
[c]Radiation therapy = 6000 rads over 6 weeks.

mg/sq m for 3 consecutive days, given every 2 months) did not lengthen median patient survival significantly as compared to surgery alone (25 weeks versus 17 weeks), whereas the addition of radiotherapy did prolong survival significantly. However, radiation therapy plus BCNU therapy did not lengthen median patient survival significantly as compared with postoperative radiation therapy alone (41 weeks versus 38 weeks).

Similar data have been obtained for therapy with CCNU. The most encouraging data for BCNU efficacy have been the higher proportion of 18-month survivors in the BCNU-plus-radiation group as compared with the radiation-alone group (23% versus 5%). The proponents of BCNU and CCNU claim that these agents also improve the quality of survival in 30–40% of patients.

   c. Nitrosourea treatment schedules. Standard treatment schedules are BCNU 80–100 mg/sq m IV for 3 days every 6–8 weeks or CCNU 130–150 mg/sq m PO every 6–8 weeks. CCNU has the advantage of being administered PO. However, both drugs can cause considerable leukopenia and thrombocytopenia, which usually occur 2–4 weeks after each treatment. Blood counts return to normal in 5–7 weeks.

If blood counts are closely monitored and subsequent dosages are appropriately adjusted, myelosuppression should not become a major problem. However, the need for frequent blood tests adds to the morbidity of these treatments.

   d. Other agents. Other agents, including procarbazine and epipodophyllotoxin, can cross the blood-brain barrier and have been evaluated against glioblastoma. However, the preliminary clinical data do not suggest that these drugs represent a dramatic therapeutic advance.

   e. Recommendation for chemotherapy. Chemotherapy (BCNU, CCNU, etc.) is not recommended as a routine postoperative procedure for all patients with glioblastoma multiforme. The data indicate that these treatments are only marginally effective and do not justify the additional patient morbidity.

However, there are several medical centers in the United States that are actively studying new agents and combinations of drugs. Thus patients who request that everything possible be done may be referred to one of these centers. It is hoped that objective data gathered at these institutions will one day result in an improved outlook for patients with glioblastoma multiforme.

B. Supratentorial astrocytomas and oligodendrogliomas in adults

   1. Biology. Astrocytoma, grades 1 and 2 (the so-called low-grade astrocytomas), and oligodendroglioma of the cerebral hemisphere occur much less commonly in adults than glioblastoma multiforme (astrocytoma, grades 3 and 4). These tumors are usually slow-growing, and symptoms (such as focal epilepsy) antedate the discovery of the tumor by years in some cases. Although cerebral astrocytomas and oligodendrogliomas in adults may remain histologically benign, over the course of months or years, many undergo dedifferentiation, assuming the terminal histologic picture and prognosis of glioblastoma multiforme. Furthermore, histologic sampling of brain tumors at biopsy can be misleading. For example, the biopsied portion of the tumor may reveal grade 1 or 2 astrocytomas, whereas other (unbiopsied) regions may be composed of glioblastoma multiforme. Consequently, the prognosis in these cases is notoriously uncertain.

   2. Surgery and radiotherapy. Most neurologists and neurosurgeons agree that the treatment of choice is the most extensive surgical resection possible, although complete removal is seldom accomplished. "Gross total tumor removal" has been associated with lower morbidity and mortality and longer postoperative survival than partial removal. When radical surgical extirpation is not possible because of the tumor location (e.g., astrocytomas of the hypothalamus or third ventricle), postoperative radiation therapy (5000–6000 rads over 5–6 weeks) is given to slow down or arrest further tumor growth. There is some clinical evidence that radiotherapy modestly improves the chances of long-term survival following subtotal resection.

When gross total removal is surgically possible, the role of radiotherapy is controversial. Some radiotherapists advocate routine postoperative cranial irradiation for all cases of supratentorial astrocytoma in grades 1–2 and oligodendroglioma. Others recommend that radiotherapy be withheld until there is clinical evidence of postoperative recurrence of the tumor.

There are some uncontrolled retrospective data suggesting that survival is improved by routine postoperative radiotherapy even after gross total removal, and this is the currently recommended mode of treatment.

3. **Prognosis.** As mentioned previously, the prognosis for supratentorial astrocytoma, grades 1–2, and oligodendroglioma is highly variable. Statistics taken from a large heterogeneous series of cases suggest a median survival of 3–5 years following surgery and radiotherapy, and the range in survival is quite great. A fair number of patients die within the first year, whereas a small number survive over 10 years without further symptoms. The vast majority of patients eventually suffer recurrent progressive neurologic symptoms. In many cases this represents a malignant histologic and prognostic change in the nature of the neoplasm.

Patients in whom the recurrent tumor is in a surgically accessible location, such as the anterior frontal region, often benefit substantially from repeat craniotomy and tumor resection. Antineoplastic chemotherapy has not been shown to be of value in these cases, but experience with this procedure is limited.

C. **Reticulum cell sarcoma (histiocytic lymphoma)**

1. **Biology.** Primary reticulum cell sarcoma (histiocytic lymphoma) of the brain is usually a subacutely evolving mass lesion that is clinically similar to glioblastoma multiforme and has been thought by some to arise from brain microglia (microglioma). The brain tumor often occurs without any lymph node or visceral involvement. Therefore it may be a clinically distinct entity from systemic reticulum cell sarcoma, which often infiltrates the epidural space but very rarely causes metastases within the brain parenchyma.

Primary reticulum cell sarcoma of the brain is a relatively uncommon tumor. Its peak incidence is in the fifth and sixth decades, and most reticulum cell sarcomas occur in patients who are otherwise healthy. However, considerable interest has been focused on the increased incidence of these tumors in renal transplant recipients and in association with dysglobulinemias (e.g., Waldenström's macroglobulinemia and the Wiskott-Aldrich syndrome).

2. **Surgery and radiotherapy.** Our current recommendation for treatment is craniotomy with extensive tumor resection followed by cranial irradiation (5000–6000 rads over 5–6 weeks). There is some clinical evidence suggesting that these tumors, like other proliferations of the lymphoreticular system, may be sensitive to radiation therapy.

However, several patients who were given radiotherapy to one lobe later developed recurrent tumors in adjacent areas. Pathologically, the site of previous radiotherapy was often tumor-free. This observation underscores the fact that reticulum cell sarcoma is an invasive, sometimes multifocal, tumor. Therefore irradiation of the whole brain is necessary to cover subclinically involved areas.

3. **Prognosis.** Data are limited, but the median survival following this treatment is approximately 2–3 years. Unfortunately, there are very few cures and survival beyond 5 years of diagnosis is uncommon. The role of antineoplastic chemotherapy has not been evaluated in this disease.

D. Meningiomas

1. **Biology.** Meningiomas are histologically benign tumors that arise from arachnoidal cells. They are the second most common primary intracranial tumors in adults. Their peak incidence is in the fourth and fifth decades and, unlike other primary brain tumors, meningiomas occur more commonly in women than in men (a ratio of about 2:1).

   Meningiomas may arise wherever arachnoidal cells are present, but the chief sites of origin are over the cerebral convexity (50%—parasagittal, falx, or lateral convexity) or base (40%—olfactory groove, sphenoid wing, or suprasellar). Meningiomas of the foramen magnum, posterior fossa, or ventricular system also occur but are relatively uncommon.

2. **Surgery.** Meningiomas are well circumscribed, slowly growing tumors. They may infiltrate the dura, dural sinuses, or bone, but they generally do not invade the underlying brain parenchyma. These histologic features mean that complete surgical removal and surgical cure are often possible in cases of meningioma, unlike the tumors previously discussed.

3. **Radiotherapy.** The role of cranial irradiation in the treatment of meningiomas is controversial. If a meningioma can be completely resected, surgical excision alone is the treatment of choice. Some radiotherapists contend that if resection is incomplete, radiation therapy (5000–6000 rads) may prevent or delay recurrence. Similarly, some contend that recurrent meningiomas may be controlled occasionally for extended periods by irradiation. As mentioned previously, the natural course of meningioma is long and variable.

   At present there are insufficient data to clearly define what role, if any, radiation therapy plays in the treatment of unresectable or recurrent meningioma. A reasonable recommendation is to withhold radiotherapy except for those patients with recurrent meningioma in whom repeat surgical therapy is inadequate or contraindicated.

4. **Prognosis.** The prognosis is generally favorable, and prolonged survival after surgical resection is the rule rather than the exception. Nevertheless, the rate of tumor recurrence and life expectancy may vary depending on whether complete surgical resection is possible.

   In a large series of patients with meningioma, a macroscopically complete removal of the tumor was achieved in about 60% of cases. Also, meningiomas over the convexity of the brain were generally more accessible to complete resection than tumors at the base of the brain. The vast majority of patients in this group were permanently cured. There was a 10% rate of tumor recurrence in the patients with "complete tumor removal," probably due to residual untreated nests of tumor; and the average time that elapsed between primary operation and confirmation of recurrence was 4–5 years (range, 1–13 years). Many of these patients benefited from a second tumor resection.

   In the group of patients in whom the resection of intradural tumor was frankly incomplete, there were clinical recurrences in half the cases. However, there were many satisfactory results even in this group; 25% survived more than 10 years after only partial resection.

   The major histologic subtypes of meningiomas are endotheliomatous, transitional, and angioblastic. The prognosis with these tumors is the same except for the rare hemangiopericytoma and malignant meningioma, both of which recur with significantly higher frequency and after shorter intervals than the other types of meningiomas.

E. Acoustic schwannoma

1. **Incidence.** Schwannomas, tumors of the Schwann cells of peripheral nerves, commonly occur in the intracranial cavity, originating from the acoustic nerve at the cerebellopontine angle. Schwannomas are by far the most common cerebellopontine-angle tumors, but meningiomas, gliomas, and cholesteatomas may also occur in this location.

Acoustic schwannomas account for 8% of all brain tumors. They occur mainly in middle adult life and are rare in childhood. About 5–10% of patients with acoustic schwannoma have the "central form" of von Recklinghausen's neurofibromatosis. In these patients the acoustic tumors are often bilateral and may be associated with multiple cranial and spinal schwannomas, meningiomas, and gliomas.

2. Clinical features. The earliest symptoms of acoustic schwannoma are caused by impairment of the acoustic nerve (deafness, tinnitus, and unsteadiness), with trigeminal dysfunction (loss of corneal reflex and facial numbness), facial weakness, and ataxia, which usually occurs later.

3. Treatment. Schwannomas are slow-growing, and symptoms are usually present for months to years before the diagnosis is made. The tumors are usually encapsulated and compress the adjacent neural tissue without invading it. Tumors less than 2 cm in diameter can usually be completely removed, but this is seldom possible with large tumors. Thus complete surgical excision and cure are often possible with early diagnosis (see Chapter 4).

The surgical mortality has also been directly related to the size of the tumor, being less than 5% for tumors smaller than 2 cm in diameter, and more than 20% for tumors greater than 4 cm in diameter. If left untreated, these tumors ultimately cause increased intracranial pressure and fatal brainstem compression. This result underscores the importance of early diagnosis and treatment to reduce the morbidity and mortality of this disease.

With recent advances in diagnostic and surgical techniques, the operative risks have been greatly reduced. In a recent series of 46 consecutive patients treated at Massachusetts General Hospital, total tumor removal was possible in 70% and radical subtotal removal was possible in 10% of patients. Forty-one patients (90%) were able to return to their previous level of activity after surgery, and damage or severance of the facial nerve, a well-known operative risk, was avoided in most cases. After 1–2 years from the initial resection, tumors recurred in 33% of patients who underwent partial resection only. There were no recurrences in cases of total or radical subtotal removal after 2–7 years of follow-up. However, the technical difficulties of subsequent operations are increased in cases of recurrent schwannoma, and the prognosis is often poor.

Postoperative radiotherapy has not been of value in the treatment of acoustic schwannoma.

F. Pituitary adenomas

1. Classification. Pituitary adenomas can be divided into three histologic and clinical groups.

a. Tumors that do not secrete hormones (usually chromophobe adenomas);

b. Tumors that secrete growth hormone (usually acidophil adenomas); and

c. Tumors that secrete corticotrophin (usually basophil adenomas).

2. Clinical features of chromophobe adenomas. The vast majority of pituitary tumors (about 80%) are chromophobe adenomas. These tumors do not secrete clinically significant amounts of hormones, although the recent development of sensitive immunoassays has revealed hyperprolactinemia in one-third of the patients.

The initial symptom of patients with chromophobe adenoma is usually failure of vision due to compression of the optic chiasm. Bitemporal hemianopia, first involving the superior quadrants, is the most common pattern of visual loss. Chromophobe adenomas may also produce hypopituitarism by compressing the adenohypophysis. All the hormones are not equally depressed, and the order of susceptibility is as follows:

a. Growth hormone.

    b. Gonadotropins.

    c. Corticotrophin.

    d. Thyroid stimulating hormone.

    Since chromophobe adenomas occur exclusively in adults, stunted growth due to growth hormone deficiency is not encountered. The most common clinical endocrine manifestation is amenorrhea or loss of libido due to gonadotropin deficiency. Advanced cases of chromophobe adenoma can spread beyond the sella turcica and invade the hypothalamus, third ventricle, cavernous sinus, frontal lobe, or temporal lobe. Recent data suggest that some chromophobe adenomas secrete prolactin, so measurement of elevated levels of this hormone in the blood may help to make the diagnosis.

3. Clinical features of acidophil adenomas. The pituitary tumors that secrete excess amounts of growth hormone and cause acromegaly are usually acidophil adenomas. They are usually diagnosed before there is suprasellar extension or visual-field deficit (unlike chromophobe adenomas), due to the prominent somatic signs and symptoms associated with acromegaly.

    In a recent series at the Massachusetts General Hospital, fewer than 25% of patients with acidophil adenomas had visual deficits at the time of diagnosis.

4. Clinical features of basophil adenomas. The pituitary tumors that secrete corticotrophin and cause Cushing's syndrome are usually basophil adenomas. These tumors are small and, at the time of clinical diagnosis, usually have not deformed the sella turcica or involved the optic chiasm.

5. Therapy of chromophobe adenomas. The treatment of choice for chromophobe adenomas includes surgery or radiotherapy or both. The approach to therapy must be determined in accordance with the nature of the neurologic or endocrinologic disturbances or both produced by the tumor.

    a. Surgery. Signs of significant extrasellar extension, such as involvement of the optic chiasm or cranial nerves, are indications for surgery. The principal reason for surgery in most cases is to promptly restore lost vision, avoid further loss, or both.

    Modern microsurgical technology has reduced the risk of operative mortality in patients with pituitary tumors to 1%. Following surgical decompression and tumor resection, visual improvement occurs in about 70–80% of patients, and vision may return to normal in up to 50%. The prognosis for visual recovery is best when the history of impairment has been brief. The endocrine status after surgery is also occasionally improved (e.g., menstruation may return), but more commonly there is no change or even worsening.

    During surgery for pituitary tumors patients are treated with corticosteroids as prophylaxis against adrenal insufficiency. The degree of pituitary impairment is reassessed postoperatively so appropriate replacement therapy, if indicated, can be administered. Diabetes insipidus is an occasional consequence of surgery, but it is usually transitory.

    Despite meticulous effort, it is often impossible to completely remove pituitary adenomas that have extended beyond the sella turcica. In about one-quarter to one-half of patients the tumor will ultimately recur within 1–10 years postoperatively.

    b. Postoperative irradiation. Radiation therapy has proved to be a useful adjunct in significantly reducing the rate of postoperative recurrence. In one series of patients the recurrence rate was decreased from 42 to 13% by postoperative irradiation. Current practice is to administer 5000–6000 rads over 5–6 weeks. The field size is determined by the radiographic and surgical findings.

    c. Radiation alone. Treatment by radiation therapy alone is reserved for patients with clinical and radiographic evidence of chromophobe adenoma with **no extrasellar extension.** This is one of the few situations in which radiotherapy is indicated without histologic confirmation of the lesion. When the diagnosis is in serious question, surgery is performed.

Conventional irradiation of small chromophobe adenomas will eliminate the tumor in one-half to one-third of patients. However, close post-irradiation follow-up of these patients, including careful serial visual-field examinations, is important for early detection of recurrent tumors, because radiation failure is common with cystic tumors. Thus a patient who is not successfully treated with irradiation alone should undergo surgical resection. If the lesion is cystic, additional radiotherapy is unnecessary unless there is a residual solid tumor.

Surgery is successful in controlling recurrent chromophobe adenomas after radiation failure in the majority of cases.

d. **Proton beam therapy.** A recent advance in the radiation therapy of pituitary adenomas has been the introduction of proton beam therapy. The advantages of proton beam therapy, compared to conventional radiotherapy, are the sharp collimation of beam edges and the increased amount of radiation at the end of the beam range. This feature allows for focal concentration of the radiation dose within the pituitary fossa with minimal radiation to the skin or adjacent brain structures. Doses of 10,000 rads or more can be safely administered to a patient with a pituitary adenoma in one session, although a single dose of 2000–4000 rads is adequate to induce growth arrest in chromophobe adenomas, while maintaining normal pituitary function in most cases. Such high doses cannot be given to patients at a single sitting by conventional radiation techniques without serious risk of radiation-induced brain damage.

After proton beam therapy, the incidence of recurrence of chromophobe adenomas without suprasellar extension is only 3%.

The efficacy, relative low cost, low morbidity, and no mortality make proton beam therapy the **treatment of choice** for most pituitary adenomas without extrasellar extension. Unfortunately, facilities for proton beam therapy are available at only two centers in the United States (the Harvard cyclotron and the Berkeley cyclotron). Patients are referred to these centers from all over the country.

6. **Treatment of acidophil adenomas.** Much of the disability caused by acidophil adenomas is the result of the active secretion of growth hormone. In most cases conventional radiotherapy (4000–5000 rads) can arrest the continued rise in hormone levels. For example, the secretion rate of plasma growth hormone gradually declines by a mean of 50% after 1 year of therapy and 75% after two years. Proton beam therapy can also induce focal radionecrosis in acidophil adenomas if high doses of radiation (up to 15,000 rads) are used. Growth hormone levels gradually fall, and the metabolic disabilities of acromegaly are thereby avoided. Also, the acral growth and glucose intolerance of acromegaly resolve after radiation therapy. However, the crippling arthritis, severe hypertension, and cardiomyopathy associated with acromegaly are usually irreversible.

In the Harvard cyclotron series of 179 patients with acromegaly, 85% underwent remission or improved, 8% were "arrested," and only 7% worsened after proton beam therapy. Thus results of conventional radiation and proton beam therapy are roughly equivalent. Acidophil adenomas with **suprasellar extension** should be resected surgically, and patients with these tumors are not candidates for conventional radiation or proton beam therapy.

7. **Treatment of basophil adenomas.** Proton beam therapy also provides a safe and effective treatment for Cushing's disease due to basophil adenoma of the pituitary. In the Harvard cyclotron series of 45 patients, 89% showed remission or improved and treatment failed in only 11%.

8. **Secondary empty sella.** Deterioration of visual function after treatment for pituitary adenoma is generally assumed to indicate tumor recurrence. How-

ever, in a small number of cases there is progressive visual dysfunction without tumor recurrence. This rare complication can occur after any form of treatment—surgery, x-ray, or proton beam. The pathophysiology of the visual loss is uncertain, but it is related to the appearance of an empty sella turcica on pneumoencephalogram (the "secondary" empty sella syndrome). Consequently, the presence of a recurrent tumor is **documented on pneumoencephalogram or CT scan** before further treatment (surgery, radiation) is undertaken in patients with previously treated pituitary adenoma.

9. **Pituitary apoplexy.** Pituitary apoplexy is another uncommon complication of pituitary adenoma. The pituitary hemorrhage is usually spontaneous, but sometimes it develops during radiotherapy. The onset is sudden, with headache, vomiting, stiff neck, and visual disturbances being the most common symptoms. In severe cases consciousness is impaired, and the CSF is bloody in most patients with pituitary apoplexy. Corticosteroids are started immediately to prevent signs of adrenal insufficiency; and after radiographic confirmation of the diagnosis (angiography or PEG or both), surgery is undertaken to decompress the optic chiasm and preserve the patient's vision.

10. **Asymptomatic enlarged sella turcica.**

   a. **Empty sella.** Occasionally, when skull x-rays are taken for unrelated reasons (e.g., after a minor head injury), asymptomatic patients are discovered who have enlargement of the sella turcica. Many, if not most, of these patients have the so-called primary empty sella syndrome.

   The etiology of this condition is not well understood. The primary empty sella syndrome is a benign condition that is sometimes associated with mild endocrine deficiencies but only rarely with visual loss. Thus the condition requires no treatment, although a few of these patients may require hormone replacement.

   b. **Evaluation.** It is important to determine which patients with asymptomatic sella enlargement have an early chromophobe adenoma. Certainly, an abnormality in the visual fields or in endocrine function (particularly gonadotropin or growth hormone deficiency) raises the index of suspicion in favor of a pituitary tumor. Since some chromophobe adenomas secrete prolactin silently, a prolactin assay might prove to be a useful test for detecting early tumors.

   At present one must resort to a **pneumoencephalogram** (PEG) in most cases to distinguish between an empty sella and an early pituitary adenoma. A dose of hydrocortisone 50 mg is usually given before the PEG as prophylaxis against stress-induced adrenal insufficiency in patients whose pituitary reserve may be marginal. The examination must include tomographic views, with the patient's head extended in the "brow-up" position, to adequately establish whether the subarachnoid space extends below the clinoid process (empty sella syndrome) or whether there is an intrasellar mass.

   If the PEG demonstrates the presence of an asymptomatic pituitary adenoma, the custom of following patients with serial skull x-rays and visual-field examinations does little to protect the patient from later suprasellar extension of the tumor. Therefore if a tumor is found, it is better to employ proton beam therapy, which is a minimal risk, than to deal with the chiasmal syndrome by craniotomy at a later date.

G. **Cerebral metastases.** Metastasis to the brain or meninges, or both, is a common complication of systemic cancer. Approximately 15–20% of patients dying of cancer will have brain metastases at the time of autopsy. The frequency of brain metastases varies considerably with the histology of the cancer (Table 11-3). Bronchogenic carcinoma, breast carcinoma, and malignant melanoma are the cancers most likely to metastasize to the brain. However, any malignant neoplasm may potentially involve the brain.

Table 11-3. Brain Metastases

Type	Number of Autopsied Cases	Cases with Brain Metastases	Percent
Disseminated melanoma	24	22	92
Bronchus and lung	656	218	33
Breast[a]	27	10	37
Testis	34	10	29
Kidney	72	15	21
Thyroid	14	2	14
Osteogenic sarcoma	15	2	13
Urinary bladder	84	7	8
Ovary	13	1	8
Colon	260	18	7
Esophagus	59	4	7
Stomach	207	7	3
Prostate	159	2	1

[a]The relatively small number of cases of breast cancer reflects the fact that these statistics were gathered at veterans hospitals. Breast cancer is the most common source of cerebral metastases in women.

There are two major patterns of cerebral metastasis: the formation of a solid tumor mass lesion within the CNS parenchyma and diffuse sheetlike infiltration of the leptomeninges by tumor cells (meningeal carcinomatosis). These two entities may sometimes coexist in an individual patient, but their clinical picture and therapy differ considerably, so they are considered separately.

1. **Intraparenchymal metastases**

   a. **Clinical features.** The formation of a solid mass lesion is the most common type of cerebral metastasis, and it may occur in any lobe of the cerebrum, the cerebellum, or brainstem. The frequency of metastasis in these structures is roughly in proportion to the relative size of the region (cerebral hemispheres > cerebellum > brainstem).

   These lesions cause symptoms due to increased intracranial pressure, destruction of neurologic structures, cerebral edema, or seizures (just as do primary brain tumors).

   b. **Cancer presenting with brain metastases.** In patients with a known history of malignancy, the development of neurologic signs or symptoms prompts immediate investigation for evidence of CNS metastases. However, perhaps as many as 10% of patients with brain metastasis will have neurologic symptoms before the diagnosis of the primary tumor has been made. Therefore the possibility of metastasis from an occult primary tumor must be considered in every case of brain tumor.

   Thorough general physical examination and routine screening tests (e.g., urinalysis, stool guaiac, CBC, liver function tests, chest x-ray, and xeromammography) are always performed before craniotomy for a (presumed) primary brain tumor. Lung tomograms and cytologic examination of sputum are also indicated in patients who are heavy smokers.

   c. **Surgery for solitary metastases.** The therapy for brain metastases depends on the location and number of metastases as well as the general condition and prognosis of the patient. In the majority of cases there is more than one cerebral metastasis present at the time of diagnosis. However, in perhaps one-third of cases the brain metastasis is solitary. If the tumor is in a relatively accessible location (e.g., frontal lobe, parietal lobe, or cerebellar hemisphere), total surgical excision of a solitary metastasis is often possible. The tumor resection is then followed by radiotherapy of the whole brain (2500–4000 rads over 2–4 weeks) to suppress any residual tumor or "micrometastases" that escaped clinical detection.

In a recent series, 30% of patients survived longer than 1 year after craniotomy for a solitary metastasis, and the neurologic quality of survival was good to excellent in the great majority of cases. In addition, there were several patients suspected of having a solitary metastasis who were found at surgery to have resectable "benign" lesions (subdural hematoma or meningioma). Thus if the patient's general condition and prognosis warrant the morbidity of craniotomy, there is substantial reason for considering resection of suspected solitary metastases.

d. **Radiotherapy.** Patients with multiple cerebral metastases and those with solitary metastases who are not candidates for surgery should undergo cranial irradiation. This is one of the few instances in which radiotherapy is justified without a histologic diagnosis of the lesion. The presence of intracerebral metastases is documented on CT scan or radionuclide brain scan before starting radiotherapy. The radiation dose is generally 2500–5000 rads delivered to the whole brain over 2–4 weeks.

The response to therapy varies somewhat with the histology of the underlying tumor. For example, metastases from breast cancer and lung cancer generally respond better than metastases from melanoma or sarcomas. These patients are quite ill, and 20–30% may die within 1 month of radiotherapy or before therapy is completed. Nevertheless, most patients who complete the intended course of cranial irradiation experience at least some relief of symptoms. Also, the 6-month survival rate in this group is 33%; the 1-year survival rate is 10%. Death is usually due to disseminated metastases rather than to brain disease per se.

Patients who suffer recurrent cerebral metastases after radiotherapy may benefit from a second course of treatment. Recently, radiotherapists have tried treating cerebral metastases with a single dose of 1000 rads to the whole brain. However, the results have not been as satisfactory as those following standard fractionated radiotherapy. Further information is needed to assess the role of single-dose irradiation.

e. **Corticosteroids.** High-dose corticosteroids are often extremely useful in the palliation of symptoms from cerebral metastases. The use of corticosteroids should not be withheld in patients with progressive neurologic deficits, intractable headache, etc. (See sec II on corticosteroids for edema that is related to brain tumor.)

f. **Systemic chemotherapy.** Systemic anticancer chemotherapy (e.g., methotrexate, 5-FU, nitrogen mustard, vincristine, and cyclophosphamide) has not proved useful in the treatment of intracerebral metastases. For example, cerebral metastases often continue to grow despite the administration of chemotherapy that is effective against systemic metastases.

The difficulty has probably been related to the inability of most effective drugs to cross the blood-brain barrier. Although nitrosourea derivatives, BCNU and CCNU, can cross the blood-brain barrier in therapeutic concentrations, few solid tumors are sensitive to the nitrosoureas. Thus to date these drugs have not been of great general value in treating patients with brain metastases.

2. **Meningeal carcinomatosis and lymphomatosis**

a. **Incidence.** Infiltration of the leptomeninges by neoplastic cells (meningeal carcinomatosis or lymphomatosis), once believed to be rare, is now recognized as a common complication of cancer. Meningeal carcinomatosis occurs most often in cases of lymphoma, breast cancer, lung cancer, malignant melanoma, and gastrointestinal neoplasms.

  b. **Clinical features.** The neurologic signs of meningeal carcinomatosis are caused by focal infiltration of cranial or spinal nerves (e.g., radicular pain and weakness, facial palsy, or oculomotor palsy), or cerebral symptoms (headache, change in mental status).

  This clinical picture is quite different from that generally associated with intraparenchymal metastases, in which tract findings (e.g., hemiparesis and hemianopia) are prominent.

  c. **Diagnosis.** The diagnosis of meningeal carcinomatosis or lymphomatosis is confirmed by demonstrating the presence of malignant cells in the cerebrospinal fluid. In some cases multiple CSF specimens must be examined before malignant cells are successfully identified, because they do not appear in the CSF until the tumor has disseminated in the meninges. They are not apparent when the tumor is strictly intraparenchymal.

  CSF protein is often elevated and CSF glucose is often diminished in meningeal carcinomatosis. Perhaps one-third to one-half of patients with meningeal carcinomatosis will have a concomitant intraparenchymal brain metastasis (or metastases).

  d. **Treatment.** Since the tumor is seeded throughout the meninges, treatment must encompass the entire neuraxis. Craniospinal irradiation (e.g., 4000 rads to the brain and 3000 rads to the spine over 6–8 weeks) might successfully control the disease. However, most cancer patients do not have adequate bone marrow reserve to tolerate such extensive radiotherapy. Even in those patients with adequate bone marrow reserve, craniospinal irradiation limits their ability to tolerate future systemic chemotherapy, so this treatment is not recommended. Since the tumor is located in the meninges, this is the one situation in which injection of antineoplastic drugs directly into the subarachnoid space makes therapeutic sense.

  The current approach to treatment of meningeal carcinomatosis is **focal irradiation** delivered to areas where there are major symptoms (e.g., focal irradiation for a facial palsy) and frequent **intrathecal injections of methotrexate or cytosine arabinoside or both.** Most patients require irradiation of the whole brain, especially when a concomitant intraparenchymal metastasis is suspected. A typical schedule of intrathecal treatment is methotrexate 10–20 mg every other day or cytosine arabinoside 35–50 mg every other day. When clinical and CSF cytologic improvement occur, the response is generally seen after the first two to four doses of intrathecal chemotherapy. Then intrathecal therapy is continued until the CSF is devoid of malignant cells, following which two or more "booster treatments" are administered. (For further details on intrathecal chemotherapy, see sec **IV.A** on leukemia).

  e. **Prognosis.** Early and vigorous treatment are often successful in reversing neurologic symptoms and prolonging life. Approximately 50% of patients with meningeal carcinomatosis from breast or lung cancer show substantial clinical improvement following this therapy, and over 80% of patients with meningeal lymphoma respond favorably. However, a course of intrathecal chemotherapy and radiotherapy involves considerable patient morbidity. This treatment should therefore be reserved for patients whose general condition and prognosis warrants aggressive therapy.

  This disease is inexorably progressive and leads to death from neurologic dysfunction within a month in patients who are untreated or fail to respond to treatment.

IV. CENTRAL NERVOUS SYSTEM TUMORS IN CHILDHOOD. Cancer is the second leading cause of death in children in the group from age 1 to 15 years; and brain tumors are the second most common type of cancer in children.

A. Leukemia

1. **Biology and clinical features of acute lymphocytic leukemia.** The leukemias (and lymphomas) less often produce intraparenchymal mass lesions (as do solid tumors). Rather they have a propensity to infiltrate the leptomeninges diffusely (meningeal leukemia). The clinical symptoms of meningeal leukemia relate mainly to diffuse cerebral dysfunction or infiltration of cranial or spinal nerve roots or both. The diagnosis is made by finding leukemic cells in the CSF.

   In the early 1960s the majority of children with acute lymphocytic leukemia (ALL) ultimately developed meningeal leukemia, even when systemic chemotherapy was successful in inducing hematologic remission. It seemed as though the central nervous system were a "pharmacologic sanctuary," where leukemic cells could not be eradicated. Thus, by increasing the survival in acute lymphocytic leukemia by systemic chemotherapy, a higher incidence of meningeal leukemia was created. To correct this problem prophylactic CNS treatment was given before clinical manifestations became apparent to prevent the seemingly inexorable development of meningeal leukemia. Thus **prophylactic CNS therapy** is one of the great advances that has dramatically increased the length and quality of survival of children with acute lymphocytic leukemia.

2. **Prophylaxis of CNS leukemia.** At present there is no drug that crosses the blood-brain barrier following systemic administration that will successfully prevent or treat meningeal leukemia. Thus the treatment protocols for prophylaxis against meningeal leukemia have utilized:

   a. Intrathecal methotrexate;

   b. Intrathecal methotrexate plus cranial irradiation; or

   c. Craniospinal irradiation.

   The prophylactic CNS therapy is started as soon as possible after the diagnosis of acute lymphocytic leukemia has been made. Typical treatment schedules are:

   a. Intrathecal methotrexate 12 mg/sq m/wk for six doses;

   b. Intrathecal methotrexate 12 mg/sq m/wk for six doses plus 2400 rads cranial irradiation; or

   c. 2400 rads craniospinal irradiation.

   These treatment programs seem to have equal effectiveness, but studies are underway to determine whether one program is superior. The use of CNS prophylaxis has reduced the prevalence of CNS involvement to fewer than 5% of patients with leukemia after prolonged follow-up periods.

3. **Acute myelogenous leukemia.** The incidence of meningeal leukemia in acute myelogenous leukemia (AML) of adulthood has also shown a steady increase. CNS prophylaxis is not currently part of most standard treatment protocols for acute myelogenous leukemia. However, as newer systemic therapeutics result in a higher proportion of long-term survivors, it seems likely that CNS prophylaxis will become necessary in acute myelogenous leukemia as well.

4. **Treatment of active meningeal leukemia**

   a. **"Induction" of meningeal remission.** The treatment of active meningeal leukemia is similar in both acute lymphocytic leukemia and acute myelogenous leukemia. Radiotherapy is administered to sites of focal involvement (e.g., to the course of the seventh nerve if there is facial palsy). Methotrexate (12 mg/sq m) is injected into the subarachnoid space by means of lumbar puncture every other day or twice a week. Then intrathecal methotrexate is continued until leukemic cells have disappeared from the CSF, following which two or more additional doses are usually given.

A reduction in the number of leukemic cells in the CSF and clinical improvement usually occur after the first few doses. The initial episode of meningeal leukemia is successfully controlled in over 90% of cases by this treatment.

   b. Maintenance of meningeal remission. Unfortunately, the length of CNS remission is short, and there is a median duration of only 3 months before leukemic cells reappear in the CSF. Consequently, maintenance therapy is necessary to prolong the remissions of CNS leukemia.

Intrathecal methotrexate (12 mg/sq m), if given every 6–8 weeks after control of the acute episode of meningeal leukemia, will prolong the CNS remission to a median duration of 15 months. Recurrent episodes of meningeal leukemia may be treated again with an intensive course of intrathecal methotrexate.

   c. Alternative intrathecal therapy. Intrathecal cytosine arabinoside (35–50 mg) is a useful alternative to methotrexate. Although clinical experience with intrathecal cytosine arabinoside is less extensive, it is probably as effective as methotrexate. Also, it has the advantage of not causing leukopenia, because the drug is deaminated to an inactive form before it enters the systemic circulation from the CSF. Conversely, intrathecal methotrexate ultimately enters the systemic circulation and can cause leukopenia, especially in previously myelosuppressed patients.

5. Method of subarachnoid injection. After multiple lumbar punctures, the opening pressure is often very low (possibly due to CSF leakage), and it is often difficult to determine whether the drug is actually administered into the subarachnoid space. Also, the distribution of drug throughout the CSF is often erratic, even when lumbar subarachnoid injection is successful. However, administration of medications through an indwelling intraventricular catheter (e.g., an Ommaya reservoir) will ensure an adequate distribution of drug throughout the CSF.

Several treatment centers advocate routine use of Ommaya reservoirs for the treatment of meningeal leukemia or meningeal carcinomatosis. In most instances, these intraventricular devices can be used safely by experienced clinicians but, unfortunately, at most centers the morbidity associated with indwelling catheters (e.g., infection, misplaced cannula) remains prohibitive (25%). Consequently, lumbar injection is generally the safest mode of administration.

6. Side effects of intrathecal chemotherapy. In the majority of cases there is little or no morbidity associated with intrathecal methotrexate or cytosine arabinoside (other than the trauma of lumbar puncture itself). Headache, transient meningismus, paresthesias, nausea, or mild CSF pleocytosis occur in 5–50% of patients. Serious complications, such as paraplegia or drug-related encephalopathy, have fortunately been rare.

Encephalopathy is thought to be more frequently encountered in patients who have received both intrathecal methotrexate and radiotherapy. However, the true incidence and pathophysiology of this disorder are unknown. For example, a recent follow-up study of children with acute lymphocytic leukemia who received cranial irradiation and intrathecal methotrexate revealed no impairment of neurologic or psychological functioning when they were compared to controls. The search for newer, safer methods of treatment continues. At present the value of intrathecal methotrexate or cytosine arabinoside in the prophylaxis or treatment of meningeal leukemia far outweighs the risks.

B. Cerebellar astrocytoma

1. **Incidence.** The most common brain tumor in childhood is cerebellar astrocytoma, accounting for 25–30% of cases. These tumors are generally slow-growing and, if treated properly, may have an excellent prognosis. This is in great contrast to the most common brain tumor in adulthood—malignant astrocytoma (glioblastoma multiforme)—which is supratentorial in location and uniformly fatal.

2. **Clinical picture.** Cerebellar astrocytomas occur most frequently in children from the ages of 5 to 10 years. In younger children the only signs may be irritability, vomiting, and an enlarging head (due to obstructive hydrocephalus). More commonly, the presenting symptoms include those of a cerebellar hemisphere lesion, namely, incoordination and ataxia.

3. **Surgery.** Cerebellar astrocytomas occasionally occupy the vermis, but most often they are located in the cerebellar hemisphere. At least one-half these tumors have an associated cyst, and the neoplastic mass is sometimes confined inside a relatively small mural nodule. When this occurs, surgical excision of the nodule is curative. On the other hand, noncystic cerebellar astrocytomas are often large and infiltrative, and a small number of these tumors invade the brainstem by way of the cerebellar peduncles. Total tumor removal is impossible in this situation.

   In a recent review of 26 cases of childhood cerebellar astrocytoma, gross total tumor removal was achieved in 17 patients (65%). The operative mortality is low (4%), and the cerebellar dysfunction that persists after surgery is usually mild. Subsequent tumor recurrence is uncommon in patients who have "gross total tumor removal," even after decades of follow-up. Thus successful removal of an astrocytoma of the cerebellum often results in a complete and permanent cure.

4. **Radiotherapy.** Some cerebellar astrocytomas have relatively little potential for sustained growth, and even incomplete removal can be followed by an apparent tumor arrest and prolonged survival. More commonly, however, incomplete removal of cerebellar astrocytoma is followed by continued growth that can prove fatal. Thus we advocate the routine use of postoperative radiation therapy (5000 rads over 5–6 weeks) in children with incompletely resected cerebellar astrocytomas. The treatment fields should encompass the suspected tumor volume plus a margin of several centimeters; irradiation of the whole brain is not necessary.

   In a recent series of children with incompletely removed cerebellar astrocytomas who received postoperative irradiation, 65% were alive and "disease free" after 10 years of follow-up. The majority of survivors were neurologically normal or very nearly so.

C. Medulloblastoma

1. **Incidence.** Medulloblastoma is the second most common brain tumor in childhood, accounting for 20–25% of cases. The tumor occurs mainly between the ages of 2 and 10 years. However, about 30% of cases of medulloblastoma occur during adolescence and early adulthood.

2. **Clinical picture.** Medulloblastomas arise from primitive germinative cells in the cerebellum, and the majority of tumors originate in the midline of the cerebellum, occupying the vermis and fourth ventricle. Therefore initial clinical features are often due to noncommunicating hydrocephalus and increased intracranial pressure. In older (over age 6) age groups, medulloblastoma is more likely to occupy a lateral lobe, and signs of cerebellar involvement (staggering gait, ataxia) are more prominent.

3. **Metastasis.** Medulloblastomas that arise from the vermis often fill the cavity of the fourth ventricle and infiltrate into the brainstem. The tumor may also

spread *en plaque* over the surface of the cerebellum. Infiltration of the sub-arachnoid space with metastatic spread of medulloblastoma through the CSF pathways (to the spinal cord, base of the brain, or cerebral hemispheres) is also common. Malignant cells can be demonstrated in CSF cytology in about 40% of specimens taken by means of lumbar puncture.

4. **Surgery.** Due to the unfavorable location, invasiveness, and metastatic potential of medulloblastoma, complete surgical resection with cure is rarely, if ever, achieved. The goal of surgery is to provide the correct histologic diagnosis, to resect the tumor mass to whatever extent possible, and to reestablish the patency of the CSF pathways. In some cases a ventricular shunt may be necessary for decompressive purposes.

5. **Radiotherapy.** Unlike most other primary brain tumors, medulloblastoma is a **highly radiosensitive neoplasm.** However, radiation is not delivered without **histologic confirmation of the presence of a medulloblastoma,** since an alternative childhood posterior fossa tumor, cerebellar astrocytoma, can often be cured by radical surgery.

   Local irradiation is followed by a marked regression of signs and symptoms and, apparently, complete clinical recovery in most cases. Unfortunately, the dramatic response is temporary, with recurrent medulloblastoma and death occurring in the next 2 or 3 years. It is now recognized that irradiation of the entire neuraxis (spine and brain) is necessary in all cases, due to the marked propensity of medulloblastoma to metastasize by means of the CSF.

   The current trend in treatment has been to increase the radiation to the maximum tolerable dose (5000–6000 rads to the brain and posterior fossa and 4000 rads to the spinal cord over 1 month, but with reduced doses for children under 3 years old). Following histologic diagnosis, one radical course of craniospinal irradiation is preferable to multiple short courses.

6. **Prognosis.** Recent studies indicate that an aggressive approach to the treatment of medulloblastoma will result in survival rates, without recurrence, of approximately 35% and 25% in 5- and 10-year follow-ups, respectively. The majority of patients in the latter category have presumably been permanently "cured" of medulloblastoma. Over 80% of the long-term survivors have no serious neurologic disability and lead normal lives. These results are in striking contrast to the uniformly gloomy prognosis associated with medulloblastoma in the past.

7. **Morbidity of craniospinal irradiation.** It is difficult to assess the radiosensitivity of the nervous system in very young children. Most radiotherapists decrease the dose of radiation significantly in children under the age of 3 years to avoid possible radiation damage to the immature brain. Despite this precaution, craniospinal irradiation is not without certain adverse sequelae.

   a. **Radiation-induced leukopenia** occurs transiently during therapy but, fortunately, is seldom a serious clinical problem.

   b. **Decreased physical stature** due to retardation of vertebral growth is often observed following spinal irradiation over 2500 rads in children.

   c. The total **epilation** that follows cranial irradiation is reversible, and the regrowth of scalp hair is usually satisfactory.

   d. Radiation therapy can **induce malignancies** (e.g., thyroid cancer, leukemia, and sarcomas). However, to date this complication has not been a problem in patients with medulloblastoma. As more patients survive into adulthood, the incidence of second malignancies is likely to be increased relative to the general population.

   e. There appears to be **no significant neurologic sequelae** to 5000 rads brain irradiation in most children over 3 years of age. The mental retardation that occurs in a small proportion of survivors can usually be attributed to effects of the tumor and severe hydrocephalus rather than to the radiation therapy.

D. Recurrent medulloblastoma. The management of patients with recurrent medulloblastoma in the brain or spine is difficult. Unfortunately, further treatment is only palliative; the chance for "cure" has been lost in these patients. Most of them are unable to tolerate an adequate second course in radiotherapy, because the risk of nervous system radionecrosis is prohibitive. Likewise, surgery is seldom feasible, especially when there are multiple CNS metastases.

Medulloblastoma possesses several biologic characteristics that might make the tumor susceptible to **chemotherapeutic** attack (e.g., the tumor is rapidly growing and is highly radiosensitive). There have been several reports of patients with recurrent medulloblastoma who responded to systematic chemotherapy with BCNU, procarbazine, vincristine, or intrathecal methotrexate. However, the relative value of these agents in recurrent medulloblastoma has not been clearly established.

E. Ependymoma

1. **Biology.** Ependymomas, tumors derived from ependymal cells, are a common brain tumor in childhood, accounting for 10% of cases. About 70% of childhood ependymomas arise in the fourth ventricle, 20% in the lateral ventricles, and 10% in the region of the cauda equina. The median age of onset in these sites is 2, 6, and 13 years, respectively. Ependymomas also occasionally occur in adults, in which case the spinal cord and lateral ventricles are the sites of predilection. The majority of ependymomas are histologically benign, although a few cases have an anaplastic histologic picture and are designated as malignant ependymomas (or ependymoblastomas).

2. **Surgery.** The treatment of ependymoma begins with the most **extensive surgical resection** possible. Unfortunately, ependymomas in the fourth ventricle are often attached to the floor of the medulla, making total removal impossible. Also, these tumors often have produced ventricular obstruction and hydrocephalus by the time of diagnosis. Thus if direct surgical attack on the mass cannot relieve the obstruction of CSF flow, a ventricular shunt may be necessary.

3. **Radiotherapy.** Ependymomas almost invariably recur after surgery, regardless of their initial site or "completeness" of excision. The median symptom-free interval after surgery alone is less than 1 year for ependymomas of the fourth ventricle or lateral ventricle. The addition of routine postoperative irradiation (4500–6000 rads over 4–6 weeks) has prolonged survival significantly.

The 5–10-year survival rates after surgery and radiotherapy are around 70% for histologically benign ependymomas. The less common malignant ependymomas (ependymoblastoma) have a worse prognosis, with only 20% of patients surviving 10 years after surgery and local radiotherapy.

The malignant ependymomas have a tendency to metastasize through the CSF, much as do medulloblastomas. In these cases irradiation of the entire neuraxis may reduce the risk of tumor-seeding elsewhere in the CNS, thereby improving the survival rate. For histologically benign ependymomas, the risk of metastasis through the CSF is minimal, and local irradiation to the primary tumor site is sufficient. The quality of life in the surviving patients is generally good and justifies an aggressive approach to diagnosis and treatment.

F. Brainstem glioma

1. **Incidence.** Intrinsic brainstem gliomas occur most frequently in the first decade of life and account for nearly 20% of childhood brain tumors.

2. **Clinical picture.** The pons is the site of predilection for brainstem gliomas. The typical clinical presentation of these tumors consists of progressive

cranial nerve impairment (particularly of the sixth, seventh, ninth, or tenth cranial nerves), ataxia, hemiparesis, and headache. Routine laboratory studies (EEG, lumbar puncture, and brain scan) are seldom helpful in the diagnosis of these tumors. The most reliable diagnostic test is the pneumoencephalogram, which reveals enlargement of the pons by an intrinsic mass.

3. **Surgery.** In the majority of cases surgical verification of the diagnosis is not attempted or indicated due to the inaccessible location of the tumor within the brainstem parenchyma. The diagnosis therefore rests on the characteristic clinical and radiographic picture. However, in patients with atypical clinical or neuroradiologic findings, surgical exploration is often indicated in an attempt to find a more amenable lesion (e.g., an extra-axial mass in the fourth ventricle, such as an ependymoma).

4. **Radiotherapy.** Radiation therapy to the brainstem (4000–6000 rads over 4–6 weeks) results in significant clinical improvement in about 70% of patients with presumed brainstem gliomas; and perhaps 25–30% of these patients will survive longer than 5 years without recurrent neurologic symptoms. The results are difficult to interpret, since histologic verification of tumor is lacking in most cases. Furthermore, the natural history of brainstem gliomas can be highly variable. Thus some long-term survivors following radiotherapy may truly be cured, others may still suffer late recurrence, and still others may never have really had a brainstem glioma. The majority of patients with brainstem glioma suffer recurrence of progressive neurologic deficits within 2 years of radiotherapy.

High-dose corticosteroids will reverse many of the signs and symptoms, perhaps for a few weeks or months, but will not alter the fatal outcome. Chemotherapy with BCNU or procarbazine has temporarily stabilized the neurologic deficits in a few cases of brainstem glioma.

G. Craniopharyngioma

1. **Incidence.** Craniopharyngioma is a tumor that originates from squamous cell nests in the region of the pituitary stalk. This tumor occurs in both childhood and adulthood and accounts for about 3% of all brain tumors.

2. **Clinical picture.** Craniopharyngiomas can cause symptoms by compressing the optic chiasm or tracts, depressing pituitary or hypothalamic function, increasing the intracranial pressure, or all of these. Plain skull x-rays are often diagnostic of craniopharyngioma: Calcification is seen in or above the sella turcica in more than 80% of children and 40% of adults with craniopharyngioma. CT scan will often reveal calcifications that were not seen on plain skull x-rays.

3. **Surgery.** Craniopharyngiomas are biologically and histologically benign, but their intimate relation to vital neural and neuroendocrine structure presents a formidable obstacle to complete surgical resection. With the use of the operating microscope, some tumors can be completely removed. However, the realities of unavoidable operative morbidity and almost certain postoperative dependency on exogenous hormones detract from the success of surgical "cure." In most cases only partial removal of the craniopharyngioma and its accompanying cyst is feasible. However, the resulting decompression of the optic pathways is usually beneficial for preserving vision.

4. **Radiotherapy.** After partial resection, the tumor has a propensity to recur. Most patients require a second palliative operation within 2 years; fewer than 30% of patients remain recurrence-free 5 years after partial resection alone. The tumor grows at a slower rate in adults, and long-lasting relief of symptoms occurs more commonly in adults than in children.

Postoperative radiotherapy (4500 rads or more) is effective in delaying recurrence of craniopharyngioma: 5- and 10-year follow-up studies reveal that 60% and 40% of patients, respectively, remain recurrence-free. Injection of radioactive isotopes into the cyst of craniopharyngiomas has been tried as a method for preventing recurrences. Unfortunately, these treatments have not been of great therapeutic value.

H. Tumors of the pineal region

1. **Clinical picture.** Tumors that arise in the pineal region occur mainly during adolescence and early adult life. These tumors usually produce symptoms by compressing the midbrain tectum (causing Parinaud's syndrome) or obstructing the aqueduct of Sylvius (causing noncommunicating hydrocephalus). Pineal tumors can also encroach anteriorly to involve the hypothalamus (diabetes insipidus, pubertas praecox) or optic pathways.

2. **Histology.** Several biologically and histologically distinct tumors can arise from the pineal region to produce this clinical picture. The **germinoma** (also referred to as pinealoma or atypical teratoma) is the most common pineal tumor, accounting for more than 50% of cases. Germinomas arise from primitive midline germ cells in the pineal or hypothalamic regions. Other germ cell tumors, including **teratomas** and **embryonal carcinoma,** also occasionally occur in this region; and tumors of the pineal parenchyma (the **pineocytoma** and **pineoblastoma**), **glial tumors** (astrocytoma, ganglioneuroma), and **epidermoid cysts** account for the remainder of these tumors.

3. **Radiotherapy.** When clinical findings and neuroradiologic studies establish the diagnosis of a pineal tumor, the current recommendation is to undertake a full course of cranial irradiation (5000–6000 rads) without histologic verification of the lesion. If symptomatic hydrocephalus is present, a ventricular shunt is often necessary for palliative purposes.

   Germinomas, the most common pineal tumors, are usually quite sensitive to radiotherapy. The 5-year disease-free survival after irradiation of these tumors is approximately 60%; and many of these long-term survivors are permanently cured of pineal germinoma.

4. **Metastasis.** Pineal tumors occasionally metastasize through the CSF, much as do medulloblastomas. This phenomenon occurs most often with the rare pineoblastoma, but it also occurs occasionally with germinomas. Therefore thorough cytologic examination of the CSF is important in planning treatment.

   If malignant cells are detected in the CSF, irradiation of the entire neuraxis, rather than irradiation of the brain alone, is indicated. Some radiotherapists advocate craniospinal irradiation for all pineal tumors, regardless of CSF cytology findings. At present it is unclear whether there are benefits to be gained by that approach to therapy.

5. **Surgery.** The use of the operating microscope has significantly lowered the operative morbidity and mortality of surgery in the pineal region. Yet the risks of radiation damage to the brain are small compared to the hazards of subjecting all patients with posterior third-ventricle tumors to immediate direct surgical intervention. Furthermore, the radiosensitive germinomas are infiltrative tumors, and they are seldom amenable to complete surgical resection.

   Six weeks following the completion of radiotherapy, pneumoencephalography or CT scan or both should be repeated. If the tumor has regressed, the lesion is presumed to have been a germinoma, and the patient is followed clinically at regular intervals. If the mass has increased or is unchanged, surgical intervention is indicated. Occasionally those tumors that do not respond to radiotherapy (e.g., pineocytoma or epidermoid cyst) are amenable to complete surgical resection and cure.

I. Optic glioma

1. **Incidence and clinical picture.** Optic glioma accounts for approximately 3% of all childhood brain tumors; it usually occurs in the first decade of life. Also,

perhaps one-third of cases of optic glioma occur in association with von Recklinghausen's neurofibromatosis. By the time of diagnosis the tumor commonly produces loss of vision or exophthalmos or both. In some cases the clinical picture mimics optic neuritis.

2. Treatment

a. Natural course. There is considerable controversy regarding the natural course and treatment of optic gliomas in children. Patients with gliomas confined to the optic nerve have an excellent prognosis after optic nerve excision. Tumor recurrence during long-term follow-up is rare when complete excision is performed, and vision is normal in the unaffected eye. In patients who have optic gliomas that involve the optic chiasm, complete resection is impossible in 50% or more without unacceptable operative morbidity.

Some patients have a remarkably protracted and benign course after only partial excision or even without any therapy. Also, improvement in visual acuity and proptosis occasionally occur spontaneously. Thus in some instances childhood optic gliomas behave more like congenital hamartomas than neoplasms.

b. Radiotherapy. On this basis, some experts advocate withholding surgical or radiation therapy for cases of optic glioma that involve the chiasm. However, the short-term prognosis is poor for many children with optic gliomas.

Over 30% of patients with chiasmal gliomas die from intracranial tumor within 5 years of diagnosis, many within 1 year. Therefore many radiotherapists advocate routine radiation therapy to the optic pathways soon after the diagnosis is made. There may be some benefit to vision following radiotherapy of optic chiasm gliomas, but it is unclear whether the ultimate prognosis is affected. In adults, optic gliomas are rare, aggressively invasive, lethal neoplasms. By the time the diagnosis is suspected, complete surgical resection is usually not possible. The prognosis is very poor, resembling that of glioblastoma multiforme.

V. SPINAL CORD TUMORS.

Tumors occur much less commonly in the spinal region than in the brain in both adults and children. Also, intraspinal neoplasms account for only about 10% of all primary tumors of the central nervous system. These tumors are seldom fatal, unlike their intracranial counterparts, but they are extremely disabling. Prompt recognition and treatment can do much to relieve the morbidity.

A. Spinal neoplasms

1. Clinical features. The clinical manifestations of a tumor that affects the spinal cord or cauda equina are caused by compression. If the lesion is **extramedullary** (e.g., not growing within the spinal cord parenchyma), the tumor will often produce symptoms by compression or destruction of nerve roots or bone before the spinal cord itself becomes involved. **Intramedullary** tumors often produce manifestations of disturbed spinal cord function from the outset. The clinical picture in individual cases depends on the transverse level of the tumor (cervical, thoracic, lumbar, sacral, or cauda equina), the topography of the tumor, peculiarities in the local blood supply to the spinal cord, and the speed of compression.

2. Radiologic features. The diagnosis of intraspinal tumor is suggested by x-ray evidence of bony erosion of the pedicles and intervertebral foramina (e.g., by a schwannoma) or bony destruction (e.g., by metastatic cancer or lymphoma).

Myelography is of great value in confirming the presence of an intraspinal tumor and determining its rostrocaudal extent. In some cases it is necessary to combine lumbar myelography with the instillation of contrast material by means of cisternal puncture to determine the superior extent of the tumor. From the pattern of the deformity produced in the myelogram contrast material, it is usually possible to deduce, prior to surgery, whether the tumor is intramedullary, extramedullary-intradural, or extradural.

Myelography is occasionally followed by a rapid clinical deterioration due to increased spinal compression. In these cases surgery is performed as soon as possible to avoid severe permanent neurologic deficit. Therefore myelography is undertaken only when the facilities for surgery are readily accessible.

The recent introduction of spinal cord angiography has also proved to be useful, particularly in the localization of angiomatous tumors.

B. Primary intraspinal tumors. The relative incidence of primary intraspinal tumors by histologic type differs quite markedly from that of intracranial tumors (Table 11-4).

1. Schwannoma

   a. Clinical features. The most common primary intraspinal tumor is the schwannoma. These are extramedullary-intradural tumors composed of Schwann cells, which can arise from spinal nerves at any level (cervical, thoracic, lumbar, or cauda equina) and most often arise from a posterior (sensory) nerve root. Therefore the most common initial symptom is pain of radicular distribution.

   Schwannomas are slow-growing, and pain may be present for years before the correct diagnosis is made, especially if they are in the relatively spacious lumbosacral region. However, schwannomas of nerve roots in the relatively tight cervical region compress the spinal cord early in their course.

   b. Treatment. Spinal schwannomas can usually be completely excised and cured by surgery. In some cases the tumor grows through the intravertebral foramen to form an extraspinal mass ("dumb-bell tumors"), and a second operation is often necessary to remove the extraspinal portion of these dumb-bell tumors. Fortunately, a high degree of clinical recovery can be expected, because the diagnosis is generally made before the spinal cord has been extensively damaged by pressure.

   Recurrence of schwannoma is likely only in cases in which total extirpation is impossible, such as very large tumors or tumors with extradural extension.

2. Meningiomas

   a. Clinical features. Meningiomas are the second most common primary intraspinal tumor, accounting for 26% of cases. Spinal meningiomas have a marked propensity to occur in the thoracic spinal cord, and they are rare below the midlumbar level. Like schwannomas, meningiomas are slow-

Table 11-4. Relative Incidence of Primary Intraspinal Neoplasms

Tumor	Percent of Total
Schwannomas	30
Meningiomas	26
Gliomas (ependymomas)	23
Sarcomas	11
Hemangiomas	6
Other	4

growing extramedullary-intradural tumors. The clinical picture usually evolves slowly over months to years before the diagnosis is made.

b. **Treatment.** Spinal meningiomas can usually be completely removed surgically. The neurologic deficits are at least partially reversible, and the patient is thus cured of the disease. However, complete resection is often technically quite difficult without damaging the spinal cord, especially in tumors located anterior to the cord. In these cases it may prove impossible or unwise to attempt complete tumor removal.

Recurrence is likely in patients with partially resected tumors, but it does not become clinically evident for months or years.

3. **Astrocytomas and ependymomas**

a. **Clinical features.** The most common intramedullary spinal tumors are the **gliomas,** which are comprised mainly of ependymomas and astrocytomas. The ependymomas predominate in the cauda equina and lumbar region; the astrocytomas, in the cervical region. The clinical syndrome produced by these tumors is usually indistinguishable from that produced by extramedullary tumors: Spinal gliomas are slow-growing tumors, and a history of deficits of several years' duration is commonplace.

b. **Surgery.** Most spinal gliomas are invasive as well as expansive and, unfortunately, complete surgical resection is possible in less than 20% of cases. Most intramedullary spinal tumors can be "decompressed" by means of a laminectomy, partial resection, and opening of the dura mater. Also, approximately 60% of intramedullary spinal tumors are also associated with syringomyelia; in these cases its cavity should be opened to allow drainage.

These procedures are likely to produce some recovery of neurologic function if the tumor has not caused irreversible damage to the spinal cord. The prognosis depends on the growth rate of the tumor, and in many patients the deficits progress slowly over several years.

c. **Radiotherapy.** Postoperative radiation therapy to the spinal cord is thought to delay the onset of recurrent neurologic symptoms and is therefore recommended for patients with partially resected intraspinal glioma. The spinal cord tolerance to irradiation is less than that of brain, and the maximum permissible tissue dose is 3500–4500 rads over 6–8 weeks, depending on the field size.

C. **Metastatic spinal tumors**

1. **Biology.** Metastatic tumors can reach the spinal cord by direct spread from an involved vertebra, by extension of tumor through an intervertebral foramen, or (uncommonly) by direct hematogeneous spread to the extradural fat. Therefore metastatic neoplasms of the spine are almost always contained in the extradural space. The thoracic-lumbar vertebral levels are the sites of predilection.

The tumors that are most likely to spread to the spinal canal are multiple myeloma, lymphomas, and cancers of the lung, breast, prostate, kidney, or sarcomas.

2. **Clinical features**

a. **Prodromal phase.** Perhaps 80% of patients with cancer who develop spinal cord compression pass through a prodromal phase, which is characterized by severe back pain or radicular pain or both. This pain precedes the onset of spinal cord compression by weeks to months in nearly all cases.

Unremitting back pain is always considered a serious symptom in a cancer patient. If the possibility of spinal metastasis is not considered, the opportunity for early diagnosis and treatment will be missed. Evidence of metastatic tumor (e.g., lytic or blastic lesions in the vertebrae, a paravertebral soft tissue mass, or a positive bone scan) should be sought diligently in cancer patients with back pain or radicular pain or both. If a tumor is found, a course of local radiotherapy or chemotherapy or both, depending on the histology of the primary neoplasm, might effectively relieve the pain and prevent eventual spinal cord compression.

b. **Stage of spinal compression.** The stage of spinal cord compression usually begins with subtle weakness or numbness in the legs or both. Hesitancy or urgency may lead to painless urinary retention with overflow. The tempo of neurologic progression is usually quite rapid, and over the next few days or weeks the patient becomes completely paraplegic. Metastatic lung cancers, renal carcinoma, and lymphomas are said to produce the most rapid progression to paraplegia. Thus spinal cord compression in this context is an **emergency.**

The earliest signs and symptoms of spinal cord compression should *promptly* lead to myelography. If a spinal block is found, cervical or cisternal myelography may be indicated to delineate the rostral extent of the tumor. As mentioned earlier, myelography may produce a sudden worsening of the patient's neurologic deficit, and facilities for surgery should be readily accessible.

3. **Treatment**

a. **Steroids.** Corticosteroids (e.g., dexamethasone 20 mg daily in divided doses) should be started at the time of diagnosis. There is significant clinical evidence that steroids relieve local "edema" (see sec II) and in some instances may have a significant oncolytic effect. This therapy allows the clinician to "buy time" while awaiting results of more definitive therapy (radiotherapy or surgery).

b. **Surgery and radiotherapy.** Most texts and reports advise that surgery be undertaken as soon as possible to relieve spinal cord or cauda equina compression and to prevent irreversible damage. The operation usually consists of extensive laminectomy with removal of as much tumor as possible. However, the majority of epidural metastases arise from the vertebral body and remain mainly anterior to the spinal cord. Since the surgeon approaches the spine posteriorly, it is usually not possible to remove substantial portions of the mass without damaging the spinal cord. Postoperatively, local radiotherapy is administered to arrest further tumor growth (e.g., 3000 rads given over 3 weeks, beginning about 6 days after surgery).

Unfortunately, the results of this combined surgery and radiotherapy approach are usually unsatisfactory. Surgical mortality and morbidity (e.g., poor wound healing, postoperative infection, worsening of neurologic deficits) are considerable. Large retrospective series have found that only 30–50% of patients with metastatic cancer of the spine have significant neurologic improvement (e.g., regain ambulation) following surgical decompression. The remainder are left with a stable deficit (about 40%) or continue to deteriorate (about 20%).

c. **Radiotherapy alone.** Most oncologists have realized that spinal epidural compression by "radiosensitive" tumors, such as lymphomas, could be managed effectively by radiotherapy without surgery. Recent data from the Sloan-Kettering Cancer Center reveal that radiotherapy alone is as effective (or ineffective) as decompressive laminectomy followed by radiotherapy in treating epidural spinal compression, regardless of the underlying histology (e.g., prostate, lung, breast, or renal cancer). Following both forms of treatment, the overall improvement rate was 40–50% and the duration of clinical remission was similar. Patients with rapidly progressing neurologic deficits (weakness evolving over 48 hours) did as well or better when treated with irradiation alone as compared to surgically treated patients. The Sloan-Kettering group administered 400 rads daily for the first 3 days to a port encompassing two vertebral bodies above and below the block, followed by 200 rads daily to a total dose of 2000–4000 rads, depending on the histology of the tumor. Decompressive laminectomy is indicated when (1) the histologic diagnosis is in doubt, (2) relapse occurs after radiotherapy, or (3) symptoms progress inexorably after several doses of radiotherapy.

d. Prognostic features. The stage of underlying malignancy determines the patient's overall prognosis, and in some patients with widespread systemic cancer it is appropriate to not treat spinal epidural compression at all.

When the pretreatment neurologic deficit is complete (absolutely no motor, sensory, or sphincter function below the level of the cord lesion), the likelihood of significant recovery following any form of therapy is remote. Therefore, if treatment is to be undertaken, it should be initiated as soon as spinal epidural compression is detected clinically and confirmed radiographically.

Patients with multiple myeloma, lymphoma, and breast cancer have a greater likelihood of responding favorably to treatment (whether radiation alone or surgery) than patients with other cancers. Some patients will remain ambulatory for 1 year or more following radiotherapy for spinal epidural metastasis.

VI. REMOTE EFFECTS OF SYSTEMIC CANCER ON THE NERVOUS SYSTEM (PARANEOPLASTIC SYNDROME)

A. Description. Many neurologic syndromes have been associated with systemic cancer, most often with oat cell carcinoma of the lung, but with many other tumors as well. The main ones, described in other chapters, include polymyositis and dermatomyositis, polyneuropathy, Eaton-Lambert syndrome, progressive multifocal leukoencephalopathy, and cerebellar degeneration.

B. Treatment. The incidence of all the syndromes is very low compared with the incidence of central nervous system metastases, and the only effective long-term therapy consists of successful treatment of the underlying tumor. In the short term some benefit has been found in treating patients with the Eaton-Lambert syndrome with guanidine, and there is some suggestion that adenine arabinoside may retard the course of progressive multifocal leukoencephalopathy.

SELECTED READINGS

General References on Brain Tumors
Posner, J. B., and Shapiro, W. R. Brain tumor—Current status of treatment and its complications. *Arch. Neurol.* 32:781, 1975.

Rubinstein, L. J. Tumors of the Central Nervous System, in *Atlas of Tumor Pathology*, 2nd series, fascicle 6. Washington D.C.: Armed Forces Institute of Pathology, 1972.

Corticosteroids and Tumor-related Brain Edema
French, L. A., and Galicich, J. G. The use of steroids for control of cerebral edema. *Clin. Neurosurg.* 10:212, 1962.

Gutin, P. H. Corticosteroid therapy in patients with cerebral tumors. *Semin. Oncol.* 2:49, 1975.

Matson, D. D. Treatment of cerebral swelling. *N. Engl. J. Med.* 272:626, 1965.

Renaudin, J., Fewer, D., Wilson, C. B., Boldrey, E. B., Calogero, J., and Enot, K. J. Dose dependency of decadron in patients with partially excised brain tumors. *J. Neurosurg.* 39:302, 1973.

Glioblastoma Multiforme
Hekmatpanah, J. (ed.) *Gliomas: Current Concepts in Biology. Diagnosis and Treatment.* New York: Springer-Verlag, 1975.

Jelsma, R., and Bucy, P. C.   The treatment of glioblastoma multiforme of the brain. *J. Neurosurg.* 27:388, 1967.

Walker, M. D., and Weiss, H. D.   Chemotherapy in the treatment of malignant brain tumors. *Adv. Neurol.* 13:149, 1975.

Astrocytomas and Oligodendrogliomas

Elvidge, A. R.   Long term survival in the astrocytoma series. *J. Neurosurg.* 28:399, 1968.

Shenkin, H. A.   The effect of roentgen-ray therapy on oligodendrogliomas of the brain. *J. Neurosurg.* 22:57, 1965.

Weir, B., and Elvidge, A. R.   Oligodendrogliomas—An analysis of 63 cases. *J. Neurosurg.* 29:500, 1968.

Reticulum Cell Sarcoma

Henry, J. M., Heffner, R. R., Dillard, S. H., Earle, K. M., and Davis, R. L.   Primary malignant lymphomas of the central nervous system. *Cancer* 34:1293, 1974.

Schaumberg, H. H., Plank, C. R., and Adams, R. D.   The reticulum cell sarcoma—Microgliomas group of brain tumors. *Brain* 95:199, 1972.

Schneck, S. A., and Penn, I.   De-novo brain tumors in renal transplant recipients. *Lancet* 1:983, 1971.

Meningiomas

Jellinger, K., and Slowik, F.   Histologic subtypes and prognostic problems in meningiomas. *J. Neurol.* 208:279, 1975.

Simpson, D.   The recurrence of intracranial meningiomas after surgical treatment. *J. Neurol. Neurosurg. Psychiatry* 20:22, 1957.

Wara, W. M., Sheline, G. E., Newman, H., Townsend, J. J., and Boldrey, E. B.   Radiation therapy of meningiomas. *Am. J. Roentgenol. Radium Ther. Nucl. Med.* 123:453, 1975.

Acoustic Schwannoma

Ojemann, R. G., Montgomery, W. M., and Weiss, A. D.   Evaluation and surgical treatment of acoustic neuroma. *N. Engl. J. Med.* 287:895, 1972.

Pituitary Adenomas

Kjellberg, R. N., and Kliman, B.   A System for Therapy of Pituitary Tumors, in *Diagnosis and Treatment of Pituitary Tumors*. Amsterdam: Excerpta Medica, 1973.

Pistenma, D. A., Goffinet, D. R., Bagshaw, M. A., Hanbery, J. W., Eltringham, J. R.   Treatment of chromophobe adenomas with megavoltage irradiation. *Cancer* 35:1574, 1975.

Ray, B. S., and Patterson, R. H., Jr.   Surgical experience with chromophobe adenomas of the pituitary gland. *J. Neurosurg.* 34:726, 1971.

Weisberg, L. A.   Asymptomatic enlargement of the sella turcica. *Arch. Neurol.* 32:483, 1975.

Cerebral Metastases

Deutsch, M., Parson, J. A., Mercado, R., Jr.   Radiotherapy for intracranial metastases. *Cancer* 34:1607, 1975.

Lokich, J. R.   The management of cerebral metastasis. *J.A.M.A.* 234:748, 1975.

Raskind, R., Weiss, S. R., Manning, J. J., and Wermuth, R. E.   Survival after surgical excision of single metastatic brain tumors. *Am. J. Roentgenol. Radium Ther. Nucl. Med.* 111:323, 1971.

Meningeal Carcinomatosis

Olson, M. E., Chernik, N. J., and Posner, J. B.   Infiltration of the leptomeninges by systemic cancer. *Arch. Neurol.* 31:122, 1974.

Meningeal Leukemia

Jones, B.   Prophylactic central nervous system therapy of leukemia. *Med. Prob. Pediatr.* (Basel: Karger) 16:99, 1975.

Soniss Marten, G. W., Pitner, S. E., Duenas, D. A., and Powazek, M.   Effects of CNS irradiation on neuropsychologic functioning of children with acute lymphocytic leukemia. *N. Engl. J. Med.* 293:113, 1975.

Sullivan, M. P., Vietti, T. J., Haggard, M. E., Donaldson, M. H., Krall, J. M., and Gehan, E. A.   Remission maintenance therapy for meningeal leukemia. *Blood* 38:680, 1971.

Weiss, H. D., Walker, M. D., and Wiernik, P. H.   Neurotoxicity of commonly used antineoplastic agents. *N. Engl. J. Med.* 291:75, 127, 1974.

General References—Brain Tumors in Childhood

Sheline, G. E.   Radiation therapy of tumors of the central nervous system in childhood. *Cancer* 35:957, 1975.

Wilson, C. B.   Diagnosis and surgical treatment of childhood brain tumors. *Cancer* 35:950, 1975.

Cerebellar Astrocytoma

Geissinger, J. D., and Bucy, P. C.   Astrocytomas of the cerebellum in children. *Arch. Neurol.* 24:125, 1971.

Medulloblastoma

Bloom, H. J. G.   Concepts in the natural history and treatment of medulloblastoma in children. *Crit. Rev. Radiol. Sci.* 2:89, 1971.

Wilson, C. B.   Medulloblastoma—Current views regarding the tumor and its treatment. *Oncology* 24:273, 1970.

Ependymoma

Shuman, R., and Alvord, E.   Ependymomas in childhood. *Arch. Neurol.* 32:73, 1975.

Brain Stem Gliomas

Marsa, G. W., Probert, J. C., Rubinstein, L. J., and Bagshaw, M. A.   Radiation therapy of childhood astrocytic gliomas. *Cancer* 32:646, 1972.

Craniopharyngioma

Hoff, J. T., and Patterson, R. H., Jr.   Craniopharyngiomas in children and adults. *J. Neurosurg.* 36:299, 1972.

Pineal Tumors

DeGirolami, U., and Schmidek, H.   Clinicopathological study of 53 tumors of the pineal region. *J. Neurosurg.* 39:452, 1973.

Optic Glioma

Chutorian, A. M., Schwarta, J. F., Evans, R. A., and Carter, S.   Optic gliomas in children. *Neurology* 14:83, 1964.

Hoyt, W. F., and Baghassarian, S. A.   Optic glioma of childhood. *Br. J. Ophthalmol.* 53:793, 1969.

Spinal Tumors

Gilbert, R. W., Kim, J., and Posner, J. B.   Epidural spinal cord compression from metastatic tumor: Diagnosis and treatment. *Ann. Neurol.* 3:40, 1978.

Hall, A. J., Mackay, N. N. S.   The results of laminectomy for compression of the cord or cauda equina by extradural malignant tumor. *J. Bone Joint Surg.* 55:497, 1973.

Harries, B.   Spinal cord compression. *Br. J. Med.* 1:611, 173, 1970.

Mullins, G. M., Glynn, J. P. G., El-mahdi, A. M., McQueen, J. D., and Owens, A. H., Jr.   Malignant lymphoma of the spinal epidural space. *Ann. Intern. Med.* 74:416, 1971.

Posner, J. B., Howieson, J., and Cvitkovic, E.   Oncolytic effect of glucocorticoids on epidural metastases. *Ann. Neurol.* 2:409, 1977.

Vieth, R. G., and Odom, G. L.   Extradural spinal metastases and their neurosurgical treatment. *J. Neurosurg.* 23:501, 1965.

12

Trauma
Telmo M. Aquino

I. **HEAD INJURY** is a problem of enormous magnitude. Automobile and work accidents experienced by adults and accidents at play and falls experienced by children account for most cases. Also, the patient frequently suffers multiple associated injuries. Although methods of treating head injury have improved (e.g., nursing care, respiratory monitoring, control of brain edema, and early recognition of intracranial hematoma) and the mortality has decreased, a substantial number of patients are left with varying degrees of disability. Many of these patients cannot regain their previous employment level, some are left unemployable, and some are left in what has been called a *persistent vegetative state*. Since a high percentage of these patients are in the working age group, the economic consequences of head injury are staggering.

A large number of deaths are caused by primary brain damage that cannot be treated. In other instances, death is a result of associated injuries, usually pulmonary injuries or hemorrhagic shock. Still other cases exist in which the brain damage is in itself nonlethal, but intracranial complications develop (e.g., infections, hematoma, or brain edema) that, unless treated adequately, prove fatal. Extracranial complications, such as pneumonia, pulmonary thromboembolism, and fat embolism, also may threaten life. These complications must be diagnosed and treated with some degree of anticipation, since the additive effect they have on the primary brain lesion increases the neurologic damage and resultant disability.

A. **Diagnosis**

1. **The history.** The circumstances of the injury, the nature and force of the impact, whether or not there is loss of consciousness, and changes in the degree of alertness from the moment of injury are important.

2. **Routine general examination.** Look for associated trauma and other disease processes.

3. **The neurologic examination.** Head trauma can be a rapidly changing process, and repeated examinations should be made to detect changes. The neurologic–vital signs sheet (i.e., blood pressure, pulse, respiratory rate, pupillary size and reaction, level of consciousness, and motor responses) is a very useful tool for this purpose.

   a. **The level of consciousness** is the single most important feature in detecting progression. Therefore it should be evaluated in a standardized manner at regular intervals. Descriptive terms, such as *obtundation, stupor,* and *coma* (see Chap. 1) should be qualified by more precise descriptions, such as "opens eyes and smiles to gentle calling of name," and "no response to forceful pinching of nipples."

   b. **Inspect and palpate the head and scalp,** looking for wounds and fractures. Bilateral orbital fractures will cause periorbital hematomas (raccoon eyes); and swelling and hematoma over the mastoid (Battle's sign) points to fracture of the temporal bone. Check for blood or CSF in the external auditory canal (basilar skull fracture).

   c. **Cranial nerves**

      (1) In alert patients, check **smell** (coffee; tincture of benzoin suffices in the emergency room.)

      (2) Check **vision, visual fields,** and **funduscopy.**

      (3) Unilateral dilatation of the **pupils** and sluggishness of light reaction suggests third-nerve compression due to transtentorial herniation.

(4) Check **extraocular mobility** on command and following. The doll's head maneuver may be used to demonstrate eye movements in unconscious patients, but it **should not be performed** if there is a question of neck injury. Caloric stimulation may be used in neck-injured patients or those in whom an incomplete range of eye movements is obtained using the doll's head maneuver. Ensure the integrity of the tympanic membrane and the external auditory canal before instilling liquid. (For details of the test, see Chap. 1.)

(5) **Sensation** and **motility** of the face and corneal reflexes reflect the integrity of the trigeminal and facial nerves. They may be checked in succession.

(6) **Hearing** is examined after the otoscopic examination.

(7) The **lower cranial nerves** (i.e., glossopharyngeal, vagus, spinal accessory, and hypoglossal) may be checked briefly by looking at palatal motion, swallowing, articulation of words, trapezius and sternocleidomastoid motion, and tongue protrusion.

d. Motor system. First observe spontaneous posture and movement, and then apply noxious stimuli of graded intensity to certain standard areas, such as the medial aspect of elbows and knees. Spontaneous, purposeful, or fending-off movements of a limb are consistent with good preservation of the corresponding corticospinal tract. Absence of movement, decreased tone, and diminished reflexes (in the early stages) suggest hemiparesis. Also, spontaneous decerebrate movements may occur.

Arm or leg abduction, on pinching the patient's elbow or knee, are considered high-level responses; i.e., they require intactness of the corresponding corticospinal tract. Flexion at the elbow with extension of the legs is called *decortication*. Extension of the arm with internal rotation of the forearm and wrist and extension of the leg is called *decerebration*.

e. Deep tendon reflexes and plantar responses should be recorded in all patients.

f. Sensory system, cerebellar system, stance, and gait should be investigated and recorded in all alert patients.

4. Differential diagnosis. One crucial point in the management of head injury is the decision of whether to treat the patient medically or surgically. Some criteria include the following:

a. Penetrating brain injuries and depressed skull fractures generally require surgical treatment.

b. Intracranial hematomas of such magnitude as to produce symptoms of brain compression should be evacuated surgically. CT scanning differentiates hematoma from cerebral edema, a frequent accompaniment of contusions, which in the majority of patients may be handled medically. However, progression of signs suggests an expanding intracranial hematoma. Decrease in alertness, bradycardia, hypertension, and vomiting point to acutely increasing intracranial pressure.

c. Intracranial pressure monitoring through a pressure-recording device is helpful in indicating when elevations of the intracranial pressure reach dangerous levels, thus prompting surgical intervention.

5. Ancillary studies

a. Skull x-rays (PA, Townes, and lateral views) are obtained in every case of head injury. Besides fractures, pineal gland displacements can be identified when this structure is calcified. Tangential views may be necessary to demonstrate depressed skull fractures.

b. **Cervical spine x-rays** are mandatory, given the association of cervical spine fracture in patients with head injury.

c. **Lumbar puncture** is probably not needed in the initial evaluation of head injury. Also, it may be potentially dangerous if increased intracranial pressure is present.

d. **Electroencephalography** (EEG) does not serve any useful purpose in acute head injury.

e. **Cerebral angiography.** Where CT scanning is not available, this is the diagnostic tool with which the diagnosis of intracranial hematoma is made. However, the distinction between intracerebral hematoma and cerebral edema is less clear than with CT scanning. Remember that a significant proportion (around 20%) of traumatic intracranial hematomas are bilateral.

f. **Echoencephalography** is used to detect a shift of midline structures. However, its reliability is questionable unless it is performed by experienced operators.

g. **CT scanning** has improved the quality of diagnosis and management of head injury. It is the preferred test for the detection of contusion, hematomas, edema, shift of midline structures, hydrocephalus, and so forth. A hematoma is rarely undetected with a satisfactory examination. Also, postoperative CT scanning helps detect hematomas not recognized during surgery. Its main drawback is that the patient's head must remain immobile for the duration of the test (between 10 and 20 minutes), which makes the use of sedation or even general anesthesia necessary in uncooperative, agitated patients.

h. **Burr holes** may be needed when there is rapid deterioration, which is measured by impairment of consciousness, pupillary dilatation, and contralateral hemiparesis. Three burr holes are placed (temporal, frontal, and parietal) on the **same side as the dilated pupil.** Additional burr holes should be placed contralaterally if the initial ones are negative.

B. **General therapeutic measures in the head-injured patient.** Conscious patients require only observation. The unconscious patient requires the following management:

1. Call the neurosurgical consultant.

2. Establish a good airway. Frequently, intubation and artificial ventilation are necessary.

3. Insert a large intravenous catheter.

4. Obtain vital signs at least every 15 minutes initially. Hemorrhagic shock is rarely caused by head injury. Thus other sources of bleeding must be investigated.

5. Draw blood for routine tests:

    a. CBC

    b. Electrolytes

    c. BUN

    d. Blood sugar

    e. Clotting studies

    f. Type and cross-match

6. Insert a bladder catheter and start monitoring urine output.

7. Insert a gastric tube, evacuate, and take note of gastric contents (e.g., blood).

8. Perform a baseline neurologic examination (see sec. **I.A.3**).

9. Obtain skull and cervical spine x-rays and any other additional x-rays (i.e., chest, abdomen, or extremities) that may be warranted.

10. If the patient remains **comatose:**

   a. Place the patient in the lateral decubitus position to avoid aspiration.

   b. **Turn** the patient at frequent intervals (every 1–2 hours) to avoid decubitus ulcers.

   c. **Suction** the patient hourly, taking sterile precautions.

   d. **Chlorpromazine** 10–25 mg IM every 4–6 hours may be given for agitation.

   e. **Restrain** and **bandage** the hands and feet to prevent the patient from injuring himself or pulling out tubes.

   f. **Phenytoin** (Dilantin) may be administered to prevent seizures. The loading dose is 15 mg/kg, which may be given as rapidly as 50 mg/min IV. (See Chap. 6 for details.) The maintenance dose is 5 mg/kg/day.

   g. The three-way **bladder catheter** is constantly infused with bladder irrigation (0.25% acetic acid solution). Discontinue catheters **as soon as possible.**

   h. 1000 ml/sq m of 0.45% NaCl in **2.5% dextrose in water** or its equivalent are administered daily, and KCl 20–40 mEq is added to each liter of solution. After 5–7 days, start nasogastric tube feedings.

   i. Check serum **electrolytes, osmolality,** and **BUN** frequently to monitor fluid therapy.

   j. Obtain **chest x-ray, urinalysis,** and **CBC** at least twice weekly to detect early infectious complications.

   k. If constipation develops, a **rectal examination** for disimpaction is done, followed by enemas.

   l. If coma persists longer than 1 week, consider doing **tracheostomy** and **gastrostomy.**

C. **The lesions**

1. **Scalp wounds** indicate the site of the injury. This site should be investigated further for direct and contrecoup lesions, which can cause rather severe bleeding. Also, cranial osteomyelitis, with meningeal or encephalic propagation, may originate in scalp wound infections. Treatment consists of surgical closure of the wound.

2. **Skull fractures** derive their importance from the possibility of associated infection, involvement of vascular elements intimately related to the skull (e.g., middle meningeal artery and vein, dural sinuses), brain damage, dural defects produced by bone fragments in depressed fractures, and, finally, as the source of skull defects. Fractures may be closed (simple) or open (compound).

   Involvement of the cribriform plate and the basisphenoid and paranasal sinuses, provided there is a mucosal tear, is the criterion for determining whether a basilar fracture is compound, while breach of integrity of the overlying scalp is the criterion for the diagnosis of vault fractures. Skull fractures are customarily divided between those of the base (basilar) and the vault.

   a. **Basilar fractures**

      (1) **Description.** Basilar fractures are usually associated with severe trauma. Clinically, they are manifested by CSF or blood discharge

from the ears or nose. Skull x-rays are frequently normal, but **an air level or an opacified mastoid or sinus may be seen. The complications** of basilar skull fracture are:

(a) **CSF leak** wth a resultant high probability of infection.

(b) **Injury to large basal vessels** (e.g., carotid arteries, venous sinuses), with resultant hemorrhage, arteriovenous fistula, or thrombosis.

(c) **Cranial nerve injury,** particularly optic, olfactory, auditory, or facial.

(2) **Treatment**

(a) Observation

(b) Complications may require surgical treatment.

b. **Vault fractures**

(1) **Description.** Vault fractures may assume different forms: linear, comminuted, depressed, or stellate. They may or may not be palpable. In children, because of the thinness and elasticity of the skull, a depression can be made without fracture being a frequent occurrence.

(2) **Treatment**

(a) **Linear fractures** may be treated with simple analgesics and observation.

(b) **Depressed, comminuted, and compound fractures** often need surgical treatment, although depressed fractures in children without a neurologic deficit may be treated conservatively.

3. **Concussion**

a. **Description.** Concussion is a clinical syndrome characterized by immediate and transient impairment of neural functions due to mechanical forces. Its most striking manifestation is impaired consciousness. A period of impaired memory, both for events preceding the injury **(retrograde amnesia)** and following it **(anterograde amnesia),** also occurs. Recovery from traumatic unconsciousness usually evolves through a period of restlessness and agitated confusion to gradually increasing periods of rational behavior until normality returns. In children, the syndrome often consists of lethargy, irritability, pallor, and vomiting.

b. **Pathophysiology.** Rotational acceleration produces a differential rate of movement between the skull and brain and between different areas of the brain. Thus sudden displacements (linear acceleration and deceleration) can induce rapid pressure changes in the brain substance, which are positive under the stricken area and negative in the anti-pole. This pressure will then give rise to contrecoup lesions. Although rotational acceleration is the most important mechanism, in a clinical concussion more than one type of stress is probably operative at any given moment. For example, mechanical forces acting on the brain will subject it to various stresses, which can produce strains responsible for tissue-shearing in various parts of the brain.

There is ample evidence that brainstem derangement plays a central, although not exclusive, role in traumatic unconsciousness. There is also evidence of widespread white-matter degeneration in patients who die after a severe concussion.

c. **Treatment.** If there has been a definite loss of consciousness, the patient is admitted for observation. For treatment of unconscious patients, see sec **I.B.** Children with the syndrome of lethargy alternating with irritability and vomiting are observed until definite improvement is noted. If the patient cannot be admitted, arrangements should be made for careful observation at home for the next 24–48 hours.

4. Contusion

a. Description. Contusion refers to bruised, necrotic cortex and white matter with variable amounts of petechial hemorrhages and edema. Subarachnoid bleeding is common. The clinical state in brain contusion is similar to that of concussion, but it is usually more severe and has associated focal neurologic deficits.

b. Pathophysiology. Contusion may result from direct bruising of the brain at the site of impact, fragments of bone under depressed fractures (coup injuries), or negative pressure at the pole opposite the impact (contrecoup). The orbital surface of the frontal lobes and the frontotemporal junction of the hemispheres are frequently affected, due to violent displacements of the brain against bony irregularities of the orbital roof or the lesser sphenoid wing.

c. Treatment

(1) Observation.

(2) General supportive measures (see sec **I.B.**).

(3) Steroids for the control of brain edema. Dexamethasone is usually used: a 10 mg loading dose is given, followed by 4–6 mg every 6 hours PO, IM, or IV.

(4) Phenytoin for seizure control in the usual dose.

(5) Surgery may be needed for decompression in severe cases.

5. Laceration involves actual loss of continuity of the brain tissue and is commonly associated with contusion and skull fracture. The treatment is surgical removal of necrotic tissue and control of bleeding.

6. Epidural hematoma (EDH))

a. Description. Epidural hematoma is a collection of blood situated between the skull and dura. It is usually a disease of young adult life. Early recognition of a **true neurosurgical emergency** can lead to a lifesaving operation.

(1) Lucid interval. Classically, after an initial short period of unconsciousness on impact, there is a lucid interval followed by progressive impairment of consciousness and contralateral hemiparesis. In about 50% of cases, however, there is no lucid interval, and unconsciousness is present from the moment of the injury. Progressive headache is usually present when there is a lucid interval.

The duration of the lucid interval is usually 6–18 hours, but shorter or longer intervals are common. This interval represents the time elapsed between the initial traumatic unconsciousness and the beginning of diencephalic derangement produced by transtentorial herniation. A short lucid interval suggests that the bleeding is brisk and probably arterial.

(2) Hemiparesis. The focal neurologic deficit is generally contralateral hemiparesis, due to the effect of the expanding mass on the origin of the corticospinal tract. Hemiparesis ipsilateral to the clot is less common. It is caused by compression of the contralateral cerebral peduncle against the tentorial edge (Kernohan's notch).

(3) Seizures may occur.

(4) Herniation. Unilateral pupillary dilatation is the first indication of transtentorial herniation.

b. **Evaluation.** The classic history of initial loss of consciousness, followed by a lucid interval and later by progressive obtundation and hemiparesis, is highly suggestive of epidural hematoma. When a linear skull fracture is seen across the middle meningeal groove in plain skull x-rays, cerebral angiography or CT scanning is the next step. Frequently, however, herniation has already begun by the time the patient reaches the emergency room, and exploratory burr holes (often done in the emergency room) are necessary.

c. **Pathophysiology.** Epidural hematoma usually results from low-speed blunt head injury, such as from falls or impacts with objects, and it is almost always associated with linear skull fracture. In the majority of patients the bleeding vessels are the middle meningeal artery or vein or both. The middle meningeal vessels are injured when the fracture line crosses the middle meningeal groove in the temporal squama.

d. **Treatment.** In this situation, time should not be wasted on unnecessary tests.

   (1) In herniating patients

   (a) Intubation.

   (b) Hyperventilation (aim for Pco_2 of 25 mm Hg).

   (c) Decadron 10 mg IV.

   (d) Mannitol, 250 ml of the 20% solution by rapid intravenous infusion.

   (e) While the above steps are being performed, the operating room is made ready for the patient with maximum expediency.

   (f) Avoid hypotonic intravenous fluids.

   (2) In more stable patients surgery may be postponed until after angiography or CT scan. However, in infants with open fontanelles, a subdural tap is performed immediately, since epidural hemorrhage cannot be distinguished from subdural hemorrhage clinically.

7. Subdural hematoma (SDH)

a. **Description.** Subdural hematoma is a collection of blood between the dura and the underlying brain and is more frequent than epidural hematoma. Depending on the time interval between the injury and the onset of symptoms, it is clinically divided into **acute** (up to 24 hours), **subacute** (1–10 days), and **chronic** (more than 10 days). About one-half of cases are associated with skull fracture.

   Subdural hematoma can be located anywhere within the cranial cavity, but it is most frequently over the convexity. About 20% are bilateral, and they are usually caused by blunt trauma without fracture, simple or compound fractures, birth injury, or bleeding diathesis.

b. **Pathophysiology.** Cortical veins going to the dura, dural sinuses, or vascular tears in contusions and lacerations are the most common bleeding vessels.

c. **Specific types of subdural hematoma**

   (1) Acute subdural hematomas (ASDH) are frequently the result of high-speed impacts, such as automobile accidents. Associated severe primary brain damage is the rule and, predictably, the mortality is high. Nonremitting coma from the moment of impact is suggestive of acute subdural hematoma. The distinction between an acute subdural and an epidural hematoma is difficult or impossible to make on clinical grounds. However, the course is similar in both types.

(2) Subacute hematomas are suspected when, after several days of somnolence or stupor, deterioration of consciousness develops. In all other respects, this type of hematoma resembles the acute variety.

(3) Chronic subdural hematomas (CSDH). In contrast to the preceding ones, chronic subdural hematomas may follow trivial trauma, at times unnoticed by the patient or not witnessed by family or friends. Therefore its diagnosis demands a high degree of clinical suspicion. A gradual drift into stupor or coma, preceded by headaches, is the common picture. Mental changes may be prominent and simulate dementia, psychiatric disorders, or drug toxicity. In infants, chronic subdural hematoma is most common between 2–6 months of age and often is caused by accidental or inflicted head injury. In this age group the clinical picture is one of increasing intracranial pressure with vomiting, lethargy, and irritability; an increasing head circumference; and a bulging fontanelle. Seizures and retinal hemorrhages are common as well.

Rotational acceleration can easily tear the superior cortical veins as they enter the superior sagittal sinus. Also brain atrophy associated with aging, prolonging the trajectory of these veins, probably makes them more susceptible to rupture. This would explain the significant proportion of cases of chronic subdural hematoma in elderly patients following minor degrees of head injury or with no antecedent trauma.

In nonfatal cases, the evolution is toward encapsulation of the clot in a progressively more fibrous capsule, lined with a vascular granulation tissue. The dural or parietal layer of this capsule is much thicker than the arachnoidal or visceral layer. Thus the contents of the hematoma vary from thick and tarry dark fluid with fragments of dissolving clot at the onset to thinner and clearer fluid at later stages. These contents are thought to increase in volume due to transudation of plasma and small hemorrhages from the highly vascular lining membranes.

d. Treatment

(1) Acute subdural hematoma. Surgical treatment is similar to that of epidural hematoma. In children with open fontanelles, subdural tap is performed as the first diagnostic and therapeutic maneuver.

(2) Chronic subdural hematoma

(a) Adults. Burr holes are used for drainage of fluid. Sometimes the membranes must be excised.

(b) Children with open fontanelles. The head is shaved and prepped with iodine. An 18–22-gauge short-beveled subdural needle with a stylet is introduced at the lateral corner of the anterior fontanelle, at least 3–4 mm from the midline. If the fontanelle is small, the needle is introduced through the coronal suture. The needle is advanced slowly until the dura is punctured, and it is secured by the examiner's finger against the scalp. The stylet is then removed and fluid is allowed to drain. **Suction should not be used on the needle.** Subdural taps are repeated as often as necessary to relieve symptoms or signs of increased intracranial pressure. If repeated subdural taps have failed and further treatment is necessary, then temporary shunting procedures may be indicated. Craniotomy and membrane stripping are rarely indicated and should be considered as a last resort.

8. Subdural hygroma

a. Description. This term is applied to subdural collections of yellow fluid found both in adults and infants after head injury. Since subdural hygromas resemble subdural hematomas both clinically and radiographically, diagnosis is made at operation.

b. **Pathophysiology.** Theoretically, a small subdural hemorrhage becomes diluted with CSF that seeps through a minor arachnoidal defect, acting like a ball valve.

c. **Treatment.** Occasionally a subdural hygroma has a membrane formation similar to that of a subdural hematoma and necessitates excision, but usually the drainage of fluid through burr holes will suffice.

9. **Intracerebral hematoma** (ICH)

a. **Description.** Intracerebral hematoma refers to hemorrhage larger than 5 ml within the brain substance (smaller hemorrhages are called *punctate* or *petechial*). The symptoms vary with the location of the hematoma. In the absence of prolonged initial unconsciousness, there may be a lucid interval with progressive headaches, and progressive contralateral hemiparesis may occur, provided the hematoma is in the appropriate site. Stupor that progresses to coma will develop if the diencephalon is displaced by the mass effect. Skull fracture is absent in up to 30% of cases. CT scanning is the most useful study for demonstrating intracerebral hemorrhage.

b. **Pathophysiology.** The same factors that are involved in the production of contusion lesions are observed. (These factors are also seen in association with penetrating injuries.) Intracerebral hematomas are frequently located in the temporal and frontal lobes; traumatic cerebellar hematomas are rare and difficult to diagnose. A fracture of the occipital squama may be present. Alteration of the mental state and, rarely, an ipsilateral cerebellar syndrome can help localize the lesion.

c. **Treatment** consists of observation and supportive measures in small hemorrhages. Large intracerebral hemorrhages may be removed surgically, when accessible.

10. **Cranial nerve injuries**

a. **Olfactory.** Since testing of the sense of smell requires patient cooperation, first cranial nerve dysfunction cannot be assessed until consciousness returns. Although the olfactory bulb or nerve may be involved in ethmoid fractures or in association with orbital fractures, it is most frequently affected in patients with severe concussion. Up to one-third of patients recover the sense of smell spontaneously.

b. **Optic nerve and chiasm.** Optic nerve and, more rarely, chiasmal lesions occur in approximately one-half of orbit fractures. Most frequently the nerve is affected at the level of the optic foramen. While chiasmal damage usually follows serious trauma, optic nerve damage may be caused by more trivial injuries.

Chiasmal lesions are occasionally associated with hypothalamic damage, which can be caused by diabetes insipidus; and optic nerve damage may simulate an oculomotor nerve palsy (by dilating the pupil), thus creating the impression that herniation is occurring. The pupil, however, will still react consensually (Marcus Gunn pupil).

Occasionally, surgery is helpful in decompressing the optic nerve from scars and bone fragments. The prognosis for return of vision is generally poor.

c. **Oculomotor, trochlear, and abducens nerves.** These may be affected within the orbit or at the superior orbital fissure in sphenoidal fractures. The sixth (abducens) nerve may be affected by a fracture at the apex of the petrous bone; brainstem, particularly midbrain, contusion may produce pupillary and extraocular movement abnormalities; and diplopia may be caused by orbital trauma and consequent misalignment of the visual axis.

d. Trigeminal nerve. In most cases, the trigeminal nerve is affected in its extracranial course, the maxillary branch being the most frequently damaged. The gasserian ganglion can be damaged in basilar skull fractures or penetrating injuries. Also, other neighboring structures (cavernous sinus; cranial nerves II, IV, and VI; carotid artery) are usually affected.

e. Facial nerve. Although the facial nerve can be injured extracranially, it is more frequently damaged in its intrapetrosal course. Paresis (incomplete lesion) has a better prognosis than paralysis, because the latter reflects anatomic transection of the nerve. Immediate paralysis also has a poor prognosis for the same reason. Delayed onset may be a result of hemorrhage or edema within the canalicular portion of the nerve, and it may be amenable to decompression.

To establish whether there is only physiological nerve impulse blockage or actual axonal degeneration, electric testing is required.

(1) A percutaneous nerve excitability test may be done at the bedside and is simple to perform. It can detect evidences of axonal degeneration earlier than electromyography (EMG).

(2) EMG is a useful tool for detecting evidence of axonal regeneration. It is important to determine whether the lesion is situated proximally or distally to the geniculate ganglion, because surgical approach is easier in the latter case.

(3) The Schirmer test is based on the fact that the greater petrosal nerve leaves the facial nerve at the level of the geniculate ganglion. Thus a strip of filter paper is left in the lower conjunctival sac, and the wetting by tears is compared between the two sides. Normally, the lacrimal gland can wet a minimum of 2–3 cm of the paper over 5 minutes, whereas the denervated gland will wet only a few millimeters.

f. Vestibulocochlear nerve

(1) Vestibular branch. Posttraumatic dizziness and vertigo are covered in Chapter 4.

(2) Cochlear branch. This branch is frequently damaged in temporal bone fractures, usually in conjunction with the vestibular branch. Thus evaluation of hearing is part of the examination in all alert patients, particularly when a temporal bone fracture is suspected. Audiometry is done as soon as the patient's condition permits it.

(a) Posttraumatic tinnitus may result from injuries to the cochlear nerve, labyrinth, and blood vessels supplying the inner ear. There is no known reliable treatment for traumatic tinnitus.

(b) Hearing loss is usually mixed at the onset, with both conductive and sensorineural components. In **conductive hearing loss,** the sound is impeded in reaching the receptor organ due to typanic rupture, hemorrhage in the middle ear, or disorganization of the ossicular chain. The conductive component tends to resolve spontaneously in many patients by reabsorption of edema and hemorrhage, except in cases of ossicular chain disruption.

Sensorineural hearing loss results from direct injury to the receptor organ, the cochlear nerve or its neural connections. The prognosis in this type of hearing loss is poor.

g. Glossopharyngeal, vagus, spinal accessory, and hypoglossal nerves. Injury to these cranial nerves is usually associated with severe basilar skull fracture. Most patients do not recover from this type of injury.

11. Traumatic carotid and vertebral artery thrombosis. Occasionally the carotid artery is injured in the neck during trauma and thromboses as a result; it may also be injured in or above the cavernous sinus; or the vertebral artery may be damaged in fracture-dislocations of the neck. The clinical syndromes associated with great-vessel thrombosis are covered in Chapter 10.

D. Traumatic, acutely increased intracranial pressure

1. **Cerebral edema.** Contusions and lacerations of the brain are habitually accompanied by varying degrees of focal cerebral edema (CE). Epidural and subdural hematomas are also associated with cerebral edema, both before and after surgical evacuation. In these cases, cerebral edema results from obstruction to the venous outflow by the mass, with ensuing escape of fluid to the extravascular space. The edema and the resultant increased intracranial pressure (ICP) are proportional to the severity of the insult.

   The most widely accepted mechanism of the production of cerebral edema in head injury is that the injury affects the capacitance vessels primarily, leading to venous stasis; and decrease in cerebral blood flow results in cerebral hypoxia. Then energy-dependent mechanisms that maintain fluid balance fail, with a resultant accumulation of sodium chloride and water inside the glial cells; and cerebral edema increases intracranial pressure, leading to further reduction in cerebral perfusion, causing more hypoxia. The resultant vicious cycle may be fatal if it is not treated promptly. **Treatment** of cerebral edema is covered in Chapter 6.

2. **Mass lesions and herniations**

   a. **Description.** Mass lesions, increasing the volume contained within the rigid cranial cavity, may be caused by contusion, hematoma, ventricular dilatation in cases of obstructive hydrocephalus, brain edema, and the like.

   b. **Pathophysiology.** Extra volume in the cranial cavity is initially accommodated by fluid loss from the ventricles and subarachnoid space. As the limit of this capacity is surpassed, the brain is pushed through certain weak points of the cranial cavity, giving rise to internal displacements or herniations.

   c. **Diagnosis**

   (1) Since papilledema may take up to 1 day to develop, it is not a reliable sign of **acutely** increased intracranial pressure.

   (2) **Decrease in alertness,** which may or may not be accompanied by changes in pulse (bradycardia), increase in blood pressure, or a change in respiratory pattern, is the most reliable indication of increased intracranial pressure.

   d. **Types of herniations**

   (1) **The uncal herniation syndrome** of rostrocaudal deterioration is caused by masses that compress the hemisphere laterally and push the inferomedial part of the ipsilateral temporal lobe through the tentorial incisura, compressing the midbrain. The oculomotor nerve is compressed early, giving rise to pupillary dilatation and fixation, and complete ophthalmoplegia follows along with contralateral hemiparesis, due to pressure on the ipsilateral cerebral peduncle. Consciousness soon deteriorates, often precipitously.

   Another neighboring anatomic structure that may be affected is the posterior cerebral artery, compression of which gives rise to hemorrhagic infarction of the posterior temporal and occipital lobes. Less commonly, the contralateral peduncle is crowded against the tentorial edge, producing a hemiparesis ipsilateral to the clot (Kernohan's notch). If this situation is prolonged for more than a few minutes, irreversible brainstem damage occurs due to pressure and stretching of the vasculature, with consequent hemorrhagic infarction.

(2) Central herniation syndrome. Lesions that displace the brain rostrocaudally without significant lateralization, i.e., lesions over the convexity or bilateral hematomas, produce the less-frequently seen central or diencephalic syndrome. The first sign of this syndrome is **decreasing alertness,** followed by Cheyne-Stokes respiration and small, **reactive** pupils. Eye movements remain full on doll's head maneuver or caloric stimulation, and motor impairment may begin with unilateral hemiparesis.

The contralateral limbs show paratonic resistance (Gegenhalten), while still retaining appropriate responses to noxious stimuli. This is followed in succession by bilateral decortication, bilateral pupillary dilatation and fixation, and bilateral decerebration. The latter stages of the uncal and central syndromes fuse in a common pathway, because the brainstem is progressively damaged in a caudal direction.

e. Treatment of herniations consists of attempts to decrease cerebral water content acutely, followed by surgical removal of the causative mass (see sec **I.C.6.d.(1)**).

E. Delayed complications of head injury

1. Posttraumatic epilepsy (PTE)

a. Description. A proportion of head-injured patients will develop seizures. Care must be exercised to ensure that the process is truly epileptic to distinguish it from other paroxysmal disorders, such as vasovagal syncope and anxiety attacks. The incidence of posttraumatic epilepsy varies markedly with the mode of injury, i.e., whether the injury was penetrating or blunt.

(1) Penetrating injuries. The overall incidence of posttraumatic epilepsy is about 50%. Factors that influence the likelihood of seizures are: the **extent** of the lesion, as measured by neurologic deficit (e.g., hemiparesis), **infection,** and the **location** of the lesion (lesions around the rolandic region have the highest propensity to become epileptogenic).

(2) Blunt injuries are more common in civilian practice. The incidence of posttraumatic epilepsy in this group is around 5%.

b. Pathophysiology. Seizures that occur within the first week (early seizures) reflect the initial brain damage. Early seizures are more common in children, provided that the injury is relatively minor. Also early seizures are a well-recognized antecedent of late seizures.

Besides the occurrence of early seizures, depressed skull fractures and intracranial hematomas are associated with a high incidence of late posttraumatic seizures.

c. EEG. In most cases of blunt head injury, the EEG cannot determine which individuals will develop posttraumatic epilepsy. However, its predictive capacity is much better following penetrating injuries. Early tracings habitually show alpha suppression and focal theta or delta, slowing unilaterally or generally.

d. Pattern of seizures. Although some early seizures tend to begin focally, most seizures (early and late) are generalized from the onset. The epilepsy remits (the criterion being no seizures for 2 years) in 50–75% of cases.

e. Treatment

(1) When to treat. If traumatic unconsciousness has been brief, and there is no hematoma, fracture, or neurologic deficit, no treatment is given. In cases of cerebral contusion, prolonged unconsciousness, and hematoma, many clinicians administer phenytoin prophylactically in the usual way (loading dose of 15 mg/kg, or 1000 mg in adults, over the first 24 hours; then a maintenance dose of 5 mg/kg, or 300–400 mg, daily in adults IV or by means of nasogastric tube.) Early or late seizures are treated with phenytoin or barbiturates or both in the usual way and in the usual dose (see Chap. 6).

(2) How long to treat. Since most posttraumatic epilepsy occurs within 2 years after injury, anticonvulsants are given, at least for that period if no seizures have occurred. If seizures are frequent, a seizure-free period of 5 years should be allowed before stopping anticonvulsants. If less frequent, the seizure-free interval may be shortened to 3 years. It is also important to avoid stopping anticonvulsants abruptly, since this may be associated with the recurrence of seizures. Discontinuation may be done gradually over 2–3 months.

2. Postconcussive encephalopathy. See Chapter 3.

3. Infection. Meningeal and encephalic infection may occur after head injury, especially after compound and basilar fractures. These are discussed in Chapter 8.

4. CSF leak is a frequent complication of basilar skull fractures. It has to be repaired surgically.

5. Hydrocephalus. See Chapter 3.

II. SPINAL CORD INJURY.

Since World War II, there has been an enormous advance in the understanding and management of spinal cord injuries. The creation of centers that specialize in this problem has improved the prognosis for this condition, which was almost universally fatal in the past. Automobile accidents, falls, sports (e.g., diving), industrial accidents, and gunshot and stab wounds are all causes of spinal cord injury. Therefore the paraplegic is no longer seen only in military hospitals.

Most of the lesions are in the lower cervical cord (C4–7, T1) and the thoracolumbar junction (T11–12, L1). The thoracic spinal cord is less frequently affected, as are the cauda equina and conus medullaris.

A. Immediate care of the spinal cord injured patient.
The aim is to avoid further damage to the spinal cord by all possible means. A certain proportion of spinal cord injuries are made worse by improper handling of the patient in this stage.

1. Move the patient carefully if a spinal lesion is suspected.

2. Place the patient on a firm, flat surface for transport. If a cervical lesion is suspected, a person should be assigned to ensure stability of the patient's head during movements.

3. Pillows, rolled blankets, or sandbags may be used at the patient's sides to prevent lateral displacements.

4. Cover the patient with blankets to avoid loss of heat.

5. As soon as the patient's condition permits, make arrangements for transfer to a center that specializes in spinal cord injuries.

B. The lesions

1. Spinal cord concussion

a. Description. This is a state of transient loss of cord function due to trauma without associated fracture-dislocation. The usual causes are whiplash injuries, sudden flexion or extension of the neck, and the like, and immediate flaccid paralysis occurs. Recovery is complete in a matter of minutes to hours.

b. Pathophysiology. Violent pressure waves propagated through deep tissues are believed to change the normal properties of tracts and neuronal groups.

c. Treatment. Observation.

2. Spinal cord contusion and transection

a. Description. In these conditions there is some discernible anatomic change of the spinal cord, although there may be functionally complete transection with few pathologic changes. Occasionally, the cord is completely severed.

In cord contusion, early changes include edema, petechial hemorrhages, neuronal changes, and an inflammatory reaction. In severe cases, the cord is liquefied. At later stages, the cord may be reduced to a fibrotic structure, and the pathologic changes may extend above and below the damaged segment. If paralysis is present for longer than 48 hours, the chances for functional recovery are minimal, and the spinal cord changes are assumed to be anatomic rather than physiologic.

Delayed loss of neurologic function may occur early or late. The early losses are usually caused by unrecognized fractures at the C7–T1 level, which is a difficult area to explore radiologically. Late deficits are usually a result of the formation of intramedullary cysts or syringomyelic cavities at the cervical level. The neurologic syndromes that result from spinal cord injury are varied, but a few are well established.

(1) Complete cord transection

(a) Spinal shock. At first there is immediate flaccid paralysis and sensory loss below the level of the lesion. Reflexes are lost as a rule, but a few may remain (e.g., bulbocavernous). This state lasts 3–6 weeks, but sepsis, malnutrition, or other complications may prolong it for months.

(b) Increasing reflex activity. Spinal shock is replaced by gradual return and an eventual increase of reflex activity. In cervical lesions there is an initial tendency to flexion, which is later followed by extension. The presence of internal stimuli, such as urethritis, cystitis, and decubitus ulcers, provoke flexor spasms, which if repeated tend to fix the posture in flexion.

The mass reflex is the most dramatic manifestation of increased reflex activity. It consists of contraction of the abdominal muscles, triple flexion of the lower limbs, profuse perspiration, piloerection, and automatic urination in response to stimuli below the lesion.

(c) Sensation. In incomplete lesions there may be some recovery of sensation after a variable interval of time.

(d) Pains. Radicular pain due to root involvement may be present for weeks or months. However, more frequently a more severe type of pain, commonly described as burning, occurs below the lesion level. This pain lasts longer and is resistant to narcotics. However, anesthetizing the distal stump of the proximal segment of spinal cord has been shown to abolish it. Note that pain, whatever its nature, is markedly influenced by the patient's emotional state.

(e) Autonomic disturbances occur.

Temperature regulation. Sweating is decreased or absent below the level of the lesion if it is above T9-10. If the lesion is above C8, all thermoregulation is lost. The profuse sweats seen in these patients are reflex in nature and are triggered by impulses from the bladder or rectum (distention).

Hyperhydrosis is another manifestation of this hyperreflexic state.

Blood pressure regulation. Orthostatic hypotension is caused by a lack of reflex contraction of the capacitance vessels in response to posture changes. If the patient is tilted up, a precipitous drop in blood pressure occurs, which may lead to unconsciousness. Episodes of paroxysmal hypertension also occur, which is usually in response to a distended bladder or rectum.

Bladder regulation. Disturbances of bladder function and its result, chronic renal failure, are the most frequent causes of death in these patients. (For details on neurogenic bladder, see Chap. 17.)

Immediately following cord damage, reflex bladder function, as with other reflexes in spinal shock, is abolished. There is marked atony and overdistention of the bladder, and overflow voiding occurs. This stage may last days to weeks, depending on the same factors operative in spinal shock (age, associated diseases, malnutrition, sepsis, etc.).

The second stage then occurs, which varies according to the location of the lesion. In lesions above the lumbosacral segments, reflex bladder function returns, and an automatic or reflex bladder develops. Initially the detrusor contractions are weak, and the volume of urine voided is small, although later emptying becomes more complete. Bladder distention may be heralded by hypertension, flushing, headache, nasal congestion, and other signs the patient learns to recognize as bladder fullness.

The establishment of satisfactory reflex micturition depends much on avoidance of infection and overdistention during the initial stage of bladder atony. If the lesion is at the level of the conus medullaris or cauda equina, the bladder is called **autonomic** (i.e., deprived of voluntary and reflex activity). Detrusor contractions mediated by the intramural autonomic plexus are not effective, and voiding is never complete (as in the automatic or reflex type). Intravesical pressure is high, dribbling may occur, and there is a large residual volume. If the external sphincter is surgically severed, the bladder may be emptied by abdominal compression.

In the third stage of reconditioning, the patient with an autonomic bladder, having learned the signals of bladder distention, is able to trigger micturition by such acts as abdominal pressure and pinching certain zones. The autonomic bladder may require surgical severance of the external sphincter, so abdominal compression is enough to accomplish satisfactory emptying.

Bowel dysfunction goes through the same three stages. Initially the bowel is distended and atonic, and peristalsis is abolished. Return of bowel sounds and passage of flatus signal the beginning of the second stage. Once peristalsis begins, reflex or automatic evacuation may be accomplished if the stool is kept soft (stool softeners, bulk-producing agents) and there is no fecal impaction. Reflex evacuation may be triggered by abdominal compression or the insertion of a suppository. In the autonomic type, the sphincter is patulous and rectal incontinence develops. **Reconditioning** of the bowels is easier than that for the bladder.

Sexual dysfunction varies, depending on the severity of the process, and it goes through the three stages previously mentioned. In men, penile erection during spinal shock is the result of passive engorgement of the corpora cavernosa. During the automatic phase, erection and ejaculation are possible reflexes.

(2) Anterior cord syndrome is characterized by paralysis and pain loss below the level of the lesion with some preservation of touch, vibratory, and position senses.

(3) Central cord syndrome is characterized by a greater motor deficit in the arms than in the legs, and there are variable sensory deficits. The greater arm affectation may be explained by anterior horn cell damage in the cervical cord, or involvement of the more medially placed fibers of the corticospinal tract in the lateral columns.

(4) Brown-Sequard syndrome results from damage to one-half of the cord, with resulting ipsilateral weakness, proprioceptive loss, and contralateral loss of pain and temperature. This syndrome usually follows stab injuries.

b. **Pathophysiology.** The facts that set spinal cord injuries apart from cranioencephalic injuries are the great concentration of important neural tracts and centers in a structure of relatively small diameter; the position of the cord within the vertebral column; peculiarities of the spine, such as canal size; presence of osteophytes; and variability of vascular supply.

The effect on neural tissue is most important in spinal injuries. The cord and roots are injured by four mechanisms:

(1) Compression by bone, ligaments, extruded disc material, and hematoma. The most severe damage is caused by bony compression, compression from a posteriorly displaced vertebral body fragment, and hyperextension injuries.

(2) Overstretching of tissues. Overstretching that causes disruption of tissue usually follows hyperflexion. The stretch tolerance of the cord may decrease with age.

(3) Edema. Cord edema appears soon and produces further impairment of capillary circulation and venous return.

(4) Circulatory disturbance. Circulatory disturbances are the result of compression by bone or other structures of the anterior or posterior spinal arterial systems.

C. Diagnosis

1. Shortly after the patient's arrival at the hospital, a detailed neurologic examination is carried out and recorded.

2. The spine is examined carefully for deformities, swelling, tenderness, and limitation of movement, particularly in the neck.

3. Radiologic examination should include the whole spine. Anteroposterior and lateral projections are usually sufficient, but special x-rays may be needed for certain basilar skull views.

4. CBC, chemistries, and clotting times are obtained.

5. Lumbar puncture is seldom useful.

D. Treatment. It has been shown conclusively that the best results are achieved in special centers where large numbers of these patients are seen. The treatment is determined by the interval of time that has elapsed since the injury, the presence of associated problems, the level and completeness of the injury, and several other factors. The need for an airway, ventilation, and treatment of associated injuries is self-evident.

1. **General nursing care**

   a. **Bladder care.** The aim of bladder care is to obtain a patient-controlled reflex bladder that is free of infection. To accomplish this, the technique of intermittent, sterile "no touch" catheterizations has yielded the best results. Also, maintenance of an acid urine with ascorbic acid, 1 gm four times daily helps prevent infection and urinary calculi.

      Recent evidence indicates that urine production is decreased for the first day or so after the injury. Thus the initial catheterization may then be deferred for 24 hours, depending on the size of the bladder by palpation. Thereafter it may be repeated two or three times daily, depending on the residual volume. (See Chapter 17 for details.)

   b. **Bowel care.** The aim of bowel care is to obtain a patient-controlled reflex evacuation. The initial stage of bowel distention is treated by rectal tube or enemas. Later, when peristalsis returns, bulk-producing agents, such as psyllium hydrophilic mucilloid (Metamucil) or stool softeners, such as dioctyl sodium sulfosuccinate (Colace), are used. As the bowel becomes more active, enemas are replaced by suppositories. The patient should be examined frequently for fecal impaction.

   c. **Skin care.** The patient's pockets should be emptied immediately. Blankets and sheets are drawn tight and smooth, and the patient is put on a hard flat surface, over which a mattress or foam pad is placed. The patient should be turned every 2 hours, day and night. Pillows and rubber donuts are used to protect pressure points and to maintain normal posture of body parts. Special frames can be used for turning the patient.

   d. **Nutrition.** A high-calorie, high-protein diet is essential. If the patient is unable to eat, supplements are given parenterally or by means of nasogastric tube. Fluid and electrolyte balance should be watched closely.

   e. **Pain control.** If possible, narcotics are avoided because of their addictive potential. Acetylsalicylic acid (aspirin), propoxyphene (Darvon), and, in rare cases, codeine are used. Sedative drugs can be used to control anxiety.

2. **Treatment of the vertebral injury.** If paraplegia is total and remains unchanged for over 48 hours, there is no reason for attempting to obtain perfect spinal alignment, because the cord changes are presumed to be permanent.

   a. **Cervical injuries**

      (1) Hyperextension injuries without evidence of fracture or dislocation require no traction as long as the patient remains in bed with a neck collar and sits in an erect posture.

      (2) Dislocations and fractures are treated with axial traction through skull callipers. Slight neck extension is desirable. A little pad under the nape of the neck helps to unlock the articular facets.

   b. **Thoracolumbar injuries.** Pillows or pads are placed under the lumbar curvature to produce hyperextension of the spine. In the lateral position, sandbags or pads are used to correct the deformity.

3. **Surgery.** Decompressive laminectomy is not advocated at the present time except in rare instances. Current indications for surgery are:

   a. Open reduction of dislocation, with or without fracture in the cervical region, if traction and manipulation have failed.

   b. Cervical fractures with partial cord lesions, in which a bony fragment remains compressing the anterior aspect of the cord despite adequate traction.

c. Cervical injuries with partial cord lesions, in which no bony fragment can be seen and extruded disc material is suspected of pressing the cord. Myelography may be necessary to demonstrate this condition.

d. Depressed fragments of the neural arch.

e. Compound injuries, with foreign bodies or bone fragments in the spinal canal. Clean stab wounds do not necessarily require surgery.

f. Partial cord lesions, with gradual worsening of the neurologic picture or worsening after initial improvement.

E. Complications

1. Urinary calculi are related to improper urinary drainage, infection, and hypercalciuria due to prolonged immobilization. Prevention is accomplished by acidifying the urine, promoting a high urine output, avoiding infection, and mobilizing the patient early. Upper urinary tract calculi may be treated conservatively unless they become obstructive. Vesical stones are crushed.

2. Decubitus ulcers are heralded by an area of redness in the pressure points. The incidence of decubiti has fallen dramatically since World War II, attesting to the better nutritional state and nursing care that these patients receive.

Body casts that cover pressure points are strictly contraindicated. Small decubiti often heal spontaneously, provided they are scrupulously cleansed and kept dry. Larger lesions may require plastic surgery (see Chap. 17).

3. Muscle spasms may be greatly diminished if their precipitating factors are kept at a minimum (urethritis, cystitis, decubiti, rectal or vesical distention, etc.). Also, they tend to ameliorate spontaneously after the second year.

Drugs, such as diazepam, have some value, and subarachnoid injection of absolute alcohol 10–15 ml and, most recently, phenol have been used to control spasms. With this procedure, spasms may be arrested or ameliorated for months. Sphincteric disturbance is the most serious complication of this procedure. Rhizotomy is reserved for exceptionally severe cases and is rarely done.

F. Rehabilitation

1. Physiotherapy. Massage and passive movements are started as soon as possible. Later, special exercises are devised for the development of certain muscle groups necessary for independence.

2. Occupational therapy prepares the patient for future gainful employment, while at the same time shifting his attention away from the disability. Multiple devices are available that permit patients a wide range of activities.

3. Sports. Wheelchair basketball, archery, and bag punching are available. Special hunting seasons are set for paraplegics.

4. Psychiatric therapy may be needed for suicidal or excessively depressed patients.

SUGGESTED READING

Head Injury
Gallagher, J. P., and Browder, E. J.   Extradural hematoma. Experience with 167 patients. *J. Neurosurg.* 29:1, 1968.
Grubb, R. L., and Coxe, W. S.   Central Nervous System Trauma: Cranial, in S. G. Eliasson, A. L. Prensky, and W. B. Hardin (eds.), *Neurological Pathophysiology.* Oxford: Oxford University Press, 1974. Pp. 292–309.

Jennet, B. Head injuries in children. *Dev. Med. Child Neurol.* 14:137, 1972.

New, P. J. F., and Scott, W. R. *Computed Tomography of the Skull and Orbit.* Baltimore: Williams and Wilkins, 1975.

Plum, F., and Posner, J. B. *Diagnosis of Stupor and Coma.* Philadelphia: Davis, 1972.

Youmans, Jr. (Ed.) *Neurological Surgery. Section VIII, Trauma.* Philadelphia: Saunders, 1973. Pp. 865–1049.

Spinal Cord Injury

Boshes, B. Trauma to the Spinal Cord, in A. B. Baker (ed.), *Clinical Neurology.* Maryland: Harper and Row, 1975.

Coxe, W. S., and Grubb, R. L. Central Nervous System Trauma: Spinal, in S. G. Eliasson, et al. (eds.), *Neurological Pathophysiology.* Oxford: Oxford University Press, 1974.

Crutchfield, W. D. Spinal Injury, in *Surgery of the Nervous System.* London: Blackwell, 1973.

13

Demyelinating Diseases

Daniel B. Hier

I. MULTIPLE SCLEROSIS

A. Diagnosis

1. No specific laboratory test is currently available to confirm the diagnosis of multiple sclerosis (MS). The diagnosis generally rests on two features of the illness:

   a. A history of **fluctuations in the clinical course:** either well-defined exacerbations and remissions or lesser variations in a progressive down-hill course.

   b. A physical examination consistent with that of **multiple lesions** in the white matter of the central nervous system.

2. The spinal fluid is abnormal in about 90% of patients, and about 50% of patients have a **CSF pleocytosis** with more than five lymphocytes. Pleocytosis tends to be more marked early and during acute exacerbations in the course of multiple sclerosis.

   Nearly 75% of patients have **elevated CSF gamma globulins** (with IgG making up greater than 12% of the CSF total protein). An abnormal colloidal gold curve (usually a first-zone or "paretic" curve) generally reflects the increase in CSF IgG. Mild elevations of total CSF protein are common, but elevations over 100 mg/100 ml are unusual.

   Lumbar puncture has not been shown to have any adverse effect on the course of the disease, and it should be performed diagnostically in all suspected cases.

3. When there has been no history of optic neuritis, demonstration of **abnormal pattern shift, visual evoked responses** may support the diagnosis of multiple sclerosis by demonstrating subclinical lesions in the visual pathways.

4. A number of other diseases may resemble multiple sclerosis clinically under certain circumstances:

   a. Tumors: e.g., hemispheric, brainstem, and spinal cord.

   b. Malformations: e.g., Arnold-Chiari and platybasia.

   c. Spinal cord compression: e.g., spondylosis and herniated intervertebral disc.

   d. Degenerations: e.g., spinocerebellar, motor neuron disease, and subacute combined degeneration of the spinal cord.

   e. Collagen vascular: e.g., polyarteritis and systemic lupus erythematosus.

   f. Behçet's disease.

   Myelography, brain scanning, and other ancillary tests are performed when the diagnosis is doubtful.

B. Prognosis.
After the patient has been diagnosed as having multiple sclerosis, the physician must correct any misconceptions the patient may have about the nature and prognosis of the illness. The course is highly variable.

A review of 146 persons treated at the Mayo Clinic over a 60-year period revealed a 25-year mortality of about 26% compared with 14% in the general population. After 25 years two-thirds of the survivors were still ambulatory.

C. Treatment

1. **Therapy aimed at halting the progression of multiple sclerosis.** There is no therapy currently available that has been shown to alter the overall course. Diets based on either restriction of fats or supplementation with linoleic acid are not of proven benefit. Also, long-term therapy with ACTH, corticosteroids (intrathecally or systemically administered), or immunosuppressant agents does not alter the course of multiple sclerosis.

2. **Therapy aimed at shortening the duration of acute exacerbations**

   a. Deterioration in the neurologic status of a patient with multiple sclerosis may be due to a new attack of demyelination or, less commonly, intercurrent infection (especially urinary tract), electrolyte imbalance, fever, drug intoxication, or conversion reaction. When doubt exists, demonstration of lymphocytes in the CSF may support the diagnosis of acute demyelination.

   b. **ACTH** is the only drug that has been shown to shorten acute exacerbations of multiple sclerosis in controlled studies. However, 70% of all exacerbations remit spontaneously, and there is no evidence that ACTH improves the degree of recovery. Thus ACTH should be thought of as a drug capable of hastening recovery from acute exacerbations in certain cases, rather than one that alters the overall course of the disease.

   c. The dosage of ACTH necessary to shorten an acute attack is not established. One acceptable regimen is:

   Days 1–3   Aqueous ACTH 80 units in 500 ml of 5% dextrose in water IV over 8 hours each day.

   Days 4–10   ACTH gel 40 units IM every 12 hours.

   Days 11–13   ACTH gel 35 units IM every 12 hours.

   Days 14–16   ACTH gel 30 units IM every 12 hours.

   Days 17–19   ACTH gel 50 units IM daily.

   Days 20–22   ACTH gel 40 units IM daily.

   Days 23–25   ACTH gel 30 units IM daily.

   Days 26–28   ACTH gel 20 units IM daily.

   Days 30, 32, 34   ACTH gel 20 units IM each day.

   d. **Common complications of ACTH therapy** include **fluid retention** and **hypokalemia.** Electrolytes are checked at least weekly and supplementation with KCl (20–30 mEq TID) is advisable (especially if diuretics are used). Fluid retention and associated **hypertension** can be controlled by the addition of hydrochlorothiazide (50–100 mg daily). As prophylaxis against **gastric irritation and hemorrhage,** antacids are administered between meals.

   Restlessness, anxiety, and **insomnia** generally diminish with chlordiazepoxide 20–75 mg daily. Depression or euphoria also occurs, especially if there are cerebral lesions. **Psychosis** is less commonly encountered and is managed with the assistance of a psychiatrist, if possible. A major tranquilizer (haloperidol 10–40 mg or chlorpromazine 100–1000 mg daily), coupled with reduction of ACTH dosage, is usually effective in controlling psychosis.

   Infection and **sepsis** are occasional complications and require prompt treatment with appropriate antibiotics. When the patient has a positive tuberculin test, concurrent treatment with an antituberculous drug is indicated. **Osteoporosis** and vertebral body collapse do not generally complicate short courses of ACTH.

   e. **Oral corticosteroids** may be as effective as ACTH in shortening acute attacks of multiple sclerosis, but their utility has not been shown in controlled studies. Corticosteroids have several advantages in that they can be administered PO, are less expensive, and have fewer side effects than ACTH. As with ACTH, the selection of dosage is somewhat arbitrary. An acceptable regimen is:

Days 1–10   Prednisone 60 mg daily.
Days 11–13   Prednisone 50 mg daily.
Days 14–16   Prednisone 40 mg daily.
Days 17–19   Prednisone 30 mg daily.
Days 20–22   Prednisone 20 mg daily.
Days 23–25   Prednisone 10 mg daily.
Days 26–28   Prednisone 5 mg daily.

Concurrent antacid therapy is recommended, although potassium supplementation and diuretic therapy are not generally necessary.

D. Complications of multiple sclerosis

1. **Weakness.** Physical therapy is of benefit when weakness is due to disuse, but it does not strengthen muscles weakened by CNS demyelination. It also maintains range of motion, assists in gait training, and boosts patient morale.

2. **Spasticity.** Physical therapy is of little benefit in diminishing spasticity; and drug therapy of spasticity is often complicated and limited by increased weakness.

   a. **Diazepam** (Valium) is generally the drug of first choice. Its exact mechanism of action is uncertain, but it appears to be largely central. Effective dosage ranges from 5–50 mg daily. Side effects include drowsiness, fatigue, and weakness.

   b. **Baclofen** (Lioresal) is a gamma-aminobutyric acid derivative that relieves spasticity (especially painful flexor and extensor spasms) in certain patients. It appears to be at least as effective as diazepam, and its use is not generally associated with increased weakness. The usual starting dosage is 5 mg TID, which may be increased to 40–80 mg daily.

   c. **Dantrolene** (Dantrium). When diazepam and baclofen are ineffective, dantrolene may be tried. Dantrolene always produces **increased weakness,** since its mechanism of action involves decoupling of excitation-contraction in muscle. The drug has proved useful in only a few patients with spasticity, but in responsive individuals the improvement can be dramatic.
   Dosage can be initiated at 25 mg daily and gradually increased to a maximum of 400 mg daily over several weeks. Dantrolene may produce **hepatitis,** and its use is contraindicated in the presence of hepatic disease. Thus liver function must be monitored regularly. Other side effects include drowsiness, dizziness, and diarrhea.

   d. **Intrathecal phenol, anterior rhizotomy,** and **peripheral nerve block** are considered only if spasticity or flexor spasms are refractory to drug treatment and make the patient uncomfortable. These procedures are generally reserved for patients with long-standing paraplegia with little hope for recovery, since relief of spasticity is accompanied by further paralysis.
   Intrathecal injection of 5–20% phenol in glycerol has been used widely to relieve spasticity. The procedure can be performed easily without general anesthesia. A radiopaque dye is added to the phenol solution, and the procedure is done under fluoroscopic control on a myelography table. Spasticity is relieved by the production of a **flaccid paralysis** that lasts 3–12 months. **Sensory loss** usually accompanies the paralysis and can lead to pressure sores. Also, **bladder and bowel sphincter dysfunction** commonly occur.

In patients with normal bowel and bladder function, **anterior rhizotomy** is probably the procedure of choice. Irreversible weakness is produced, but sensory loss and urinary retention are avoided. Alternatively, **peripheral nerve block** with phenol may relieve spasticity without risking bladder or bowel dysfunction.

3. **Tremor and ataxia.** About 70% of patients experience cerebellar intention tremor or ataxia at some time during their illness. Mild degrees of tremor or ataxia are often improved by **weighting** the affected limbs. However, when tremor is disabling and long-standing, and strength remains good, **thalamotomy** may be of benefit. Tremors of the head and trunk are particularly resistant to treatment.

4. **Pain.** Shooting or lancinating pains that affect the pelvic girdle, shoulders, and face are common features of multiple sclerosis. Facial pain that is indistinguishable from **trigeminal neuralgia** occurs in about 3% of patients, and most **bilateral** trigeminal neuralgia is caused by multiple sclerosis. These neuritic pains, regardless of location, often respond to **carbamazepine** (400–1200 mg daily). However, patients taking carbamazepine must be carefully monitored for the development of bone marrow depression or hepatic dysfunction. In drug refractory cases, surgical management is recommended (see Chap. 9).

5. **Bladder, bowel, and sexual dysfunction** are common. In patients with either urinary retention or incontinence, correctable anatomic lesions must be excluded. **Cystometry** is useful in distinguishing small spastic **(hyperactive) bladders** from large **atonic (neurogenic)** ones. (For detailed management, see Chapter 17.)

6. **Psychiatric complications** include depression, euphoria, emotional lability, and psychosis. **Depression** may be seen in a variety of settings.

   a. **Reactive depressions** that occur soon after diagnosis are often relieved by sympathetic, supportive psychotherapy.

   b. Depressions related to **increasing disability** are best managed by providing the patient with a positive therapeutic regimen, including physical therapy.

   c. Depression related to **cerebral lesions** may be resistant to treatment. However, antidepressant drugs are sometimes of benefit.

   Euphoria tends to occur late in the course of multiple sclerosis, and it is associated with signs of generalized intellectual deterioration and extensive cerebral demyelination. **Psychosis** is a relatively rare complication, usually related to high-dose ACTH or corticosteroid therapy. Treatment with an appropriate major tranquilizer (haloperidol 10–40 mg or chlorpromazine 100–1000 mg daily) is generally effective.

II. OPTIC NEURITIS

A. **Diagnosis.** The term **optic neuritis** (ON) refers to the abrupt (usually over 2–3 days) loss of vision that results from optic nerve demyelination. When the optic nerve head is visibly inflamed or swollen, the term **papillitis** is used. Other cases are classified as **retrobulbar neuritis,** in which visual acuity is diminished in the affected eye. There may also be a central scotoma.

A variety of other illnesses may resemble the symptoms and clinical features of demyelinative optic neuritis:

1. Vascular: e.g., giant cell arteritis (temporal arteritis), retinal ischemia, and central retinal artery occlusion.

2. Neoplastic: e.g., pituitary adenoma, intrinsic tumors, and compressive tumors of the optic nerve.

3. Hereditary: e.g., Leber's optic atrophy.

4. Nutritional: e.g., vitamin B_1 and B_{12} deficiency.

5. Inflammatory: e.g., retinitis, meningitis, encephalitis, and choroiditis.

6. Toxic and drug-related optic neuropathy.

Tumor, vascular disease, inflammatory disease, metabolic disorders, and retinal lesions must be excluded in each case. Skull x-ray examinations are obtained, and special attention is given to the condition of the optic foramina and sella turcica. Small lesions of the optic canals can be excluded only by tomography. When the diagnosis is in doubt, CT scanning, lumbar puncture, carotid arteriography, and pneumoencephalography are sometimes necessary to exclude vascular, neoplastic, or inflammatory disorders.

When the authenticity of the patient's complaints are doubted (hysteria, malingering), the demonstration of **abnormal pattern shift visual evoked potentials** can be a useful confirmation of the diagnosis of optic neuritis.

B. **Relation of optic neuritis to multiple sclerosis.** About 20% of patients with optic neuritis later develop multiple sclerosis, while nearly 40% of multiple sclerosis patients have at least one attack of optic neuritis, which is the first symptom of demyelination in 10–15% of multiple sclerosis patients. As with multiple sclerosis, both **CSF pleocytosis and increased CSF IgG may occur in optic neuritis,** but with a lesser frequency. Histocompatibility types HLA-A3 and HLA-B7, which are overrepresented in multiple sclerosis populations, occur in normal frequencies in optic neuritis patients. It is not yet certain whether elevations of CSF IgG or the presence of HLA-A3 or HLA-B7 histocompatibility types, in association with optic neuritis, puts patients at higher risk to develop multiple sclerosis.

C. The **prognosis** for spontaneous recovery of vision is quite good. About 50% of patients have recovery of vision within 1 month; 75%, within 6 months. Neither **pain** in the orbit (70% of cases) nor **papillitis** (20% of cases) alters the prognosis for recovery.

D. **Treatment.** Both **ACTH** and **corticosteroids** have been advocated in the treatment of optic neuritis. ACTH appears to shorten the course, but it does not influence the ultimate level of recovery. Controlled studies are not available concerning the effectiveness of oral corticosteroids.

Despite the generally favorable prognosis for spontaneous recovery of vision, some neurologists choose to treat all patients who develop optic neuritis with either ACTH or corticosteroids. Others reserve treatment for the following indications:

1. Loss of visual acuity below 20/80 in the affected eye.

2. Severe pain in the affected eye (this is generally relieved by ACTH or corticosteroids).

3. Bilateral optic neuritis.

4. Previous visual loss in the unaffected eye.

The dosage of ACTH or corticosteroids is the same as for an acute exacerbation of multiple sclerosis. Patients must be carefully observed for complications, which include gastrointestinal hemorrhage, infection, hypertension, fluid retention, hypokalemia, and psychosis. Concurrent antacid therapy is recommended.

III. ACUTE DISSEMINATED ENCEPHALOMYELITIS

A. **Terminology.** Acute disseminated encephalomyelitis is an uncommon demyelinating disease of the brain and spinal cord. Pathologically, it closely resembles experimental allergic encephalomyelitis, with extensive demyelination and perivascular infiltrates of lymphocytes.

Most cases develop 4–6 days after the viral exanthem of measles, chicken pox, small pox, or rubella **(postinfectious encephalomyelitis)**, or 10–15 days after vaccination against smallpox or rabies **(postvaccinial encephalomyelitis).** Acute disseminated encephalomyelitis in children must be distinguished from Reye's syndrome (a nondemyelinative postinfectious encephalopathy).

B. Clinical course. Acute disseminated encephalomyelitis is a monophasic self-limited disease of varying severity. In mild cases there may be only headache, stiff neck, fever, and confusion. However, in more severe cases convulsions, quadriplegia, cerebellar ataxia, multiple cranial nerve palsies, sensory loss, and coma may occur in varying combinations. Mortality is 10–20% in postmeasles encephalomyelitis, and as high as 30–50% in postvaccinial encephalomyelitis. Approximately 25–50% of survivors are left with severe neurologic sequelae.

C. Treatment. Uncontrolled studies have shown that **ACTH** and **corticosteroids** reduce the severity of the illness. These drugs may be used in the same dosages that are used to treat acute exacerbations of multiple sclerosis. In addition, anticonvulsants, mannitol, and corticosteroids are often needed to control seizures and cerebral edema.

SELECTED READINGS

Prognosis of Multiple Sclerosis
Percy, A. K., Nobrega, F. T., Okazaki, H., Glattie, E., and Kurland, L. T. Multiple sclerosis in Rochester, Minn. A 60-year appraisal. *Arch. Neurol.* 25:105, 1971.
Schumacher, G. A. The Demyelinative Diseases, in A. B. Baker, and L. H. Baker (eds.), *Clinical Neurology,* Vol. 2. New York: Harper and Row, 1975. Chapter 25.

Drug Therapy of Multiple Sclerosis
Cass, L. J., Alexander, L., Enders, M. Complications of corticotrophin therapy in multiple sclerosis. *J.A.M.A.* 197:173, 1966.
Millar, J. H. D. The Demyelinating Diseases, in W. B. Matthews (ed.), *Recent Advances in Clinical Neurology.* London: Churchill Livingstone, 1975. Pp. 218–233.
Rose, A. S., Kuzma, J. W., Kurtzer, J. F., Namerow, N. S., Sibley, W. A., and Tourtelotte, W. W. Cooperative study on the evaluation of therapy in multiple sclerosis: ACTH vs. placebo. Final report. *Neurology* 20 (supplement), 1970.
Sibley, W. A. Drug Treatment of Multiple Sclerosis, in P. J. Vinken and G. W. Bruyn, (eds.), *Handbook of Clinical Neurology,* Vol. 9. Amsterdam: North-Holland, 1970. Pp. 383–407.

Cerebrospinal Fluid
Link, H., and Muller, R. Immunoglobulins in multiple sclerosis and infections of the nervous system. *Arch. Neurol.* 25:326, 1971.
Sandberg-Wolheim, M. Optic neuritis: Studies on the cerebrospinal fluid in relation to clinical course in 61 patients. *Acta. Neurol. Scand.* 52:167, 1975.
Schapira, K. Is lumbar puncture harmful in multiple sclerosis? *J. Neurol. Neurosurg. Psychiatry* 22:238, 1959.

Weakness and Spasticity
Duncan, G. W., Shahani, B. T., and Young, R. R. An evaluation of baclofen treatment for certain symptoms in patients with spinal cord lesions. *Neurology* 26:441, 1976.
Gelenberg, A. J., and Poskanzer, D. C. The effects of dantrolene sodium on spasticity in multiple sclerosis. *Neurology* 23:1313, 1973.
Lenman, J. A. R. A clinical and experimental study of the effects of exercise on motor weakness in neurological disease. *J. Neurol. Neurosurg. Psychiatry* 22:182, 1959.
Levine, I., Jossman, P., Friend, D., DeAngelis, V., and Kane, M. Diazepam in the treatment of spasticity: A preliminary quantitative evaluation. *J. Chronic. Dis.* 22:57, 1969.
Liversedge, L. A., and Maher, R. M. Use of phenol in relief of spasticity. *Br. Med. J.* 2:31, 1960.

Selker, R., Greenberg, A., and Marshall, M.   Anterior rhizotomy for flexor spasms and contractures of the legs secondary to multiple sclerosis. *Ann. Surg.* 162:298, 1965.

Bladder, Bowel, and Sexual Dysfunction

Tarabulcy, E.   Bladder disturbances in multiple sclerosis and their management. *Mod. Treatment* 7:941, 1970.

Vas, C. J.   Sexual impotence and some autonomic disturbances in men with multiple sclerosis. *Acta. Neurol. Scand.* 45:166, 1969.

Psychiatric Complications

Lemere, F.   Psychiatric disorders in multiple sclerosis. *Am. J. Psychiatry* 122:55, 1966, Supplement 12.

Surridge, P.   An investigation into some psychiatric aspects of multiple sclerosis. *Br. J. Psychiatry* 115:49, 1969.

Tremor and Ataxia

Cooper, I. S.   Relief of intention tremor of multiple sclerosis by thalamic surgery. *J.A.M.A.* 199:689, 1967.

Hewer, R. L., Cooper, R., and Morgan, H.   An investigation into the value of treating intention tremor by weighting the affected limb. *Brain* 95:579, 1972.

Pain

Albert, M.   Treatment of pain in multiple sclerosis: A preliminary report. *N. Engl. J. Med.* 280:1395, 1969.

Chakravorty, B.   Association of trigeminal neuralgia with multiple sclerosis. *Arch. Neurol.* 14:95, 1966.

Optic Neuritis

Bowden, A. N., Bowden, P. M. A., Friedman, A. I., Perkin, G. D., and Rose, F. C.   A trial of corticotrophin gelatin injection in acute optic neuritis. *J. Neurol. Neurosurg. Psychiatry* 37:869, 1974.

Bradley, W. G., and Whitty, C. W. M.   Acute optic neuritis: Prognosis for development of multiple sclerosis. *J. Neurol. Neurosurg. Psychiatry* 31:10, 1968.

Feinsod, M., and Hoyt, W. F.   Subclinical optic neuropathy in multiple sclerosis. *J. Neurol. Neurosurg. Psychiatry* 38:1109, 1975.

Percy, A. K., Norbrega, F. T., Kurland, L. T.   Optic neuritis and multiple sclerosis: An epidemiological study. *Arch. Ophthalmol.* 87:135, 1972.

Rawson, M. S., Liversedge, L. A., and Goldfarb, G.   Treatment of acute retrobulbar neuritis with corticotrophin. *Lancet* 2:1044, 1966.

Acute Disseminated Encephalomyelitis

Alvord, E. C.   Acute Disseminated Encephalomyelitis and "Allergic" Neuro-encephalopathies, in P. J. Vinken, and G. W. Bruyn (eds.), *Handbook of Clinical Neurology*, Vol. 9. Amsterdam: North-Holland, 1970. Pp. 500–571.

Selling, B., and Meilman, E.   Acute disseminated encephalomyelitis treated with ACTH. *N. Engl. J. Med.* 253:275, 1955.

Scott, T. F.   Post-infectious and vaccinial encephalitis. *Med. Clin. North Am.* 51:701, 1967.

14

Steven M. Sagar

Toxic and Metabolic Disorders

I. LIVER DISEASE

A. Hepatolenticular degeneration (Wilson's disease) is a genetically transmitted autosomal recessive disorder of copper metabolism. It leads to cirrhosis of the liver and cerebral dysfunction; movement disorders, tremor, and personality changes are the usual neurologic manifestations. The therapy is discussed in Chapter 15.

B. Hepatic encephalopathy is a reversible global derangement of mental function. It is marked by depressed mental status, asterixis, and slowing of the EEG, which occurs in the presence of chronic liver disease. It is associated with portosystemic shunting that is produced either surgically or secondary to portal hypertension.

Hepatic encephalopathy is thought to result from the failure of the diseased liver to detoxify some metabolites that are toxic to the central nervous system. Since it occurs only in conditions with significant portosystemic shunts, it is thought that the toxins are produced in the gut and bypass the liver through the shunt to reach the systemic circulation. Ammonia, various amino acids, or biogenic amines may be the etiologic agents.

The treatment is:

1. Dietary protein restriction

    a. When the diagnosis of hepatic encephalopathy is first made, the patient is placed on a **protein-free diet** until neurologic function shows definite improvement.

        (1) The patient may be fed by mouth, nasogastric tube, or parenterally, depending on the clinical situation.

        (2) Enough calories (at least 500 in adults) should be provided to inhibit proteolysis; 1500 ml of 10% dextrose in water (10% D/W) provides 600 cal per day. If possible, a nasogastric tube is used instead of an IV, in which case a mixture of 10% D/W or 20% D/W and lipids may be given in sufficient quantity to provide 1500–2000 cal/day.

        (3) There are experimental programs of parenteral hyperalimentation being investigated, but these cannot be recommended for general use at this time. (See sec **I.B.6**)

    b. Cathartics are used to eliminate dietary protein in the gut on admittance. Magnesium citrate, 200 ml of the commercial solution, or sorbitol, 50 gm in 200 ml of water, may be administered PO or through a nasogastric tube.

    c. Gastrointestinal bleeding may deliver a large protein load to the gut. The protein may then be digested and reabsorbed as amino acids to precipitate hepatic coma.

        (1) The gastrointestinal bleeding is treated as vigorously as possible, bearing in mind the high surgical mortality of patients with severe liver disease.

        (2) Blood in the stomach is aspirated continuously through a nasogastric tube.

        (3) The gut is purged with an enema followed by cathartics. Repeated doses of sorbitol 50 gm in 200 ml of water are given to produce at least one loose bowel movement every 4 hours as long as the bleeding persists.

   d. Adequate vitamin supplementation is provided, with daily doses of folate 1 mg, vitamin K 10 mg, and multivitamins.

   e. NH_4Cl should never be given to a patient with hepatic encephalopathy.

   f. As the patient improves, a diet of 20 gm protein per day is provided, and the daily protein intake is then increased by 10 gm every 2–3 days until the patient's maximum protein tolerance is reached. In outpatients, it is impractical to maintain a protein intake of less than 50 gm/day.

2. Decrease gut NH_4 absorption. Bacteria in the large bowel produce a significant quantity of nitrogenous products.

   a. Neomycin, a poorly absorbed antibiotic, will decrease the number of bacteria in the gut. The dose for adults is 1 gm QID given PO or by retention enema if necessary. About 1% of orally administered neomycin is absorbed, which is enough to produce hearing loss and renal impairment. Consequently, large doses of neomycin cannot be given indefinitely. Colitis, overgrowth of the bowel by *Candida,* and malabsorption are other possible complications of neomycin therapy.

   b. Lactulose (a synthetic disaccharide that cannot be digested in the upper gastrointestinal tract) 10–30 ml TID given PO, by gastric tube, or by retention enema will acidify the stool and minimize NH_4^+ absorption from the gut. Lactulose may be used in patients who are unable to tolerate neomycin, and it may also be used on a chronic basis. There are patients who respond to neomycin but not to lactulose and, occasionally, patients who respond to lactulose but not to neomycin.

3. Fluid and electrolyte balance

   a. Hypokalemia and alkalosis increase renal NH_4^+ production and may worsen hepatic encephalopathy. These conditions should be treated promptly, and potassium-wasting diuretics should be avoided.

   b. Intravascular volume must be maintained to prevent prerenal azotemia and to maintain adequate liver perfusion.

   c. Hyponatremia from many causes may be associated with hepatic encephalopathy, and it is treated appropriately (see sec **VI.B**).

4. Tranquilizers and CNS depressants should be **avoided.**

5. Infection, anywhere in the body, is a common precipitant of encephalopathy in patients with liver disease. Moreover, the patients may fail to show the usual signs of infection. Therefore possible sites of sepsis are carefully sought and treated promptly.

6. Experimental forms of therapy. There are several modes of therapy that cannot be recommended for general use at this time. However, they may be undertaken if the patient fails to respond to the customary measures already outlined.

   a. L-dopa may be given PO, beginning with a dose of 250 mg BID and then increasing it by 500 mg each day to a maximum tolerated dose. If no effect is seen at the maximum tolerated dose, or by the time 4 gm per day is reached, then the drug is discontinued. Tolerance is usually limited by gastrointestinal side effects, movement disorders, or postural hypotension (see Chap. 15). The beneficial effects of L-dopa are usually short-lived.

   b. Parenteral alimentation with **amino acid solutions** that are high in branched-chain amino acids (leucine, isoleucine, and valine) and low in phenylalanine, tryptophan, methionine, and glycine has theoretical and experimental support.

   c. Parenteral alimentation with **alpha-keto precursors of essential amino**

acids is another technique that has theoretical support but, as yet, inadequate clinical evaluation.

7. Monitoring therapy

   a. Clinically

     (1) Hepatic encephalopathy may be divided into four stages with the following signs:

       (a) Stage I (precoma)—Mild confusion and mental slowness without asterixis or EEG abnormalities.

       (b) Stage II (impending coma)—Disorientation, drowsiness, asterixis, and possible mild EEG slowing.

       (c) Stage III—The patient is asleep most of the time and is confused when aroused; asterixis; EEG slowing.

       (d) Stage IV (coma)—The patient responds only to pain; there is hypotonia and marked EEG slowing.

     (2) In mild stages of encephalopathy a handwriting chart and tests of constructional ability (drawing a clock or constructing a star with match sticks, for instance) are sensitive indicators of clinical status.

   b. Blood NH_4^+ levels. If a group of patients with hepatic encephalopathy is studied, blood NH_4^+ level at one point in time will not correlate well with the degree of neurologic impairment. However, in a given patient, the NH_4^+ level, if followed serially, usually does correlate with that patient's status.

     Arterial levels correlate better than venous levels, but many patients with severe liver disease have coexistent coagulation defects, contraindicating repeated arterial punctures.

   c. EEG. In deeper stages of hepatic encephalopathy, the degree of EEG slowing has an excellent correlation with the patient's clinical status.

8. Chronic management. In most patients with hepatic encephalopathy, there is no specific treatment available for the underlying liver disease. Thus hepatic encephalopathy tends to be a chronic and recurrent problem that requires long-term therapy.

   a. Low-protein diet. Dietary protein is limited to the lowest practical and tolerable level (usually 50 gm/day). Vitamin supplementation is provided with folate, multivitamins, and vitamin K.

   b. Ensure at least one **bowel movement** each day.

   c. Chronic use of **neomycin** is limited by its toxicity, but 500 mg PO two to four times daily can usually be tolerated for a few weeks or even months. However, the patient must be followed closely for evidence of toxicity, especially diminished hearing. **Lactulose** 10–30 ml PO TID is safer than neomycin and is equally effective in most cases. However, it is unpalatable to many patients.

   d. As a last resort, **surgical exclusion of the colon** from the bowel may be done. However, the operation carries a high morbidity and mortality.

C. Acquired chronic hepatocerebral degeneration (ACHD). This disorder is like hepatic encephalopathy in that it is associated with portosystemic shunting. However, it is a chronic and nonreversible CNS disease. The cardinal features are dementia, dysarthria, cerebellar ataxia, tremor, and choreoathetosis. It develops in patients who are subject to hepatic encephalopathy, and it is often superimposed on recurrent bouts of that disease.

This disease is not specifically treatable in itself; and it is only preventable through appropriate management of the underlying liver disease. It is possible, but not proved, that prevention of bouts of hepatic encephalopathy may prevent the progression of irreversible CNS damage. Also, the choreoathetosis may respond to neuroleptics (see Chap. 10), and the behavioral abnormalities may respond to protein restriction. A neuropsychiatric disease with diverse manifestations may accompany acquired chronic hepatocerebral degeneration.

D. Acute liver failure. With acute hepatocellular failure, there is a severe CNS dysfunction that is similar to the hepatic encephalopathy associated with portosystemic shunting. Unless the liver disease reverses itself, coma and death occur.

The disease may be treated identically to hepatic encephalopathy, with dietary protein restriction and either neomycin or lactulose.

E. Reye's syndrome

1. Description

   a. Epidemiology. Reye's syndrome is a multisystem disease that occurs almost exclusively in the pediatric age group, and primarily in children between the ages of 1 and 12 years. It is associated with viral infection, and the vast majority of cases are related to either influenza B or chicken pox.

   b. Clinical course. Reye's syndrome is characteristically preceded by a benign viral illness. On about the seventh day of the illness, an abrupt onset of vomiting occurs, followed by agitation, delirium, and lethargy, progressing to stupor and coma within 24–48 hours. The comatose state is associated with hyperventilation and seizures. There are no focal neurologic signs, and papilledema is unusual.

   Mild cases occur without profound changes in mental status. If death results from Reye's syndrome, it is a cerebral death with brain swelling, respiratory arrest, and, finally, brain death.

   c. Laboratory abnormalities

      (1) Liver function abnormalities

         (a) SGOT and SGPT are very high, with a normal alkaline phosphatase.

         (b) Bilirubin is either normal or only mildly elevated.

         (c) The prothrombin time is moderately prolonged.

         (d) Blood ammonia is very high (up to 1000 mg/100 ml) during the first 72 hours of the illness, but then it falls to normal values whether or not the coma resolves.

      (2) CSF

         (a) There are no cells and the protein is normal.

         (b) After coma develops and the brain swells, the CSF pressure becomes elevated.

      (3) Hypoglycemia is frequent, especially in children under 5 years of age.

      (4) Acid-base disturbances

         (a) Respiratory alkalosis is frequent.

         (b) Metabolic acidosis, with an anion gap and elevated lactate levels, develops in severe cases.

      (5) Muscle enzymes. CPK and aldolase are elevated, with CPK fractionation yielding primarily muscle (MM) and heart (MB) isozymes.

   d. Diagnosis

      (1) The diagnosis is generally made on the basis of the stereotyped clinical presentation and pattern of laboratory findings.

(2) Routine liver biopsy is not necessary, but it confirms the diagnosis in questionable cases. The pathognomonic finding in the liver is **microvesicular fatty infiltration.**

(3) The differential diagnosis must include salicylate intoxication, hepatic encephalopathy, acute liver failure, and coma from any cause with hypoxic liver damage.

e. Prognosis

(1) The chance of surviving Reye's syndrome diminishes progressively with an increasing depression of the mental status. The mortality of those in coma has been reported variously from 15–80%. Those who do not develop coma always survive.

(2) The maximum elevation of blood ammonia is a good prognostic indicator. If ammonia does not rise above 300 mg/100 ml, the survival rate is virtually 100%.

2. Laboratory evaluation

a. All patients with Reye's syndrome should have the following tests on admittance.

(1) Blood glucose.

(2) CBC and differential cell count.

(3) BUN or creatinine and urinalysis.

(4) Electrolytes, including calcium and phosphorus.

(5) Arterial blood gases and pH.

(6) Complete liver function tests, including SGOT (or SGPT), LDH, alkaline phosphatase, total and direct bilirubin, total protein, and albumin.

(7) Prothrombin time.

(8) Blood ammonia.

(9) Salicylate level and screening of blood and urine for toxic substances, unless drug ingestion can be absolutely ruled out by history.

(10) Lumbar puncture, to rule out encephalitis or other CNS infection. Lumbar puncture is safe in Reye's syndrome until the stage of decerebration is reached, at which time the CSF pressure becomes elevated to such an extent that the patient is at risk of herniation.

b. If the diagnosis is confirmed, the hemoglobin, prothrombin time, and blood sugar must be followed every 4–8 hours during the first 72 hours. Ammonia, SGOT, and electrolytes must be followed at least daily. Arterial blood gases are drawn as indicated.

c. There is no therapeutic indication for attempting to identify the associated virus.

3. Acute management

a. Maintain vital functions

(1) Vital signs are monitored closely, and complications of coma are avoided. Reye's syndrome is a prime indication for placing the patient in an intensive care unit.

(2) The airway is protected with a cuffed endotracheal tube if the patient is stuporous or comatose. If the patient is in deep coma, respiratory arrest may occur, and respirator support is required. The arterial Po_2 is kept above 100 mm Hg, a value higher than is usually required in other situations, because of abnormalities of mitochondrial respiration that occur in Reye's syndrome.

b. Treat possible hypoglycemia

(1) A blood glucose is drawn before administering IV fluids, the blood glucose is followed closely.

(2) In children under 5 years of age and in all patients in coma, 25 ml of 50% dextrose in water is administered whether or not the blood glucose results are available.

(3) A constant infusion of a glucose-containing solution, e.g., 10% dextrose in half-normal saline, is maintained.

c. Treat complications of the abnormal liver function

(1) Hypoprothrombinemia may lead to hemorrhagic complications and requires vigorous treatment. Vitamin K (in 10 mg doses IV) may have to be given as often as every 6 hours. If the prothrombin time cannot be corrected to within 2 seconds of control with vitamin K, the administration of fresh frozen plasma in sufficient quantities is required.

(2) Hyperammonemia is treated with measures similar to those used in hepatic encephalopathy.

(a) No protein is administered for the first 72 hours of the illness.

(b) The gut is purged with enemas and cathartics to remove the protein in the patient's gut.

(c) If gastrointestinal bleeding occurs, the gut is kept free of blood by gastric lavage and catharsis.

(d) After about 72 hours, the ammonemia will return to normal, whether or not the patient's mental status improves.

(3) Experimental techniques are used in various centers in an effort to treat the metabolic derangements associated with Reye's syndrome. These techniques are only recommended for use by clinicians who are experienced in their use and as part of research protocols.

(a) Exchange transfusion

(b) Dialysis

(c) Intravenous citrulline infusion

(d) Infusions of glucose plus insulin

d. Treat brain swelling

(1) Fluids are restricted to 1200 ml total fluids/24 hours/sq m body surface area. The urine output, urine specific gravity, electrolytes, and serum osmolality are monitored at least daily.

(2) **Intracranial pressure monitoring devices** are useful in patients in coma. Their use allows the precise and continuous monitoring of intracranial pressure during the first 2–4 days of the illness, during which time the patient is at high risk from brain swelling.

(3) For acute increases in intracranial pressure, mannitol 1.5 gm/kg is given by IV infusion over 20 minutes. If the intracranial pressure is being monitored continuously, the mannitol may be repeated as necessary to keep the pressure under 200 cm water. Mannitol must be infused at the earliest sign of a "pressure wave" to prevent rapid and extreme increases in pressure.

(4) Glycerol may be given in chronic situations by nasogastric tube to maintain the serum osmolality in the range of 320–325 mOsm/L. If the patient is adequately fluid-restricted, the dose required may only be 1–2 gm/kg/day in 6–12 divided doses or less. As much as 8 gm/kg/day may be used if needed.

(5) There is no evidence that steroids are of benefit in Reye's syndrome for the control of intracranial pressure.

e. Treat seizures

(1) Prophylactic anticonvulsant therapy is recommended for all patients with Reye's syndrome who have significant mental status depression. Phenytoin (Dilantin) is preferred over phenobarbitol, because large loading doses have less effect on mental status and respirations. (The dose is 5 mg/kg/day given IV or PO.)

Therapy is initiated with a **loading dose** of approximately 15 mg/kg given IV or PO. If given IV, the usual precautions necessary for the IV administration of phenytoin are followed (Chap. 6). The anticonvulsants are continued until the patient's mental status returns to normal.

(2) The therapy of seizures, once they occur in Reye's syndrome, follows the principles listed in Chapter 6.

II. ENDOCRINE.
Virtually all hormone disorders have associated neurologic signs and symptoms, often as the cardinal features of the syndrome. In most of these disorders, the therapy is correction of the underlying defect. The exceptions are hyperthyroidism and pheochromocytoma, for which beta and alpha blockers, respectively, are used to control the manifestations of the autonomic nervous system while definitive therapy is being pursued. This therapy is not discussed in detail here. Clinicians must be aware of endocrinologic syndromes as diagnostic possibilities in patients with neurologic dysfunction. However, the detailed therapy of diabetes, thyroid, parathyroid, and adrenal diseases is beyond the scope of this text.

III. RENAL FAILURE

A. Uremic encephalopathy

1. Description

a. The clinical features of uremic encephalopathy are nonspecific and cannot be distinguished from those of other metabolic encephalopathies. There is a global affect of cerebral function, beginning with difficulty in concentration and subtle personality changes, progressing to confusion and then to drowsiness, stupor, and coma. Asterixis is prominent when higher cortical function becomes affected and before coma supervenes.

b. The EEG shows low-voltage slowing in early stages, with the development of generalized paroxysmal slowing in late stages.

c. The CSF is normal, with the possible exception of a mild elevation of the protein.

d. Generalized major motor (grand mal) seizures may occur during the stages of stupor and coma.

e. The more rapid the progression of the renal failure, the greater the severity of the encephalopathy for a given BUN or creatinine level.

2. Treatment

a. The underlying renal disease is treated.

b. Incapacitating mental changes or the development of asterixis is an indication for dialysis.

B. Seizures

1. In renal failure, **generalized seizures** may occur as a result of any of several mechanisms:

   a. Uremic encephalopathy

   b. Water intoxication with hyponatremia

   c. Hypocalcemia

   d. Hypomagnesemia

   e. Hypertensive encephalopathy

   f. Dialysis dysequilibrium syndrome

2. **Focal seizures** that occur in the setting of renal failure imply focal brain disease and must be investigated accordingly. These seizures may be precipitated by underlying metabolic imbalances, and they may respond to treatment of the metabolic problems.

3. **Treatment**

   a. Treatable underlying metabolic problems are managed appropriately.

   b. Seizures that result from uremic encephalopathy are in themselves an indication for dialysis.

   c. Seizures that do not respond to metabolic correction or dialysis are treated in the same manner as seizures in other situations.

   (1) **Phenytoin** (Dilantin) doses do not have to be modified in the presence of renal failure, but absorption of oral phenytoin may be erratic. Thus the patient must be observed frequently for signs of clinical toxicity. Blood levels of phenytoin may be helpful, but the percentage of phenytoin not bound to plasma proteins is higher in renal failure than in normal renal function.

   (2) **Phenobarbital** must be used in diminished doses in renal failure, but the necessary dose is difficult to determine. Moreover, in the presence of uremic encephalopathy, the toxic effects of phenobarbital may be difficult to distinguish from metabolic encephalopathy. Therefore the blood level must be measured frequently to adjust the dose.

   (3) **Diazepam** (Valium) IV may be used for emergency seizure control when seizures threaten vital functions or when status epilepticus occurs. As in other situations, diazepam IV has only a temporary effect (20–30 minutes) so more definitive therapy must be undertaken during this time to control the seizures.

   d. Hemodialysis patients may have seizures during, or up to 8 hours after, dialysis due to the dysequilibrium syndrome.

   (1) The chance of seizures occurring may be reduced by decreasing the rate and duration of dialysis and increasing its frequency.

   (2) Hemodialysis patients should be on prophylactic anticonvulsants. Dilantin 300 mg daily in adults is the usual regimen.

C. Uremic neuropathy

1. **Description.** Uremia causes a distal sensorimotor neuropathy that affects the legs before it does the arms. Also, it affects the legs more severely. The neuropathy is often painful, with "burning feet," and can be incapacitating.

2. The only effective treatment known is correction of the underlying renal

disease. A functioning renal transplant is virtually always effective in relieving the neuropathic symptoms, and it is often curative. Chronic hemodialysis is much less effective than renal transplantation.

3. There is some evidence that carbamazepine (Tegretol) 400–600 mg/day PO in divided doses may reduce the pain of uremic neuropathy.

D. Neurologic complications of hemodialysis

1. Seizures and the dysequilibrium syndrome are discussed in **B**.

2. **Subdural hematoma**

   a. There is an increased incidence of subdural hematoma among patients undergoing chronic hemodialysis. Possible predisposing factors include anticoagulation, rapid shifts in brain size, hypertension, and minor head trauma. In dialysis patients subdural hematomas are frequently bilateral.

   b. The signs of bilateral subdural hematoma may be confused with the dysequilibrium syndrome, thereby delaying diagnosis.

   c. The treatment of subdural hematoma is surgical drainage. Because of the osmotic and volume shifts that occur between body compartments during hemodialysis, it is not safe to defer surgical treatment and follow the patient clinically (as one might do with other patients with chronic subdural hematomas). During the postoperative period, the patient is managed with peritoneal dialysis to minimize rapid osmotic shifts and to avoid systemic anticoagulation.

3. **Headache**

   a. Migraine may be made worse by hemodialysis. Its treatment in the presence of renal failure is ergot, which is given in the same dosage as for other migraine headaches (see Chap. 2).

   b. The dialysis dysequilibrium syndrome produces headache during and for up to 8 hours after dialysis. Ergots may be tried in the same manner as for migraine therapy.

   c. Persistent headache suggests the presence of subdural hematoma.

4. **Vitamin deficiency**

   a. All chronic hemodialysis patients should be on supplemental multivitamins, including folate, thiamine, and pantothenic acid.

   b. Attempts to treat uremic neuropathy with therapeutic doses of various vitamins have been unsuccessful.

5. **Dialysis dementia**

   a. There is a syndrome of subacutely progressive mental deterioration, without known cause, that occurs in patients on hemodialysis. Its incidence seems to vary widely between different dialysis centers, suggesting that toxins in the local water supply may be responsible. The course is one of relentless progression to death.

   b. There is no known treatment for this syndrome. It is a diagnosis of exclusion, and other causes of dementia, including chronic subdural hematoma, repetitive subclinical seizures, and drug intoxication must be excluded.

6. **Muscle cramps** during or immediately following hemodialysis may cause severe pain. Quinine sulfate 320 mg given PO at the beginning of each dialysis has been reported to be beneficial and safe.

E. Neurologic complications of renal transplantation

1. CNS infections (see Chap. 8)

2. CNS malignancy, including reticulum cell sarcoma (see Chap. 11).

IV. PULMONARY. Both hypercapnea and hypoxemia are associated with encephalopathy. The treatment is the same as for underlying lung disease. The neurologic sequelae of sustained hypoxia need no repetition.

V. REMOTE EFFECTS OF CARCINOMA. Many paracarcinomatous syndromes are presumably caused by toxins manufactured by the tumor. They can be ameliorated in proportion to the amount of bulk tumor removed or destroyed. These syndromes include some paracarcinomatous neuropathies and the pseudomyasthenic syndrome (Eaton-Lambert syndrome) (see Chap. 16). Other paracarcinomatous syndromes are probably infectious in origin (e.g., progressive multifocal leukoencephalopathy) or result in irreversible anatomic alterations in the nervous system (e.g., carcinomatous cerebellar degeneration). These syndromes do not respond to treatment of the underlying neoplasm.

VI. HYPONATREMIA

A. Description

1. Sodium is the primary extracellular cation and the chief determinant of the osmolarity of the extracellular fluid, including the blood plasma. Consequently, hyponatremia and hypo-osmolarity generally coexist. Exceptions include the circumstances in which the sodium concentration is artifactually lowered (hyperlipidemia and hyperproteinemia) or in which an osmotic agent other than sodium makes up a significant portion of the serum solute content, producing hyponatremia with normal or elevated serum osmolality (hyperglycemia or the exogenous administration of osmotic agents, such as mannitol and glycerol).

2. The serum osmolarity can be computed approximately according to the following formula:

Serum osmolarity (mOsm/L) =

$$2 \times (Na \ (mEq/L) + K \ (mEq/L)) + \frac{BUN \ (mg/100 \ ml)}{3} + \frac{glucose \ (mg/100 \ ml)}{18}$$

This formula is only accurate in the absence of exogenously administered osmotic agents.

3. The hypo-osmolar state may be asymptomatic or it may cause a metabolic encephalopathy: confusion and agitation, progressing to lethargy and then to seizures and coma. Psychosis with hallucinations may occur and asterixis may be seen.

4. Symptoms usually do not appear unless the serum sodium is lower than 125 mEq/L; seizures generally occur only when the sodium level drops lower than 115 mEq/L. The more rapid the development of the hyponatremia, the more severe the symptoms for a given sodium concentration.

5. The differential diagnosis of hyponatremia is:

a. Loss of sodium out of proportion to water

(1) Renal sodium wasting

(a) Salt-losing nephropathy

(b) Diuretics

(c) Hypoadrenocorticism

(2) Extrarenal sodium losses

(a) Diarrhea, vomiting, gastric drainage

(b) Burns

b. Retention of water out of proportion to sodium

(1) Syndrome of inappropriate antidiuretic hormone secretion (SIADH)

(a) Bronchogenic oat cell carcinoma and other malignant tumors.

(b) CNS disease: stroke, head trauma, infection, tumors, acute intermittent porphyria (AIP), and hydrocephalus.

(c) Pulmonary disease: tuberculosis, pneumonia, and lung abscess.

(d) Unknown etiology.

(e) Drugs: chlorpropamide, vincristine, cyclophosphamide, phenothiazines, barbiturates, tricyclic antidepressants, clofibrate, acetaminophen.

(f) Guillain-Barré syndrome.

(2) Beer drinking

(3) Oliguric renal failure with overhydration with hypotonic fluids

(4) Edematous states

(a) Hepatic cirrhosis

(b) Congestive heart failure

(5) Psychogenic polydipsia

(6) Hypothyroidism

c. Shifts in water between body compartments

(1) Hyperglycemia

(2) Exogenous administration of osmotic agents: mannitol, glycerol

(3) Hypoadrenocorticism

(4) "Sick cell" syndrome

d. Pseudohyponatremia

(1) Hyperlipidemia

(2) Hyperproteinemia

B. General principles of treatment

1. Symptomatic hyponatremia requires immediate treatment to prevent permanent neurologic damage and death.

2. The more rapidly the hyponatremia develops, the more rapidly it must be corrected. Symptomatic hyponatremia that develops within less than 12 hours should be corrected to a serum sodium of greater than 125 mEq/L within 4–8 hours of diagnosis.

C. Specific situations

1. Dilutional hyponatremia occurs in patients who are volume-depleted and who are given access to hypotonic fluids. This is a frequent iatrogenic disease.

a. The clinical picture is one of volume depletion with a low urine sodium concentration.

b. The treatment consists of the replacement of volume and sodium deficits.

A water diuresis will then ensue, and the serum sodium will be returned to normal. In mild cases a liberalization of the sodium content of the diet or a reduction of dosage in a diuretic agent may be adequate therapy. When the patient is symptomatic or when the serum sodium level is lower than 125 mEq/L, intravenous isotonic saline is given.

c. In calculating the amount of sodium required to correct the deficit, assume that the sodium will be distributed throughout the total body water (TBW), which is about 60% of body weight. Therefore the amount of sodium to be administered can be calculated as follows:

Amount of sodium required (in mEq) = body weight (in kg) × 0.6 × (desired Na − measured Na)

d. Usually, in correcting the deficit with IV saline, sufficient NaCl is administered to correct the deficit halfway to normal by using the above calculation. Then the serum sodium is remeasured and recalculated for the additional amount required.

e. In elderly patients and those with compromised hearts or kidneys, the overly enthusiastic administration of saline may lead to congestive heart failure. Therefore careful attention must be paid to the patient's volume status. A central venous pressure (CVP)-monitoring catheter is often helpful.

2. Water retention

a. Patients may retain water out of proportion to sodium in oliguric renal failure, hypothyroidism, and, very rarely, with psychogenic polydipsia.

(1) The treatment in most cases is to restrict the water intake to the amount of calculated insensible losses (800 ml per day in a normothermic adult) until the sodium is within the normal range.

(2) In very rare circumstances, in which the patient has symptoms of severe water intoxication, it may be necessary to administer hypertonic saline in the form of 3% NaCl to raise the serum sodium to a level greater than 125 mEq/L. This should generally be done with the aid of a CVP line; furosemide (Lasix) may be administered if volume overload occurs.

b. Syndrome of inappropriate antidiuretic hormone secretion (SIADH)

(1) SIADH occurs in a variety of circumstances (see sec **VI.A.5.b.(1)**). The pathophysiology of the hyponatremia involves both water retention with volume expansion and sodium wasting. The patient is normovolemic or mildly hypervolemic but is not characteristically edematous. The following criteria must be met to verify the diagnosis:

(a) Serum hyponatremia and hypo-osmolality.

(b) Renal sodium wasting. Generally, with a normal sodium intake, the urine sodium concentration is greater than 25 mEq/L. Occasionally, when the patient is sodium restricted and a steady state has been reached, the urine sodium may be lower.

(c) The urine osmolality is inappropriately high for the serum osmolarity.

(d) The patient is not volume-depleted.

(e) Normal renal function.

(f) Normal adrenal function.

(2) In asymptomatic and mildly symptomatic cases, water restriction is the treatment of choice. The patient's daily fluid intake is restricted to calculated insensible losses until the serum sodium is within normal limits. The water intake may then be limited to daily maintenance levels.

(3) In severe hyponatremia from SIADH, the serum sodium can be corrected to 125–130 mEq/L within 4–8 hours by using Schrier's method (*Ann. Intern. Med.* 78:970, 1973).

(a) An initial diuresis is induced with furosemide (Lasix) 1 mg/kg IV, and hourly urine collections are taken and analyzed for sodium and potassium content. The hourly sodium and potassium losses thus measured are replaced by the IV infusion 3% NaCl with the appropriate amount of KCl added.

(b) Subsequent doses of furosemide are given to achieve the desired water loss over 4–8 hours. The desired negative fluid balance may be calculated by means of the following formulas:

Total body water (TBW), in liters = body weight (kg) $\times$ 0.6

TBW $\times$ plasma osmolality (mOsm/L) = total body solute (mOsm)

$$\frac{\text{Total body solute}}{x} = \frac{\text{desired plasma osmolarity}}{1\text{ L}}$$

(If the desired plasma osmolarity is taken as 270 mOsm/L, then

$$x = \frac{\text{total body solute}}{270})$$

The desired negative water balance (in L) = TBW $-$ x.

(c) The serum sodium and potassium are measured no less often than every 2 hours during the infusion of hypertonic saline. Central venous pressure should be monitored in patients over 35 years of age and those with abnormal cardiac or renal function.

(4) The inciting cause of SIADH should be eliminated if possible; i.e., offending drugs are discontinued, bulk tumor is removed if possible, or CNS or pulmonary infections are treated appropriately.

(5) The therapy of chronic SIADH is water restriction. However, water restriction is extremely unpleasant for the patient, so various means may be used to allow a more liberal water intake.

(a) Dietary sodium supplementation allows greater water intake, but it may lead to congestive heart failure in the presence of compromised cardiac or renal function.

(b) Lithium carbonate 300 mg TID PO will partially inhibit the action of ADH on the kidney, and it may allow significantly liberalized fluid intake.

(c) Demeclocycline 300 mg TID PO will also cause a partial renal diabetes insipidus and allow liberalized fluid intake.

(d) Phenytoin (Dilantin) acts centrally to inhibit ADH release, but in practice it has been of no benefit in the management of SIADH of central origin.

VII. ACUTE INTERMITTENT PORPHYRIA (AIP)

A. Description. Acute intermittent porphyria is an inherited disease of porphyrin metabolism, manifested by recurrent attacks of abdominal pain and neurologic dysfunction. It is genetically transmitted as an autosomal dominant trait, and it probably results from a deficiency of uroporphyrinogen I synthetase (Uro I synthetase).

1. Symptoms rarely appear until the onset of puberty, and in most cases they begin in the second to fourth decade of life. Females outnumber males in symptomatic cases, and asymptomatic carriers of the defect exist.

2. Acute attacks are usually heralded by abdominal pain and constipation followed by neurologic disease. Peripheral neuropathy, which may progress to quadriplegia and respiratory paralysis, cranial nerve palsies, psychosis, depression, confusion, coma, and seizures may all occur during an acute attack. Attacks may leave the patient with residual peripheral nerve or psychiatric dysfunction. Even with optimum management, a severe acute attack of acute intermittent porphyria carries a significant mortality.

3. **Diagnosis.** During acute attacks of acute intermittent porphyria, and usually between attacks as well, patients have elevated urinary excretion of delta-aminolevulinic acid (δ-ALA) and porphobilinogen (PBG). The latter can be qualitatively measured by the Watson-Schwartz test. The definitive test for this disease is to compare the activity of uroporphyrinogen I synthetase in the patient's erythrocytes with that of his relatives. Family members with this disease have Uro I synthetase levels that are about half those of unaffected family members. No definite sporadic cases of acute intermittent porphyria have ever been documented.

B. Prophylaxis against acute attacks. The mainstay of the management of this disease is the avoidance of factors known to precipitate acute attacks. Asymptomatic family members are identified by erythrocyte uroporphyrinogen I synthetase levels, so an appropriate measure can be taken to keep them in the asymptomatic class.

1. **Drugs.** The most common precipitant of an acute attack of acute intermittent porphyria is the administration of a drug that induces liver δ-ALA synthetase activity. Drugs that affect AIP may be divided into four classes.

    a. Drugs definitely known to precipitate attacks and are absolutely contraindicated:

    (1) Barbiturates

    (2) Sulfonamides

    (3) Griseofulvin (Fulvicin, Grifulvin)

    (4) Chlordiazepoxide (Librium)

    (5) Meprobamate (Miltown)

    (6) Isopropylmeprobate (Soma)

    (7) Phenytoin (Dilantin)

    (8) Methsuximide (Celontin)

    (9) Dechloralphenazone (Midrin)

    (10) Glutethimide (Doriden)

    (11) Pyrayolone compounds: aminopyrine, antipyrine, isopropylantipyrine, and dipyrone

    (12) Methylprylon (Noludar)

    (13) Imipramine (Tofranil)

    (14) Ergot preparations

    (15) Eucalyptol

    (16) Sylfonal

(17) Trional

(18) Tolbutamide (Orinase)

(19) Alcohol

b. Drugs that have been experimentally shown to induce δ-ALA synthetase, but which have not been definitely implicated in attacks are:

(1) Mephenytoin (Mesantoin)

(2) Phensuximide (Milontin)

(3) Chloramphenicol

(4) 2-Alkyloxy-3-methylbenzamide

c. Drugs known to be safe are:

(1) Opiates, including morphine, methadone, codeine, propoxyphene (Darvon), and meperidine (Demerol)

(2) Hyoscine

(3) Chloral hydrate

(4) Penicillins

(5) Streptomycin

(6) Tetracyclines

(7) Furadantin

(8) Mandelamine

(9) Corticosteroids

(10) Rauwolfia alkaloids (e.g., reserpine)

(11) Guanethidine

(12) Diphenhydramine (Benadryl)

(13) Promethazine (Phenergan)

(14) Phenothiazines

(15) Meclizine (Bonine, Bonadoxin)

(16) B vitamins

(17) Ascorbic acid

(18) Digoxin

(19) Mersalyl

(20) Atropine

(21) Prostigmin (Neostigmine)

(22) Tetraethylammonium bromide

d. For drugs not listed, there is inadequate information on which to make a judgment.

2. **Hormones.** Estrogen, progesterone, and testosterone have been shown to induce δ-ALA synthetase activity.

a. Pregnancy has been reported to precipitate acute attacks and therefore carries an increased risk in the presence of acute intermittent porphyria.

b. Exogenous administration of estrogens and oral contraceptives has been reported to precipitate acute attacks and, with the exception to be discussed in **c,** should be avoided in these patients.

    c. There are women with acute intermittent porphyria who experience regular cyclical attacks, usually mild, during the few days immediately preceding menstruation. Oral contraceptives have been successfully used to prevent these cyclical attacks and should be tried in women with this syndrome. Oral contraceptives do not prevent attacks and are contraindicated in patients who do not have this cyclical syndrome.

    d. Corticosteroids can be used safely.

  3. Infections. Although fever and leukocytosis may occur as a manifestation of an acute attack of acute intermittent porphyria, they are more often manifestations of infection. Infections in these patients must be diagnosed and treated promptly.

  4. Starvation and dieting. A high-carbohydrate intake can suppress the induction of liver δ-ALA synthetase activity. Conversely, δ-ALA synthetase activity rises during periods of low-carbohydrate intake, and starvation may precipitate an acute attack of acute intermittent porphyria. Thus these patients should be maintained on a relatively high-carbohydrate diet, ingesting over half their calories as carbohydrates.

C. Treatment of the acute attack

  1. Suppression of porphyrin synthesis

    a. High-carbohydrate intake. The patient is provided with 450–600 gm of carbohydrate daily, either PO or parenterally, during the attack. If parenteral glucose solutions are used, the serum electrolytes are followed closely because of the frequent association of SIADH with porphyria.

    b. Hematin, like carbohydrate, lowers hepatic δ-ALA synthetase levels experimentally. In several reports it has shown promising results when administered parenterally to patients with attacks of acute intermittent porphyria. However, it is not generally available.

  2. Management of complications of the acute attack

    a. Abdominal pain

      (1) Chlorpromazine (Thorazine) is highly effective for the abdominal pain. It probably works through the autonomic nervous system to control the disordered intestinal motility.

        Doses must be titrated for the individual patient to avoid oversedation. An initial dose of 50 mg IM is a reasonable starting point, and it may be repeated every 3–4 hours as needed.

      (2) Opiates may be added to chlorpromazine as necessary. One must be careful not to depress respiration excessively in patients with severe neuropathies and respiratory compromise.

      (3) Fecal disimpaction is frequently necessary.

    b. Respiratory failure and **bulbar paralysis** may require tracheal intubation, respiratory support, or gastric feeding.

    c. Hyponatremia is a frequent occurrence during acute attacks, either as a result of vomiting and dehydration or of SIADH. Since hyponatremia may worsen the central nervous system manifestations, it must be carefully avoided and vigorously treated if it occurs. (See sec **VI**).

    d. Hypomagnesemia may occur and should be treated to avoid contributing to seizures. Calcium levels are generally normal; occasionally they are either mildly elevated or depressed due to unknown mechanisms. The disorder of calcium regulation generally requires no acute treatment, but coexisting disorders of calcium metabolism should be ruled out.

e. Psychosis. Chlorpromazine (Thorazine) or other phenothiazines may be used safely to control the psychiatric manifestations. Acute and chronic depression may concur, and with these patients suicide is a risk.

f. Seizures. Because of the many drugs that cannot be used in these patients, including barbiturates, hydantoins, and succinimides, the treatment of seizures may be extremely difficult. If the seizures are only associated with the acute attack, diazepam (Valium) may be sufficient, although repeated IV doses may be required until the attack is aborted. Clonazepam has not been shown to be definitely safe in these patients, but it is probably the first-line drug for long-term use. As is mentioned in secs c and d, hyponatremia and hypomagnesemia should be treated promptly.

g. Labile hypertension or postural hypotension may accompany the autonomic nervous-system disorders associated with acute intermittent porphyria. The former usually requires no treatment, although reserpine and guanethidine are both known to be safe, if needed. Postural hypotension requires careful maintenance of intravascular volume.

3. Chemical abnormalities. There are several endocrinologic abnormalities that occur in association with acute intermittent porphyria.

a. The oral glucose tolerance test is frequently abnormal during an acute attack, but it usually requires no treatment.

b. The free T_4 and PBI may be elevated, but they do not require specific therapy.

c. Patients often have type IIA hyperlipoproteinemia that persists between attacks and, in the absence of information to the contrary, may be treated like any other case of hyperbetalipoproteinemia.

VIII. INDUSTRIAL AND ENVIRONMENTAL TOXINS

A. Lead

1. Sources of exposure. Lead is present in a large number of commonly encountered materials of everyday life. It is present in paints—both interior paints, which may still line the walls of older buildings, and modern exterior paints. Tetraethyl lead is a gasoline additive, which is present in high concentrations in the atmosphere around tanks used to store gasoline and in dirt collected from urban areas near heavily traveled intersections or expressways. Lead poisoning has occurred from drinking liquids stored in improperly glazed pottery, illicit whiskey distilled through lead pipes or through automobile radiators containing lead solder, and from inhaling the fumes of burning storage batteries.

2. Clinical manifestations of toxicity

a. Encephalopathy

(1) Epidemiology. Lead encephalopathy occurs in children who ingest large amounts of lead salts. It occurs only rarely in adults, and then only in those exposed to tetraethyl lead, which is lipid-soluble and reaches high levels in the CNS. In children it is usually accompanied by pica, and it is most frequent between the ages of 1 and 3 years. For unexplained reasons, lead encephalopathy is more common in summer than in winter.

(2) Signs and symptoms. The usual symptoms of lead encephalopathy are personality change, lethargy and irritability progressing to somnolence and ataxia, and, finally, seizures, coma, and death. In children, acute episodes of lead encephalopathy may recur, superimposed on a state of chronic lead intoxication.

(3) The mortality of acute lead encephalopathy is less than 5% in the best of hands, but 40% are left with permanent and significant residual neurologic deficits, which may include dementia, ataxia, spasticity, and seizures.

b. Lead colic is the most frequent manifestation of lead poisoning in adults. The patient is anorectic and constipated, often with nausea and vomiting. There is abdominal pain but no tenderness. Characteristically, the patient presses on his abdomen to relieve the discomfort. Lead colic generally accompanies lead encephalopathy in children.

c. Neuromuscular form. Slowing of motor nerve conduction velocity is an early sign of lead poisoning in children; symptomatic neuropathy is rare. In adults, however, symptomatic neuropathy is frequent in lead poisoning. Typically, lead neuropathy produces weakness, but paresthesias and sensory changes may occur. Extensors are weakened before flexors, and the most used muscle groups (usually the extensors of the wrist) are involved earliest.

d. It is suspected, but not yet proved, that chronic lead exposure in children that is insufficient to produce overt encephalopathy may cause the "hyperactive syndrome."

3. Making the diagnosis

a. Physical examination. The only characteristic physical finding of lead poisoning is the presence of lead lines around the gum margins. These occur in a minority of cases and only in patients with poor dental hygiene.

b. Blood smear. In chronic lead exposure, there is usually a microcytic anemia that may be superimposed on an iron-deficiency anemia. Basophilic stippling is seen in a minority of cases, and the bone marrow may show ringed sideroblasts.

c. Urine. There is proximal renal tubular dysfunction associated with lead toxicity, with glycosuria, phosphaturia, and amino aciduria.

d. X-rays. Lead lines may be seen in the long bones. In children who have recently ingested lead-containing paint, radiopaque flecks may be seen in the abdomen.

e. Laboratory evidence of increased body lead burden

(1) The serum lead level is useful as a screening test, but in many circumstances it does not reflect the total body lead burden accurately. Lead levels that are measured on capillary blood (obtained from a finger stick with a capillary tube) are subject to contamination by lead on the skin. The 24-hour urinary lead excretion test has the same limitations as the serum lead level test.

(2) An EDTA test measures total body lead burden more accurately than does a single serum or urinary level test. However, this test is dangerous in children with high lead burdens, because EDTA may mobilize lead from the tissues and precipitate encephalopathy. Therefore it should not be performed in a child who has a serum lead level higher than 80 mg lead/100 ml or who has symptoms of early encephalopathy.

The test is performed by administering calcium EDTA in either one or three doses of 25 mg/kg at 8-hour intervals. Then a 24-hour urine is collected, and the total lead excreted in 24 hours is measured. A positive test consists of greater than 500 mg of lead excreted per 24 hours, or greater than 1 mg lead excreted per 24 hours/mg EDTA administered.

(3) There are several tests that measure the toxic effects of lead on porphyrin metabolism. These tests are generally the most sensitive and reliable measures of lead toxicity.

(a) δ-ALA dehydratase activity in erythrocytes is the most sensitive test of lead poisoning, but it is not readily available.

(b) Urinary or serum δ-ALA levels higher than 20 mg/100 ml are indicative of lead toxicity.

(c) Urinary coproporphyrin excretion greater than 150 mg/24 hours is indicative of lead toxicity.

(d) Erythrocytic protoporphyrin (EP) levels higher than 190 mg/100 ml of whole blood are diagnostic of lead poisoning in the absence of either iron deficiency or erythropoietic protoporphyria, both of which may also elevate erythrocytic protoporphyrin levels. (See sec **3.a**)

4. Therapy

a. Encephalopathy

(1) According to recent guidelines by the Center for Disease Control, children may be divided into four classes, depending on serum lead levels and erythrocytic protoporphyrin levels (Table 14-1). The recommended management is as follows:

(a) Class IV. Hospitalize for immediate chelation therapy with British anti-lewisite (BAL) plus EDTA. Lumbar puncture should be avoided because of the possibility of increased intracranial pressure.

(b) Class III. If there are symptoms of lead encephalopathy present or if there is metabolic evidence of lead toxicity (abnormal erythrocyte δ-ALA dehydratase activity, urinary δ-ALA levels, or urinary CPG excretion), then treat as class IV. If there are no symptoms, an

Table 14-1. Classification of Children with Suspected Lead Intoxication

Test	Class I (Normal)	Class II (Minimally Elevated)	Class III (Moderately Elevated)	Class IV (Extremely Elevated)
Serum Pb (mg/100 ml[a])	29	30–49	50–79	80
Erythrocyte protoporphyrin (EP)[a]	59	60–109	110–189	190

Test Results	EP 59	Ep 60–109	EP 110–189	EP 190
Pb 29	I	I[b]	I[b]	I[b]
Pb 30–49	I	II	III	IV
Pb 50–79		II	III	IV
Pb 80				IV

[a] If there is a discrepancy between the classes, as determined by serum lead level and by EP concentration, in general the EP concentration is considered to be more reliable.
[b] These children generally have increased EP concentrations due to iron deficiency. EP = erythropoietic protoporphyria.

EDTA test is performed. If positive, the patient is treated as in class IV or, rarely, may be suitable for outpatient chelation therapy with close follow-up if the social circumstances permit. If the EDTA test is negative, the patient may be treated as in class II.

(c) Class II. The environment is thoroughly screened for sources of lead exposure and all these sources are eliminated. The child is evaluated for iron deficiency and followed no less frequently than every 3 months with repeat examinations, and erythrocytic porphyrin or serum lead levels are determined.

(d) Class I. Patients are normal and receive routine follow-up care.

(2) Adults may develop lead encephalopathy occasionally from ingestion of lead salts, but it is more frequent from the inhalation of fumes, particularly if they contain tetraethyl lead rather than lead salts. Adults with signs of lead encephalopathy are treated with chelation therapy with BAL and EDTA in a manner identical to that in which children are treated.

b. Lead colic and lead neuropathy in adults

(1) These conditions require immediate attention, but they are not the acute emergencies involving lead encephalopathy. The cornerstone of therapy is removal of the patient from the offending environment and elimination of sources of future lead exposure.

(2) Depending on the severity of the symptoms and the body burden of lead, one of two approaches may be used:

(a) In individuals who are very symptomatic and in those with serum lead levels of 100 mg/100 ml or greater (or erythrocytic porphyrin levels greater than 190 mg/100 ml whole blood), a course of chelation therapy with BAL plus EDTA is given and followed with a course of oral penicillamine (see sec **d.(2)**).

(b) In individuals who are mildly symptomatic without markedly elevated serum lead or erythrocytic porphyrin levels, a course of oral penicillamine is probably adequate.

(3) Patients with lead colic may respond dramatically to calcium. Thus calcium gluconate may be given at a dose of 1 gm IV and repeated as necessary.

c. Chelation therapy

(1) The immediate medical needs of the patient, which may include seizure control and protection of the airway, are attended to.

(2) A cathartic is administered to purge the gut of any unabsorbed lead if there is either a history or x-ray evidence of recent lead ingestion.

(3) A urine flow of 350–500 ml/sq m/24 hours is established. However, overhydration, especially with large amounts of free water, endangers the patient with increased intracranial pressure and should be avoided.

(4) Initially a dose of BAL is given IM at a dose of 5 mg/kg in children under age 10 years and 3 mg/kg in adults.

(5) Four hours after the initial BAL injection, simultaneous injections of BAL and EDTA are given. BAL is given IM at the same dose as the initial injection, and EDTA is given at a dose of 12.5 mg/kg every 4 hours either IM or IV (by rapid infusion, dissolved in 5% D/W).

(6) The usual course of therapy is 5 days.

(7) **Supportive therapy.** Because of the danger of vomiting with BAL, food is withheld for the first 3 days at least, and it is then given only if the patient is fully alert and has shown no gastrointestinal upset from the BAL. Iron therapy is not given along with BAL. Electrolytes, including calcium and phosphate levels, are measured daily. SIADH is a frequent accompaniment of lead encephalopathy.

(8) **Increased intracranial pressure.** The role of steroids and mannitol in the control of CSF pressure in lead encephalopathy is unclear. There is some experimental evidence that steroid and EDTA may have an adverse interaction, so some experts avoid their use together. Mannitol may be used when necessary and in the usual manner.

(9) **Side effects of chelation therapy**

   (a) BAL may produce lacrimation, blepharospasm, paresthesias, nausea, vomiting, tachycardia, hypertension, and hemolysis in the presence of G6PDH deficiency.

   (b) EDTA may produce renal injury, cardiac conduction abnormalities, and electrolyte disorders. The renal function, calcium, and electrolytes are followed daily, and urine output is carefully monitored and maintained.

d. **Long-term therapy**

   (1) A course of BAL plus EDTA longer than 5 days may be expected to remove about 50% of the soft tissue stores of lead from the body and reduce the serum lead by a corresponding amount. However, after the chelation therapy is stopped, lead may be mobilized from bone, and the soft tissue and serum lead levels may rise and endanger the patient again. Consequently, the serum lead or erythrocytic porphyrin or both should be checked every few days after completion of the chelation therapy, and another course should be given if the serum lead rises above 80 mg/100 ml or if the erythrocytic porphyrin rises above 190 mg/100 ml whole blood. Some patients may require three or four courses of chelation therapy.

   (2) Penicillamine is not approved by the Federal Drug Administration for use in lead poisoning, and its precise role is not defined. It is widely used, however, and it is undeniably effective for milder cases of lead poisoning. Some situations in which it has been used are:

      (a) After completing a course of chelation therapy with BAL plus EDTA, oral penicillamine, at a dose of 2–3 mg/kg, will bring the serum lead to normal levels faster than if it is not given. Also, it may obviate the need for repeat courses of parenteral chelation therapy. Note that pyridoxine 50 mg PO daily should be given along with penicillamine. This therapy must be continued for 3–6 months to achieve adequate diuresis of body lead stores.
      Toxic reactions to penicillamine include a nephrotoxic syndrome, optic neuritis, and blood dyscrasias.

      (b) Some clinicians have successfully used penicillamine as the only chelating agent in some class III children and in adults with mild symptoms.

B. **Mercury**

1. **Sources of exposure**

   a. Mercury salts and mercury vapor are potential environmental toxins in the chemical, paint, and paper industries, especially in chlorine production. Mercury vapor and dusts are absorbed through the skin and lungs, and ingested mercury salts are absorbed from the gut. Elemental liquid mercury is poorly absorbed from the gastrointestinal tract unless it is divided finely.

b. Organic mercury compounds have become an important source of environmental contamination in recent years. It is these compounds that pose the greatest threat to the CNS.

(1) Phenotic and methoxy methyl mercury are degraded to inorganic mercury in the body and are metabolized as inorganic mercury salts.

(2) Alkyl mercury, primarily methyl and ethyl mercury, is produced as a waste product in the plastics and agricultural fungicide industries. It is well absorbed through skin and is highly lipid-soluble, reaching high concentrations in the CNS.

Large numbers of people in Japan have been poisoned by eating fish that were contaminated by methyl mercury discharged into Minamata Bay. People have also been poisoned from eating grain contaminated with alkyl mercury-containing fungicides.

2. Clinical manifestations

a. Acute mercury poisoning from a brief exposure to a large amount of mercury produces stomatitis and a metallic taste in the mouth; a sensation of constriction of the throat; ulcers on the tongue and palate; gastrointestinal upset with nausea, vomiting, and bloody diarrhea; abdominal pain; acute renal failure; and circulatory collapse. CNS manifestations include lethargy, excitement, hyperreflexia, and tremor.

b. Chronic inorganic mercury poisoning produces stomatitis and a metallic taste, loss of appetite, a blue line along the gingival margin, hypertrophied gums, tremor, chorea, ataxia, nephrotic syndrome, and the syndrome of erythrism, which is marked by personality change, with shyness and irritability. Pink disease, or acrodynia, occurs in infants. It is characterized by irritability, insomnia, stomatitis, loss of teeth, hypertension, and erythema.

c. Organic mercury intoxication produces a syndrome of fatigue, apathy, memory loss, emotional instability, ataxia, dysarthria, tremor, dysphagia, paresthesias, and, characteristically, constriction of the visual fields. This may progress to seizures, coma, and death. Organic mercury also crosses the placenta and may produce retardation and paralysis in the offspring of asymptomatic mothers. Renal lesions with proximal tubular dysfunction also occur.

3. Diagnosis and treatment

a. Acute mercury poisoning must be diagnosed by the history of exposure and the clinical picture. The aims of therapy are to remove unabsorbed mercury from the gastrointestinal tract, to remove mercury that has already been absorbed by chelation therapy, and to prevent acute renal failure.

(1) Emesis or gastric lavage is used to empty the stomach, which is then rinsed with a proteinaceous solution (egg whites, albumin, or skim milk) or charcoal. Because of the locally corrosive nature of mercury salts, the trachea is intubated if the patient is not fully alert.

(2) Sodium formaldehyde sulfoxylate reduces mercuric salts to the less-soluble form of mercury; 250 ml of a 5% solution may be instilled into the duodenum through a tube, which may decrease mercury absorption.

(3) BAL can be given at a dose of 4–5 mg/kg every 4 hours, with no dose exceeding 300 mg. After the first 24 hours the frequency of doses is reduced to every 6 hours for 2–3 days and then every 8 hours for the remainder of a 10-day course. N-acetyl-D,L-penicillamine may be the best chelating agent for mercury compounds, but it is not generally available.

(4) Fluids are pushed immediately to maintain urine flow, and mannitol 1 mg/kg IV is given if the patient is oliguric. Dialysis may be necessary if the kidneys have shut down and the patient is severely intoxicated.

Electrolyte management may be difficult due to the diuresis induced early by mercury salts, with both sodium and potassium losses as well as volume depletion occurring.

b. Chronic inorganic mercury poisoning generally does not present the severe emergency that acute poisoning presents. Removal from exposure and a course of BAL, as described in sec a.(3), or a course of n-acetyl-D,L-penicillamine, if available, are the cornerstones of therapy. Total body sodium, potassium, and intravascular volume may need to be repleted.

c. Alkyl mercury poisoning is most often a chronic process. There is an enterohepatic circulation of alkyl mercury, so excretion can be promoted by binding the mercury compound in the small intestine with an unabsorbable resin. Cholestyramine 16–24 gm/day in divided doses may be given along with enough of an osmotic cathartic (e.g., sorbitol) to prevent constipation. The dosage of cholestyramine in children has not been established.

C. Arsenic

1. **Sources of exposure.** The primary cause of arsenic poisoning today is pesticide ingestion, either accidentally in children and agricultural workers, or intentionally through suicide or homicide. Arsenic-containing rat poison is no longer in widespread use, but it may still be stored in some homes and farms. Occasionally, iatrogenic poisoning occurs from arsenic-containing antiparasitic agents used in the treatment of trypanosomiasis (e.g., tryparsamide, carbarsone, and senite).

2. **Clinical manifestations**

   a. **Acute poisoning.** Acutely, arsenic produces capillary endothelial damage with leakage, especially in the splanchnic circulation. Nausea, vomiting, abdominal pains, and muscle cramps also occur. With somewhat larger doses, intravascular hemolysis may occur, which can lead to acute renal failure. ECG abnormalities are present and stomatitis appears. With lethal doses, a sequence of shock, coma, and death occurs in 20–48 hours.

   b. **Chronic poisoning.** Gastrointestinal symptoms are less prominent than with acute poisoning, but weight loss, anorexia, nausea, and diarrhea or constipation may occur. Neurologic toxicity may be manifested by a sensorimotor neuropathy, excessive salivation and sweating, and encephalopathy. The latter, in its early stages, consists of fatigue, drowsiness, headache, and confusion, but it may progress to seizures, coma, and death. Rarely, there may be increased CSF protein and a mild pleocytosis along with fever, so the picture may be mistaken occasionally for an infectious process. Dermatologic signs can be diagnostic, with arsenical keratoses and transverse lines in the nails (Mee's lines) being characteristic. Hepatic and renal damage may occur.

3. **Diagnosis**

   a. Acute arsenic intoxication must be recognized by a history of ingestion and by the clinical presentation. Following acute intoxication, the urinary arsenic excretion may be extremely high.

   b. **Chronic arsenic poisoning**

      (1) Chronic arsenic poisoning is suggested by the clinical picture, especially the dermatologic manifestations.

(2) The upper limits of normal of urinary arsenic excretion are not sharply defined, but levels higher than 0.1 mg/L are suggestive of abnormally high exposure. Concentrations of arsenic in the nails or hair that are greater than 0.1 mg/100 ml are indicative, but not diagnostic, of arsenic poisoning. Apparently, some individuals who are chronically exposed to arsenic may harbor large amounts in their tissues and excrete large amounts without developing symptoms of toxicity.

(3) With chronic arsenic ingestion, there is increased urinary coproporphyrinogen III, but normal urinary δ-ALA excretion.

4. Treatment

a. Removal from exposure and elimination of unabsorbed arsenic from the gastrointestinal tract by the use of emesis or gastric lavage and osmotic cathartics are the initial steps.

b. BAL is an effective chelating agent for arsenic. The usual course consists of 4–5 mg/kg IM every 4 hours for 24 hours; then the same dose is given at 6-hour intervals for 2–3 days, followed by tapering doses to complete a 10-day course. Although occasionally a patient with encephalopathy will have a dramatic response as a result of BAL, the neuropathy may require months to resolve.

c. Fluid and electrolyte disturbances must be rapidly repaired, and intravascular volume must be protected with electrolyte and albumin solutions. Pressors may be required in cases of acute poisoning.

d. The abdominal pain of acute arsenic poisoning may be severe and require large doses of narcotics.

D. Antimony

1. Antimony poisoning is rare, but it may occur from ingestion of an acidic food that is stored in improperly made enamelware or from parasiticidal drugs (e.g., tartar emetic) used in the therapy of leishmaniasis, schistosomiasis, and filariasis.

2. The clinical manifestations are similar to those of arsenic poisoning.

3. The treatment is identical to that of arsenic poisoning, including use of BAL.

E. Thallium

1. Sources of exposure. Thallium is the primary ingredient of some depilatories and rat poisons. Poisoning usually occurs as a result of accidental ingestion of these materials.

2. Clinical manifestations. Atopecia is the hallmark of thallium intoxication. Neurologic manifestations are prominent: ataxia, chorea, restlessness, and hallucinations, progressing to coma and death. Blindness, facial paralysis, and peripheral neuropathy may occur. Nausea, vomiting, constipation, and liver and renal damage may also occur.

3. Treatment

a. Removal from exposure and elimination of unabsorbed thallium from the gastrointestinal tract with emesis or gastric lavage and catharsis are the primary modes of therapy.

b. Prussian blue (potassium ferric hexacyanoferrate) may be introduced by tube into the duodenum and may decrease thallium absorption. The dose is 250 mg/kg given over 24 hours in two to four divided doses.

IX. CARBON MONOXIDE

A. Sources of exposure. Carbon monoxide (CO) is produced by the incomplete combustion of hydrocarbons. Such combustion is hazardous when it takes place in a limited space with poor ventilation. Clinically significant CO inhalation typically occurs when automobile engines are run in closed garages, when automobile exhausts leak into a closed car, in house fires, and when gasoline engines exhaust their products of combustion into poorly ventilated working spaces, such as tunnels or below decks in ships. Carbon monoxide is colorless, odorless, and does not irritate the mucous membranes. It may therefore reach high concentrations without warning. Occasionally it is an agent of suicide.

B. Clinical manifestations

1. The acute manifestations of carbon monoxide inhalation are those of hypoxia without cyanosis (typically the patient has a "cherry red" appearance). The brain is the organ most sensitive to hypoxia, and the earliest neurologic dysfunction is lethargy, which may progress to coma. As hypoxia becomes more severe, brainstem functions fail. The heart may show signs of ischemia, and acute myocardial infarction may occur.

2. The patient may either recover completely from the acute episode, if he or she is rescued in time, or be left with residual neurologic dysfunction; characteristically, the basal ganglia are the most sensitive structures. There is also a syndrome in which the patient recovers completely from the acute intoxication only to succumb to a massive subacute demyelination of the cerebral white matter that begins 1–3 weeks following exposure.

C. Diagnosis

1. The history is usually sufficient to give the diagnosis. However, the cherry red appearance may also give a clue. Generally, if the patient has inhaled smoke or flame, rather than air contaminated by carbon monoxide, the damage to the respiratory epithelium by heat or oxides of nitrogen is of more concern than carbon monoxide poisoning.

2. Many blood gas laboratories can measure carbon monoxide saturation of blood directly. (Note that venous blood is adequate for direct carbon monoxide determinations). In the absence of lung disease or a right-to-left shunt, arterial O_2 saturation, while the patient is breathing 100% oxygen, will give an estimate of the carbon monoxide saturation. The arterial Po_2 is of no use in estimating carbon monoxide saturation, because the Po_2 will not be affected by the combination of hemoglobin with carbon monoxide.

D. Treatment

1. The only available therapy for carbon monoxide intoxication is to remove the patient from exposure as rapidly as possible and to administer 100% oxygen. Any patient with symptoms of hypoxia or carbon monoxide saturation greater than about 40% should be observed in the hospital for at least 48 hours and maintained on supplemental oxygen until the carbon monoxide concentration falls below 20%.

2. Any maneuvers that reduce the tissue demand for oxygen should be undertaken. The patient is kept at rest and tranquilized if he or she is hyperactive from encephalopathy or other causes. Hyperthermia is treated vigorously.

3. Residual movement disorders are common after severe carbon monoxide poisoning. Choreoathetosis, myoclonus, and a parkinsonlike syndrome may occur. These disorders are treated symptomatically in the same manner as movement disorders of other etiologies (Chap. 10).

4. There is no known treatment for, or specific means of preventing, the late-onset massive demyelination that may follow carbon monoxide poisoning.

X. ACETYLCHOLINESTERASE-INHIBITING COMPOUNDS

A. Source.
The only source of acetylcholinesterase (ChE) inhibitors is organophosphorus insecticides. In the past, beverages and cooking oils have been contami-

nated with triorthocresyl phosphate (TOCP), which, when ingested, produces a chronic, severe peripheral neuropathy, known as Jamaica ginger palsy. Chronic TOCP poisoning is not discussed here. However, acute poisoning may occur through ingestion, inhalation, or absorption through the skin.

B. Clinical manifestations of acute ChE-inhibitor poisoning are a combination of local effects, muscarinic effects, nicotinic effects, and CNS toxicity.

   1. Local effects

      a. Inhalation exposure produces symptoms referable to the eyes, mucous membranes of the nose and pharynx, and the bronchial smooth muscle. Also, pupillary constriction, conjunctival congestion, watery nasal discharge, wheezing, and increased respiratory secretions are all prominent.

      b. Ingestion of ChE inhibitors produces anorexia, nausea, vomiting, abdominal cramps, and diarrhea.

      c. Skin exposure produces localized swelling and muscle fasciculations.

   2. Muscarinic effects include salivation, sweating, lacrimation, bradycardia, and hypotension. Severe poisoning will produce involuntary urination and defecation.

   3. Nicotinic effects are referable to the neuromuscular junction and include muscle fatigue, weakness, and fasciculations that progress to paralysis. The most immediate life-threatening effect of ChE-inhibitor intoxication is respiratory paralysis, which is especially dangerous when combined with bronchospasm and copious bronchial secretions.

   4. CNS toxicity is manifested by confusion, ataxia, dysarthria, and diminished deep tendon reflexes, all of which progress to seizures and coma.

C. Diagnosis

   1. The clinical presentation along with a history of exposure are the key elements of diagnosis.

   2. Some clinical laboratories are prepared to assay ChE activity in plasma and erythrocytes. Although the normal range for ChE activity is broad, patients with significant systemic ChE-inhibitor toxicity all have extremely low levels.

D. Therapy

   1. General measures

      a. Termination of exposure by removal of the patient from contaminated air, washing the skin copiously with water, or gastric lavage as indicated.

      b. The airway must be protected, especially if gastric lavage is required, and respiratory assistance must be provided if necessary. Frequent suctioning of respiratory secretions must also be done.

      c. Circulatory collapse is treated with fluid volume alone if possible, and pressors are added if necessary.

      d. Seizures may require treatment by the usual methods (see Chap. 6).

   2. Specific measures

      a. Muscarinic effects may be blocked with atropine in large doses. Therapy should begin with 2 mg IV, and then be repeated every 3–5 minutes until muscarinic symptoms disappear and bradycardia is reversed. If the patient is alert, he or she may then be given doses of atropine PO as required. IV doses will need to be repeated every few hours in comatose patients.

      b. Reversal of peripheral ChE may be achieved with pralidoxime (PAM) for the proportion of the enzyme that has not "irreversibly" bound the inhibitor. The initial dose for adults is 1 gm infused IV over 2 or more minutes. If improvement is not noted within 20 minutes, the dose is repeated.

The earlier pralidoxime is administered in the course of intoxication, the greater its effect. There is no purpose in giving additional doses beyond 2 gm. Pralidoxime does not reach CNS ChE, and compounds that do so are not available in the United States. Pralidoxime has no important side effects. It is metabolized in the liver and the products are excreted by the kidney.

XI. ALCOHOL

A. Acute intoxication

1. Pharmacokinetics of ethyl alcohol (EtOH, ethanol).

   a. Ethanol is rapidly absorbed from the gastrointestinal tract, being 100% absorbed within 2 hours. It is absorbed less rapidly if there is food in the stomach at the time of ingestion.

   b. It is metabolized by the liver, and it is more rapidly metabolized in those who drink regularly and heavily than in occasional users of the drug.

   c. The rate of ethanol metabolism is approximately 7–10 gm/hour, which represents about 1 ounce of 90-proof spirits or 10 ounces of beer per hour.

   d. The lethal blood level of alcohol is about 5000 mg/L. Thus in a 70-kg man, this represents about 1 pint of 90-proof spirits distributed throughout total body water.

   e. The resultant toxicity experienced from a given dose of ethanol depends on the maximum blood EtOH level obtained, the rapidity with which that level is obtained, the patient's prior experience with alcohol, and the presence of other drugs.

2. Management of acute alcohol intoxication

   a. With cases of mild intoxication, the most important aspect of management is to see that the patient can get home safely, without endangering himself and others by attempting to drive. There is good evidence that analeptics, such as caffeine, amphetamines, and theophylline, do not help "sober up" the patient or improve his driving performance.

   b. Moderate intoxication with alcohol poses no danger to the patient if he is merely observed and cared for until he is ready to make his own way home. If there has been ingestion within the preceding 2 hours, emesis, gastric lavage, and catharsis may be used to prevent further absorption. As is the case with mild intoxication, analeptics are of no use.

   c. The chief danger in cases of severe ethanol intoxication is respiratory depression. As long as adequate supportive care is provided before significant hypoxia occurs, the outlook is excellent, because within 24 hours, the alcohol will be metabolized by the patient.

      (1) The blood alcohol level may be measured directly or estimated by measuring the serum osmolarity. Each 100 mg/L of blood ethanol raises the serum osmolarity by approximately 2 mOsm/L.

      (2) Tracheal intubation and respiratory support are provided at the earliest sign of respiratory depression. Respiratory support should be continued until the patient is fully awake.

      (3) Gastric lavage (purgation of the gut) is performed if there is a possibility of alcohol or other drug ingestion within the preceding 2 hours. If

the patient is not fully awake, the trachea is protected with a cuffed endotracheal tube before gastric lavage is undertaken.

(4) Frequently, life-threatening ethanol ingestion is accompanied by ingestion of other CNS depressants. This possibility should be considered if the patient's mental status is depressed out of proportion to the blood ethanol level or if unexpected neurologic signs are present.

(5) Fluids are given to maintain adequate blood pressure and urine output, but there is no need to induce a forced diuresis.

(6) If the patient is suspected of being a chronic alcoholic or of having severe liver disease, thiamine 50 mg IV and 50 mg IM and glucose 25–50 gm by IV push are administered immediately in the event of complicating Wernicke's encephalopathy or hypoglycemia. A blood glucose level should, of course, be drawn first.

(7) Chronic alcoholics are frequently potassium-depleted and may require replacement with KCl. Acid-base balance is maintained, and alcoholic ketoacidosis is either ruled out or treated appropriately with IV glucose and fluids.

(8) If the blood ethanol level is extremely high (over 6000 or 7000 mg/L) peritoneal dialysis or hemodialysis may be justified to reduce the ethanol level rapidly.

(9) Although fructose administration hastens ethanol metabolism, its risk does not justify the benefit obtained.

B. Ethanol withdrawal

1. Mild withdrawal syndrome

a. Clinical manifestations of mild ethanol withdrawal are anxiety, weakness, tremulousness, sweating, and tachycardia.

b. Therapy

(1) In the absence of other intercurrent illness, such as coronary artery disease or an infection that is precipitated by the withdrawal, these patients may be treated at home if the social situation is appropriate.

(2) The patient is given thiamine 50 mg IM and a prescription for multivitamins if he is malnourished. He or she is instructed to maintain adequate hydration and food intake during the period of withdrawal.

(3) A benzodiazepine tranquilizer minimizes the symptoms of withdrawal. In general, one may begin with chlordiazepoxide (Librium) 25–50 mg PO every 4 hours for the first 48–72 hours and then taper the dose over 5–7 days. Diazepam (Valium) is equally effective. The initial dose is 5–10 mg PO every 4–6 hours.

2. Moderate and severe withdrawal syndromes

a. If the patient is febrile, irrational, hallucinating, or extremely agitated, he must be hospitalized until the severe manifestations of ethanol withdrawal are gone.

b. General medical therapy

(1) The patient is frequently dehydrated, and total body potassium is depleted. Those deficits are replaced with appropriate electrolyte solutions. Vascular collapse may occur, but it usually responds to rigorous volume replacement.

(2) Ethanol withdrawal is often precipitated by an intercurrent illness, often infection. Such illnesses must be detected and treated appropriately.

(3) Chronic abusers of alcohol are subject to bleeding disorders from liver disease or thrombocytopenia. Consequently, acetaminophen 600 mg or 1.2 gm PO or PR is preferred to aspirin to treat hyperthermia.

(4) The patient is usually magnesium-depleted. There is no good evidence that replacing magnesium has any effect on the course of the withdrawal syndrome, but many physicians elect to administer magnesium if the patient is admitted early in the course of the withdrawal. $MgSO_4$ may be given in a 50% solution, 1–2 ml IM, or the same amount may be mixed with IV electrolyte solutions.

(5) Severe liver disease may result in hypoglycemia, and starvation may result in ketoacidosis. Consequently, glucose is administered early either as a bolus of 25–50 gm, if the patient is comatose, or as a dextrose-plus-electrolyte solution.

Thiamine 50 mg IV and 50 mg IM are always administered to chronic alcoholics prior to glucose because of the risk of precipitating Wernicke's encephalopathy.

c. **Tranquilization.** Virtually every medical and neurologic service has its own favorite regimen of tranquilizers for treating alcohol withdrawal. Antihistamines, barbiturates, hypnotics, phenothiazines, and paraldehyde have all had their champions. The benzodiazepines are at least as effective as any other drug, or combination of drugs, and are safe when used in moderate doses with frequent observations of the patient.

(1) Diazepam and chlordiazepoxide are essentially identical in their therapeutic effect when used in equipotent doses. Both have a prolonged duration of action (12–36 hours), are well absorbed PO, are erratically absorbed when administered IM, and have a rapid and predictable effect when given by rapid IV injection. The primary danger from both drugs is excessive CNS depression after repeated doses, due to the cumulative effect of successive doses given within 24 hours of each other. Respiratory arrest may occur occasionally with rapid IV injection of either drug, but generally this does not happen with small doses.

(2) Diazepam (Valium) may be administered by the IV route in 2.5-mg or 5-mg doses every 5 minutes until the patient is calm, and then 5–10 mg PO or by slow IV injection every 2–6 hours as necessary. Chlordiazepoxide (Librium) may be used in an identical manner, chlordiazepoxide 12.5 mg being equivalent to diazepam 2.5 mg.

(3) The most important aspects of managing alcohol withdrawal with IV benzodiazepines are careful, frequent observation of the patient to prevent cumulative toxicity and avoidance of large doses (greater than diazepam 5 mg or chlordiazepoxide 25 mg) in any one IV injection. It is essential that each patient be individually titrated with tranquilizer and repeatedly reevaluated rather than being put on any fixed schedule.

d. **Withdrawal seizures**

(1) There are many possible causes for seizures that accompany ethanol withdrawal: head trauma, subdural hematoma, metabolic derangements, intercurrent CNS infection, and true withdrawal seizures are the most frequent. True withdrawal seizures occur between 12 and 30 hours after cessation of regular ethanol ingestion, are generalized major motor convulsions, and are usually brief, one or two in number. Ethanol withdrawal seizures can be prolonged, however, and status epilepticus may occur. The interictal EEG is normal and, except for periods of drug withdrawal, the patient is no more likely to have a seizure than a normal person.

The diagnosis of ethanol withdrawal seizure can only be made if the seizure fits the typical clinical pattern and there is no other possible cause to account for it. Seizures from other causes are apt to be precipitated by ethanol withdrawal and should be treated appropriately (see Chap. 6).

(2) **Phenytoin** (Dilantin) has been shown to protect against ethanol withdrawal seizures, although the protection is only partial. Assuming the patient has not been taking an antiepileptic, he or she can be given a 1-gm loading dose, either IV or PO divided into two or three doses given 1–2 hours apart. Then the patient is maintained on 300 mg/day PO or IV for 3 days, and the dose is tapered to 0 over about 1 week after the risk of withdrawal seizures has passed. Ethanol withdrawal seizures are not an indication for long-term anticonvulsant therapy.

(3) Experts differ over the indications for phenytoin prophylaxis of withdrawal seizures. Some would administer phenytoin to all patients seen during the first 24 hours of withdrawal from heavy ethanol use. Others would limit its use to those with a history of withdrawal seizures or with an underlying seizure disorder.

(4) If a patient is seen after a withdrawal seizure has occurred, it is reasonable to merely observe the patient without therapy as long as other causes for the seizure have been ruled out. The probability is high that the seizure either will not recur or, if it does recur, will be brief. Some would argue that the risk of phenytoin is sufficiently low that it should be used in this situation until the patient is out of danger.

(5) If the patient is allergic to phenytoin, the choice of an alternative drug is difficult. Barbiturates are likely to be effective, but the combination of benzodiazepines, which are used to treat withdrawal symptoms, and barbiturates is likely to produce respiratory depression. Therefore unless the patient is in immediate danger from the seizures, the best line of therapy is to manage the patient with benzodiazepine alone. If a barbiturate must be added to control the seizures, the patient should be constantly observed for signs of respiratory depression.

(6) If status epilepticus occurs as a manifestation of ethanol withdrawal seizures, it is important to avoid overmedicating the patient. Withdrawal seizures are a self-limited phenomenon, and they will cease as long as the patient is supported through the first 36 hours of withdrawal. If reasonable doses of benzodiazepines and phenytoin (or a barbiturate) do not bring the seizures under control, the patient may be paralyzed with pancuronium (Pavulon) and put on a respirator until the seizures cease.

C. Wernicke's encephalopathy

1. Wernicke's encephalopathy is a thiamine-deficiency disease that occurs in chronic alcoholics or patients with chronic malnutrition. It has an acute onset, and its cardinal manifestations are confusion and memory loss, nystagmus, extraocular movement deficits (most often unilateral or bilateral sixth-nerve palsies), and ataxia, occurring in any combination. Drowsiness, stupor, and even coma may occur.

   With prompt treatment, the ocular abnormalities usually clear within days, but about one-quarter of patients will be left with **Korsakoff's psychosis,** which is characterized by a deficit in higher cortical function whereby the ability to form new memories is impaired far out of proportion to other functions. Any patient with an appropriate predisposition who has any sign of ataxia, confusion, or extraocular movement abnormality should be treated for Wernicke's encephalopathy.

2. **The treatment** is to give parenteral thiamine immediately. The dose required is not known, but it is customary to give 50 mg IM immediately and then 50 mg/day PO or IM for 3 days thereafter. There is no doubt that this is far more thiamine than is necessary, but except for extremely rare immediate hypersensitivity reactions to commercial thiamine/HCl preparations, the drug causes no toxicity.

3. The administration of glucose before thiamine in a severely thiamine-deficient patient may precipitate Wernicke's encephalopathy. It is therefore recommended that thiamine be given before a glucose infusion is begun in any patient in whom thiamine deficiency is a possibility, including patients with coma of unknown cause.

4. The diagnosis is usually obvious clinically, but it can be confirmed with erythrocyte "transketolase" levels if the test is available. The blood sample must be drawn before the administration of thiamine in order to be diagnostic.

D. **The long-term management of chronic alcoholism.** There is no known generally effective treatment for chronic alcoholism. The following suggestions are offered as possible modes of therapy that may be useful in the setting of more general medical and psychiatric care.

1. It is useful for the physician to view alcoholism as a chronic disease, with periods of exacerbation and remission similar to chronic obstructive pulmonary disease. Only in a rare patient can a cure be found for the underlying disease, but appropriate management will decrease its morbidity and mortality.

2. Benzodiazepine tranquilizers are useful in treating withdrawal and in the short-term treatment of anxiety. There is no good evidence that long-term therapy with tranquilizers affects the course of the disease.

3. If a patient has been regularly consuming large quantities of alcohol and wants to stop drinking, either in an attempt to abstain from alcohol or because of elective surgery, the patient is weaned from his usual daily ethanol over 5–7 days. Withdrawal symptoms with such a program are usually mild and can be controlled with low doses of oral benzodiazepines.

   Some clinicians argue that patients should not be weaned from ethanol, but rather should be suddenly withdrawn and treated with high doses of benzodiazepines. The reasons usually given for this view are that it is difficult to judge the initial dose of ethanol to use, and that the administration of ethanol by a physician does psychological harm to the patient. The first problem may be overcome by eliciting a careful history of exactly how much ethanol the patient has been consuming regularly and by allowing the patient to judge his or her own intake for the first day of the program, with periodic observations by medical personnel to prevent overintoxication. On the first day a dose is found that leads neither to excessive intoxication nor to withdrawal. Then that dose is reduced by 10–20% each day until the patient has withdrawn from ethanol. This technique is at least as efficient as trying to determine a benzodiazepine dose to achieve the same goal.

   There is no evidence that careful withdrawal of patients from ethanol under medical supervision does any more psychological harm than supervised withdrawal from barbiturates, heroin, or any other abused drug. Obviously, if the patient is suffering any progressive injury from the ethanol, such as acute liver disease, cardiomyopathy, or ongoing gastrointestinal bleeding, ethanol is withdrawn suddenly and the ensuing withdrawal is managed as well as possible with benzodiazepines.

4. Depression may be manifested by alcoholism. In this instance, appropriate therapy with tricyclic antidepressants, lithium, or electroshock therapy may relieve the underlying predisposition to alcoholism.

5. Most centers that deal with chronic alcoholism believe that Alcoholics Anonymous offers the greatest chance for prolonged abstention of all therapies available.

XII. OPIATES

A. Addiction. The management of opiate addiction traditionally falls outside the practice of the neurologist and is not discussed here.

B. Overdose

1. Depressed mental status, respiratory depression, and pinpoint pupils are the typical symptoms of acute opiate poisoning. The body temperature may be subnormal, the blood pressure may be low, and the limbs and jaw are generally flaccid. With very high doses, convulsions and pulmonary edema may occur.

2. Emergency therapy is directed at respiratory depression.

   a. If the patient is cyanotic, has a respiratory rate below 10/minute, or cannot protect his own airway, he is intubated with an orotracheal or nasotracheal tube and given respiratory assistance with positive-pressure ventilation.

   b. A narcotic antagonist is administered in sufficient amount to reverse the respiratory depressant effects of the opiate. Naloxone (Narcan), the drug of choice, is given in 0.4-mg increments by rapid IV injection until the patient is respiring normally, or until 10 mg total have been given, at which point the diagnosis must be called into question. Several aspects of the pharmacology of narcotic antagonists should be borne in mind:

      (1) The duration of action of naloxone is only 1–4 hours, depending on the dose, which is shorter than the duration of commonly available opiates. Therefore after the action of an opiate is reversed with naloxone, the patient requires close observation in the event that he slips back into coma. Repeated doses of naloxone may be required, especially in the case of methadone intoxication, because the effects of methadone may last for 24–36 hours.

      (2) Paradoxically, opiate addicts are more sensitive to narcotic antagonists than patients who are not tolerant of opiates. Therefore narcotic antagonists are administered in small IV doses (naloxone 0.4 mg) repeated every 2–3 minutes until the desired effect is achieved or until 10 mg total have been given.

      (3) When given to opiate addicts, narcotic antagonists may precipitate severe acute withdrawal within minutes of IV injection if given in sufficient doses. Once the antagonist is administered, the withdrawal syndrome will be extremely resistant to reversal by the administration of opiates until the effect of the antagonist has passed.

      This phenomenon is another reason for administering narcotic antagonists in small increments. Furthermore, in narcotic addicts, one should not attempt to reverse all the narcotic effects immediately with naloxone. Rather, the aim is to return the patient's spontaneous respirations and restore his level of consciousness to the point where he can protect his own airway and make spontaneous postural adjustments in bed.

      (4) Narcotic antagonists, including naloxone, have an emetic effect. Therefore they should not be administered to comatose patients unless the trachea is protected by a cuffed endotracheal tube.

C. Acute opiate withdrawal

1. Although many of the symptoms of opiate withdrawal are dramatic, the only potentially dangerous manifestation of the syndrome is dehydration due to

nausea, vomiting, sweating, and diarrhea, combined with failure to take in oral fluids. Consequently, the essential aspect of management of severe narcotic withdrawal is the administration of appropriate electrolyte solutions to maintain intravascular volume and electrolyte balance.

2. At any point in the course of the syndrome, as long as a narcotic antagonist has not been administered, the symptoms may be rapidly relieved by narcotic administration. For example, morphine sulfate may be administered by IV injection in small incremental doses of 2–5 mg every 3–5 minutes until the desired effect is achieved.

XIII. BARBITURATES

A. **Acute intoxication.** Barbiturate overdose is the best-studied type of sedative-hypnotic intoxication. It is a significant public health problem, especially among health professionals with ready access to drugs. Barbiturates are not known to do any permanent damage to the nervous system, so every patient who reaches medical attention before the development of CNS damage from hypoxia or shock has the potential to recover completely with adequate supportive therapy.

1. **Initial evaluation of the patient**

a. A classification of the level of barbiturate intoxication is useful in determining the prognosis.

(1) **Class 0.** Patients who are asleep, but who can be aroused to purposeful activity (following verbal commands or in answer to questions).

(2) **Class I.** Patients who are unconscious, but who withdraw from noxious stimuli and whose muscle stretch reflexes are intact (the corneal reflex may be depressed).

(3) **Class II.** Patients who are unconscious and do not respond to painful stimuli, but who retain muscle stretch reflexes and have no respiratory or circulatory depression.

(4) **Class III.** Patients who are unconscious with loss of some or all reflexes, but with spontaneous respirations and normal blood pressure.

(5) **Class IV.** Patients with respiratory depression, cyanosis, or shock.

b. A complete history of the events surrounding the ingestion is obtained. In particular, the ingestion of alcohol, other sedatives, or tranquilizers along with barbiturates is frequent, which accounts for neurologic depression that is out of proportion to the dose or serum level of barbiturate taken.

c. The physical examination includes a search for any coincident condition that might influence management.

d. The initial laboratory evaluation of patients in classes III and IV should include:

(1) Hemogram (hematocrit, white cell count, and differential).

(2) BUN or creatinine or both.

(3) Electrolytes.

(4) Glucose.

(5) Chest x-ray.

(6) Urinalysis.

(7) Arterial blood gasses.

(8) If available, a screen of the serum and urine for toxic substances is performed.

    e. Serum barbiturate levels are helpful, but they must be interpreted in the context of the clinical situation.

        (1) A high barbiturate level confirms the diagnosis of barbiturate intoxication.

        (2) Prognostically, the serum level correlates with the duration of coma (Table 14-2). However, the usual method of measuring barbiturates does not distinguish between the different varieties of barbiturates, so the level must be interpreted with a knowledge of the compound ingested.

        (3) The drug level may not correlate with the clinical status of the patient in several situations:

            (a) In mixed ingestions, the patient's nervous system may be more depressed than would be predicted from the barbiturate level.

            (b) Patients who take barbiturates habitually, either therapeutically or as drugs of abuse, can tolerate much higher levels of barbiturates than those who have no tolerance for the drug.

            (c) CNS stimulants (analeptic agents) may temporarily elevate a patient's mental status.

2. Supportive therapy. All patients who reach a hospital before developing irreversible damage from hypoxia or shock should recover completely if optimum supportive therapy is provided. The only exceptions to this would be patients with coexistent life-threatening disease. In fact, the lowest mortality reported (0.8%) was achieved at a Scandinavian center that employed only supportive measures in the treatment of barbiturate intoxication.

    a. Respiration. Patients in class IV clearly need immediate endotracheal intubation and respiratory assistance. Patients in classes 0–III require a cuffed endotracheal tube if gastric lavage is to be undertaken, if the gag or cough reflex or both are absent, or if there is any doubt as to the adequacy of respirations.

        Arterial blood gases must be monitored closely to maintain the P_{CO_2} greater than 80 mm/Hg (O_2 saturation greater than 94%). The minimum

Table 14-2. Important Serum Levels of Commonly Used Barbiturates

Drug	Trade Name	Hypnotic Dose (gm)	Fatal Dose (gm)	Fatal Plasma Concentration (mg/100 ml)
Long-acting (6 hours)				
Barbital	Veronal	0.1–0.2	10	15
Phenobarbital	Luminal	0.3–0.5	5	8
Intermediate-acting (3–6 hours)				
Amobarbital	Amytal	0.05–0.2		
Butabarbital	Butisol	0.1–0.2		
Short-acting (3 hours)				
Pentobarbital	Nembutal	0.05–0.2	3	3.5
Secobarbital	Seconal	0.1–0.2	3	3.5

Data from Henderson, L. W., and Merrill, J. P., Treatment of barbiturate intoxication. *Ann. Intern. Med.* 64:876, 1966.

necessary concentration of inspired oxygen is used to prevent the development of oxygen toxicity. In the absence of underlying lung disease, room air should suffice. In class III patients, care must be exercised in administering oxygen without respiratory assistance, because removal of the hypoxic drive to ventilation may lead to more pronounced hypoventilation.

b. Cardiovascular. Hypotension occurs in barbiturate poisoning from decreased intravascular volume, from hypoxia with acidosis, and, at extremely high doses, from the direct myocardial depressant effects of barbiturates. The decreased intravascular volume is caused by dehydration and the escape of fluid from the capillaries because of increased capillary permeability, which results from both barbiturate toxicity and hypoxia. The venous pooling of blood that follows may impair cardiac output further.

(1) The chief therapy of hypotension consists of correction of hypoxia, if it exists, and replacement of vascular volume. A CVP line is placed, and volume-expanding solutions are infused at about 20 ml/min until the CVP reaches 2–6 cm H_2O.

(a) The initial 1000 ml of volume replacement may be in the form of a 5% albumin solution, because it will not only expand intravascular volume rapidly, but it will bind some of the circulating barbiturates. However this latter effect is only significant for long-acting and intermediate-acting compounds.

(b) An isotonic electrolyte solution may be used after the initial liter of albumin is infused.

(2) Pressors are rarely necessary, but they may be required in patients with severe intoxication in which the blood pressure does not respond to volume replacement. In general, the pressor chosen is infused at a rate that is sufficient to maintain systolic blood pressure at about 90 mm Hg, but the urine output is the ultimate guide. In cases of ingestion of long-acting and intermediate-acting barbiturates, which are excreted primarily in the urine, dopamine is the pressor of choice.

c. Other supportive measures

(1) Frequent turning, attention to skin care, and other supportive measures are necessary for comatose patients.

(2) Frequent suctioning of intubated patients, pulmonary physical therapy, and prompt antibiotic treatment of respiratory infections are also required.

3. Removal of unabsorbed drug from the gastrointestinal tract is only helpful if the patient is first seen within 3 hours of ingestion. The only exceptions are the rare patients who ingest large amounts of barbiturates and develop a resultant ileus. Because of their intestinal hypomotility, these patients retain unabsorbed drug in the gut for many hours.

a. Emesis should only be induced in patients with mild ingestion, who are awake and able to protect their own airways from aspiration.

b. Gastric lavage may be undertaken in patients who are seen within 3 hours of ingestion, but it should only be performed with a cuffed endotracheal tube in place.

c. After the stomach is evacuated, if bowel sounds are present, an osmotic cathartic may be administered.

(1) Sorbitol 50 gm mixed with about 200 ml of water or magnesium citrate, 200 ml of the standard commercial solution, may be used.

(2) Activated charcoal will bind barbiturates and may be given along with the cathartic; the usual dose is 30 gm.

4. Removal of already-absorbed barbiturate from the body

a. Forced diuresis may increase the clearance of long-acting barbiturates two to fourfold, but it has a relatively minor effect on the excretion of short-acting barbiturates. Obviously, the patient must have good renal function and renal perfusion for this therapy to be effective.

(1) Diuresis can usually be induced merely by the infusion of isotonic saline at a rapid rate. Urine output is maintained at about 10 ml/min.

(2) The administration of large amounts of free water (e.g., as 5% dextrose in water) is avoided, because SIADH may accompany barbiturate intoxication.

(3) If the patient is in danger of fluid overload from the rapid infusion of isotonic saline, diuresis can be induced with furosemide (Lasix) 0.5–1.0 mg/kg or ethacrynic acid (Edecrin) 50–100 mg/kg IV. Fluid and electrolyte losses must then be carefully measured and replaced with appropriate IV fluids. The diuretic dose may then be repeated as necessary to maintain the diuresis.

In managing elderly patients and those with impaired cardiac function, there is no evidence that forced diuresis improves mortality from barbiturate overdose. Therefore the physician should not jeopardize the patient's vital functions to hasten barbiturate excretion.

(4) An indwelling bladder catheter is necessary when inducing a forced diuresis in comatose patients.

b. Alkalinization of the urine increases the excretion of phenobarbital, but it is of no significant benefit with other barbiturates. Alkalinization may usually be achieved by the addition of one standard ampule (44 mEq) $NaHCO_3$ to each liter of IV fluids, but the urine pH should be checked to ensure that the pH is greater than 7. Also, $NaHCO_3$ infusion results in potassium wasting, so 10–20 mEq KCL is also added to each liter of IV fluids, and the serum potassium is measured frequently.

If urinary pH greater than 7 cannot be achieved in the face of a rapid diuresis with $NaHCO_3$ infusion alone, acetazolamide (Diamox) 250 mg every 6 hours may be given by IV injection to adults.

The infusion of $NaHCO_3$ subjects the patient to a large sodium load and, like forced diuresis, should not be used in patients with impaired cardiac reserve.

c. Hemodialysis is roughly equivalent in effectiveness to forced diuresis or peritoneal dialysis. It is also more effective for long-acting and intermediate-acting barbiturates than for short-acting compounds. However, hemodialysis has its own complications in comatose patients, and centers that use hemodialysis in a relatively large proportion of patients have not achieved the low mortality reported from the use of conservative measures alone. Nevertheless, there are generally accepted indications for the use of hemodialysis (*Arch. Intern. Med.* 117:224, 1966).

(1) Renal or hepatic insufficiency in degrees that prevent the elimination of drug through normal means.

(2) Shock or prolonged coma that does not respond to usual measures.

(3) Ingestion of a lethal dose of drug (3 gm of a short-acting compound or 5 gm of a long-acting compound).

(4) A blood level from which prolonged coma can be predicted (higher than 3.5 mg/100 ml for short-acting compounds or higher than 8 mg/100 ml of phenobarbital).

5. Complications of barbiturate intoxication primarily result from prolonged coma, but pneumonia and bladder infections are encountered most frequently. Acute renal failure due to acute tubular necrosis or to nontraumatic rhabdomyolysis can also occur.

6. Psychiatric evaluation and care are provided to all patients who ingest overdoses of drugs intentionally.

B. Barbiturate addiction

1. Elective withdrawal of barbiturates in patients addicted to a drug should be carried out in the hospital. Most addicts can be withdrawn over 2–3 weeks without precipitating withdrawal symptoms.

   a. The patient's usual daily dose (generally 1.5 to 2 gm) is estimated from the history and pentobarbital (Nembutal) is given in six doses at 4-hour intervals.

   b. The patient is examined for signs of toxicity, primarily atoxia, and drowsiness within 30–60 minutes after the first dose. If symptoms are present, the next succeeding doses are reduced by 25–50%, depending on the degree of toxicity. If withdrawal symptoms occur, an additional dose of 50–100 mg of pentobarbital is administered, and each succeeding dose is adjusted accordingly. The patient is then examined every 30–60 minutes until a baseline dose is reached.

   c. After a baseline dose of pentobarbital is obtained, the patient is withdrawn at a rate of about 100 mg pentobarbital per day. If withdrawal symptoms occur, the rate of withdrawal may be slowed. In general, if enough drug is administered to give the patient nystagmus, withdrawal symptoms will not be present.

   d. During and after elective barbiturate withdrawal, the patient is provided psychiatric and medical evaluation to minimize the chances of recurrence of the addiction.

2. Acute barbiturate withdrawal presents a clinical picture that is strikingly similar to that of alcohol withdrawal, with tremor, delirium, and seizures being prominent. Symptoms may be aborted by the IV administration of barbiturates. Pentobarbital (Nembutal) may be given in 25-mg increments every 5–10 minutes until symptoms abate.

   Unlike ethanol withdrawal, the seizures associated with withdrawal from short-acting barbiturates may be severe. IV barbiturate is the treatment of choice. Diazepam (Valium) is generally effective, but the combination of barbiturate and diazepam frequently produces respiratory depression. After the acute symptoms are under control, the patient may be withdrawn from barbiturates gradually. As with ethanol withdrawal, careful attention is directed toward fluid and electrolyte balance, antipyrexis, and prevention of infectious complications.

XIV. POISONING WITH NONBARBITURATE CNS DEPRESSANTS

A. The basic therapy of acute intoxication with all CNS depressants is similar to that of barbiturate intoxication. The respiratory and cardiovascular systems must be stabilized, unabsorbed drug is removed by lavage and catharsis, and the elimination of the drug from the body is speeded by whatever techniques are feasible for each drug.

B. Individual drugs

1. **Glutethimide** (Doriden) is notorious for its high mortality associated with overdose. The fluctuating course, which used to be attributed to enterohepatic circulation of the drug, is probably caused by delayed absorption of drug, which is a result of paralytic ileus. The signs are similar to those of barbitu-

rate intoxication, except that the drug also possesses anticholinergic activity, producing dilated pupils.

The therapy is primarily supportive, and elimination of the drug may be hastened by forced diuresis. Hemodialysis against a lipid-containing dialysis should be employed if the patient has renal failure, fails to respond to conservative measures, or has ingested a potentially lethal dose (more than 10 gm total, or if the blood level is greater than 3 mg/100 ml).

2. **Chloral hydrate** (Noctec, Somnos) and **ethchlorvynol** (Placidyl) intoxication resemble barbiturate intoxication, except that chloral hydrate may produce constricted pupils.

The therapy is identical to that of barbiturate overdose, although forced diuresis is of less benefit. Hemodialysis is effective in eliminating both drugs. It should be used with the same indications as with barbiturate overdose. Lipid dialysis increases the rate of elimination.

3. **Benzodiazepines.** Diazepam (Valium) and chlordiazepoxide (Librium) taken alone PO generally do not produce life-threatening intoxication in medically sound patients. Respiratory depression is only of significance in patients with intrinsic lung disease or in cases of mixed ingestions. The management of benzodiazepine intoxication consists of eliminating unabsorbed drug from the gastrointestinal tract and supporting the patient until he or she awakens.

XV. AMPHETAMINES

A. Acute toxicity produces psychosis, hyperpyrexia, hypertension, dilated pupils, vomiting, and diarrhea. Life-threatening effects of severe intoxication include cardiac arrythmias, seizures, coma, and respiratory arrest. The lethal dose in children is about 5 mg/kg; in adults, it is about 1.5 gm. The serum half-life is a matter of days, so toxic symptoms may persist for longer than a week.

1. Sedation with phenothiazines controls psychotic manifestations. Chlorpromazine 50 mg PO or IM may be given initially and every 30 minutes until the patient is calm. Then it is given every 4–6 hours as necessary.

2. Hyperpyrexia can be controlled with a cooling blanket and vigorous wetting with towels soaked in tepid water.

3. Arrhythmias are treated with appropriate drugs.

4. Seizures are a short-term problem if no irreversible CNS damage occurs from hypoxia or cardiac arrest. They should be treated with the usual measures (see Chap. 6).

5. Unabsorbed drug is removed with emesis, lavage, catharsis, or all three, as appropriate. Lavage may be of benefit even several hours after ingestion.

6. Acidification of the urine hastens the excretion of amphetamines and should be employed in the event of severe intoxication. NH_4Cl may be administered PO or IV at a total dose of 8–12 gm/day, and the urine pH is checked frequently. NH_4Cl is contraindicated in shock, systemic acidoses of any cause, and in hepatic failure or portosystemic shunting.

7. Severe hypertension is best treated with an alpha-blocking agent, such as phentolamine (Regitine). Moderate hypertension responds to chlorpromazine.

B. Chronic amphetamine abuse should be treated psychiatrically. Acute amphetamine withdrawal produces no medical complications, so there is no need to taper doses. After sudden cessation of habitual amphetamine ingestion, a prolonged sleep generally occurs, requiring only observation and maintenance of hydration.

C. Cocaine intoxication is clinically similar to amphetamine overdose, and the supportive treatment is identical. Cocaine has a much shorter half-life than amphetamines, and it is metabolized rapidly by the liver. Consequently, forced diuresis or acidification of the urine is of no benefit.

XVI. TRICYCLIC ANTIDEPRESSANTS

A. The acute toxic effects of the tricyclics relate primarily to their anticholinergic effects. These symptoms resemble atropine poisoning, with hyperpyrexia, dilated pupils, hypertension, tachycardia, and dryness of the skin and mucous membranes. The life-threatening manifestations are coma, seizures, cardiac arrhythmias, and cardiac conduction defects.

B. Supportive therapy

1. The initial emergency treatment is the same as for any overdose: stabilization of respiratory and cardiac status and elimination of unabsorbed drug from the gastrointestinal tract.

2. Cardiac conduction defects and arrhythmias are prominent in tricyclic intoxication. The patient should be on a cardiac monitor, a temporary transvenous pacemaker should be readily available, and the patient should be placed in an intensive or coronary care unit. Lidocaine is effective for ventricular arrhythmias. Propranolol should be used with extreme care if a conduction defect is present.

3. Hyperpyrexia can be controlled in patients by using a cooling blanket or by giving them vigorous rubdowns with towels soaked in tepid water. Chlorpromazine may increase the effectiveness of hypothermic methods.

4. Severe hypertension will respond to the administration of an alpha blocker, such as phentolamine (Regitine).

C. Physostigmine is reported to antagonize the CNS toxicity of tricyclics and other anticholinergics.

1. Physostigmine injection may serve as a diagnostic test to confirm anticholinergic ingestion. Physostigmine 1 mg is injected subcutaneously, IM, or slowly IV, which will produce peripheral cholinergic signs within 30 minutes of injection if no anticholinergics have been ingested. These signs include bradycardia, increased salivation and lacrimation, and pupillary constriction. In a patient who has ingested anticholinergics, the injection will produce no significant effect.

2. For the treatment of anticholinergic overdose, 1-mg doses of physostigmine are injected IM or slowly IV at 20-minute intervals until 4 mg have been administered or cholinergic signs appear.

3. Physostigmine is most effective against the toxic delirium of anticholinergic overdose. It will occasionally awaken a comatose patient.

4. If excessive physostigmine is administered, cholinergic side effects may, in themselves, exert harmful effects. Excessive respiratory secretions, salivation, and bronchaspasm may interfere with pulmonary function; and vomiting, abdominal cramps, and diarrhea may also occur. Excessive cholinergic effects may be counteracted with atropine.

5. The duration of action of physostigmine is only 1–2 hours in the serum, whereas tricyclics persist over 24 hours. Therefore the patient must be monitored after the initial therapy, and repeated doses are administered as necessary.

D. Tricyclic antidepressants are cleared mainly by the kidneys, so forced diuresis is effective. Dialysis is of no additional benefit beyond that of forced diuresis except in renal failure.

XVII. SALICYLATE INTOXICATION

A. Description

1. In the United States salicylate is the medicine that most frequently produces clinically significant intoxication. The most common source is aspirin, but sodium salicylate and oil of wintergreen are also common causes.

   a. Adult aspirin tablets, by agreement among drug manufacturers, all contain 5 gr (325 mg) of aspirin, whereas children's tablets contain 1¼ gr (80 mg).

   b. Oil of wintergreen contains methyl salicylate at a concentration of about 0.7 gm/ml. It is highly toxic and 1 or 2 teaspoonfuls may be a fatal dose for a small child.

2. The toxic dose of salicylate is about 250 mg/kg in a healthy person. Lower doses of both methyl salicylate and aspirin, in a patient who is dehydrated or in renal failure, may be intoxicating.

3. **Pharmacokinetics**

   a. Salicylates are well absorbed from the gastrointestinal tract, over 50% of a therapeutic dose being absorbed within 1 hour of ingestion. Also, poisoning has occurred from oil of wintergreen, applied in large quantities, as a result of cutaneous absorption.

   b. Once absorbed, aspirin is rapidly hydrolyzed to salicylic acid.

   c. Salicylic acid is variably bound to albumin. At toxic levels, the serum albumin binding sites are essentially 100% saturated.

   d. Salicylic acid is glucuronidated by the liver. It is excreted both unchanged and as its glucuronidated product in the urine. Salicylic acid has a pK_a of about 3, so it can be "trapped" in an alkaline solution. Thus alkalinization of the urine may increase salicylic acid excretion as much as fivefold.

4. **Signs and symptoms of toxicity**

   a. CNS abnormalities dominate the clinical picture.

   (1) The earliest signs are tinnitus and impaired hearing.

   (2) Agitation progressing to delirium, stupor, and coma results from severe intoxication.

   (3) Seizures may occur as a direct effect of CNS salicylate toxicity or as a secondary manifestation of hypoglycemia or effective hypocalcemia (see **4.b**).

   (4) Salicylates in toxic doses act centrally to stimulate respirations and produce hyperpnea, usually with tachypnea and respiratory alkalosis.

   (5) In extremely high doses, respiratory depression occurs.

   b. Metabolic derangements.

   (1) Salicylates interfere with carbohydrate metabolism.

   (a) Hypoglycemia may occur in young children.

   (b) The brain uses glucose inefficiently and may experience a "relative hypoglycemia," even with a normal blood glucose.

   (c) Mild to moderate hyperglycemia is frequent.

   (2) In severe intoxication, metabolic acidosis occurs with an increased anion gap and organic aciduria.

(3) The organic aciduria, with or without glycosuria, produces an osmotic diuresis, which in turn produces dehydration.

(4) The respiratory alkalosis, when prolonged, has secondary effects on electrolyte metabolism.

(a) There is sodium and potassium wasting by the kidneys. The hypokalemia renders the metabolic acidosis unresponsive to alkali therapy until the potassium is repleted.

(b) The respiratory alkalosis produces decreased unbound serum calcium levels, which can lead to tetany and seizures.

(5) SIADH has been reported in association with salicylate poisoning.

  c. Effects on blood clotting.

(1) Salicylate in toxic concentrations exerts an antiprothrombin effect, with prolongation of the prothrombin time and diminished factor VII activity.

(2) Salicylates interfere with platelet function, even in nontoxic doses.

(3) Salicylates are locally irritating to the gastric mucosa and may lead to gastrointestinal hemorrhage.

  d. Hepatotoxicity may elevate the liver enzymes, which can lead to confusion with Reye's syndrome in children or to hepatic encephalopathy in adults.

  e. Noncardiac pulmonary edema has been reported.

5. Making the diagnosis

  a. Salicylate intoxication occurs frequently in three groups:

(1) Children under 5 years of age, as a result of accidental ingestion.

(2) Adolescents and young adults, as a result of intentional overdose in a suicide gesture or attempt.

(3) Unintentional overdose in patients taking salicylates for rheumatic disease.

  b. The diagnosis is obvious with an adequate history of ingestion. However it is frequently masked by chronic therapeutic overdose if the physician is unaware that the patient is on salicylates or does not consider the diagnosis.

  c. The diagnosis is considered in patients with mental status changes, hyperpnea, and respiratory alkalosis, with or without superimposed metabolic acidosis.

  d. Serum salicylate levels are generally available and confirm the diagnosis. A level higher than 30 mg/100 ml may produce early symptoms of salicylism: mental changes and hyperpnea occur at levels higher than 40 mg/100 ml. With chronic ingestion, blood levels correlate poorly with the clinical status of the patient, but will nevertheless serve to make or to rule out the diagnosis.

  e. The **ferric chloride test** may be performed on the urine at the bedside and serves as a rapid screening test for the presence of salicylic acid.

(1) The test is performed by adding a few drops of a 10% solution of $FeCl_3$ to 3–5 ml of acidified urine. A purple color indicates a positive result.

(2) The test is extremely sensitive, so a positive result is not diagnostic of salicylate intoxication.

(3) $FeCl_3$ reacts only with salicylic acid, not with aspirin. Therefore it cannot be used to test for the presence of aspirin in gastric contents.

(4) Phenothiazines react with $FeCl_3$, but they tend to give a pink rather than a purple color.

(5) Acetoacetic acid, present in ketosis, will react with $FeCl_3$. It may be eliminated, however, if the urine is boiled and acidified before adding the $FeCl_3$.

B. The initial laboratory evaluation of a patient with salicylate intoxication should include the following:

1. Serum salicylate level is of prognostic importance and gives a baseline value with which to judge the effects of therapy.

2. Patients with intentional overdoses should have blood or urine or both screened for the presence of other toxic substances.

3. CBC, including platelet count.

4. Stool and gastric contents are tested for the presence of occult blood.

5. Arterial blood gases and pH.

6. BUN (or creatinine), electrolytes, calcium, and phosphorus.

7. Liver function tests, including SGOT, LDH, alkaline phosphatase, total bilirubin, total protein, and albumin.

8. Prothrombin time and partial thromboplastin time.

9. Chest x-ray.

10. ECG, giving particular attention to signs of hypokalemia or hypocalcemia.

11. Urinalysis with specific gravity. If the serum sodium is low and SIADH is a possibility, then urine sodium concentration and osmolality are measured.

C. Acute management

1. Routine emergency measures for the treatment of drug intoxications

a. Protect the airway and support respiration, if necessary.

b. Empty the gastrointestinal tract of unabsorbed drug.

(1) Forced emesis is done if the patient is alert.

(2) Gastric lavage is done after tracheal intubation with a cuffed endotracheal tube if the patient is stuporous, in coma, or unable to protect his own airway.

(3) Activated charcoal is given as 200–300 ml of a thick suspension to bind unabsorbed salicylates effectively.

(4) Cathartics are administered after the charcoal has been given.

2. Fluid and electrolyte management are used to treat shock if it is present, achieving and maintaining good urine output, and restoring electrolyte and acid-base balance.

a. Resuscitative measures for patients in shock

(1) All patients in shock or coma require an indwelling Foley catheter. Adults over 35 years old and patients with impaired cardiac or renal function require a CVP line.

(2) Volume deficits are corrected with the rapid infusion of albumin solutions or plasma. The end point is a normal systolic blood pressure and adequate peripheral perfusion.

(3) After the blood pressure is stabilized, isotonic saline with 5% dextrose is infused at a rate of 500 ml/sq m/hour (20 ml/kg/hour) until urine

begins to flow at a rate of 50 ml/sq m/hour or until the CVP exceeds 10 cm H_2O.

(4) If the CVP exceeds 10 cm H_2O and adequate urine output has not been established, then oliguric renal failure has occurred. Furosemide (Lasix) 0.5 mg/kg by IV push is given to verify the diminished urine output.

If little or no response is obtained with the diuretic and the patient is significantly intoxicated with salicylates, then immediate dialysis is the treatment.

(5) Extreme metabolic acidosis (pH 7.20) requires the administration of boluses of $NaHCO_3$ to maintain the arterial pH above 7.20. The overuse of $NaHCO_3$ can result in hypernatremia and sodium overloading. No attempt is made to adjust the pH to normal with alkali therapy alone.

b. Maintenance fluid management

(1) 50% normal saline (or 25% normal saline) with 5% dextrose at 100–150 ml/sq m/hour may be used. The urine output should be maintained at a level higher than 2000 ml/sq m/24 hours.

(2) SIADH may occur with salicylate intoxication and prevent the use of large amounts of free water. Thus the electrolytes should be checked after the first 4 hours of therapy.

(3) Potassium losses must be replaced vigorously, especially in the face of metabolic acidosis. If more than 10 mEq KCl per hour is infused, the patient should be on a cardiac monitor, and precautions are taken to ensure that the infusion does not run too rapidly. No more than 40 mEq/hour should be infused IV. KCl may also be given by nasogastric tube to supplement IV administration, if necessary.

(4) Elderly patients and those with abnormal cardiac function may not be able to tolerate the rapid rates of fluid administration recommended. These patients should have a CVP line, and they may require repeated administration of diuretics to achieve a brisk urine output without the risk of congestive heart failure.

(5) Alkalinization of the urine by the infusion of $NaHCO_3$ hastens the excretion of salicylic acid. However, in practice the technique has no use.

(a) In elderly patients and those with abnormal hearts, the risks of increased sodium load are not justified by the expected benefits of alkalinization of the urine.

(b) In patients with metabolic acidosis, the urine cannot be alkalinized except with massive and dangerous quantities of alkali.

(c) In patients with respiratory alkalosis and alkalemia, the administration of alkali is contraindicated.

3. Hypoglycemia

a. In young children, after blood has been drawn, 50% dextrose in water (0.5 ml/kg) is administered immediately by IV push.

b. Only glucose-containing fluids are used for maintenance.

4. Hemorrhagic complications

a. In severe salicylate poisoning, vitamin K 50 mg IV is given after an initial prothrombin time has been done. The vitamin K is repeated as necessary to maintain a normal prothrombin time.

   b. If bleeding occurs or if the prothrombin time is found to be longer than twice the control value, fresh frozen plasma or concentrates of clotting factors (Konyne) are given.

   c. Platelet transfusion may be required to achieve control of hemorrhage, because the patient's own platelets will have a disordered function.

   d. In comatose patients, antacids may be given by nasogastric tube in an effort to prevent gastric hemorrhage. However, there is no firm evidence that antacids are of benefit in this circumstance.

5. Tetany may be treated with the IV infusion of calcium gluconate in 1-gm doses, and it may be repeated as often as necessary.

6. Seizures

   a. Hypoglycemia and hypocalcemia are either ruled out or treated appropriately (secs **3** and **5**). Other metabolic causes of seizures, such as hyponatremia and hypoxia, must also be considered.

   b. Seizures that occur as a direct toxic effect of salicylate are a poor prognostic sign, generally indicating hemodialysis to hasten elimination of the salicylate. Diazepam (Valium), given IV, or muscle paralysis and respiratory support may be used for the temporary control of seizures until the salicylate level is lowered.

7. Hypothermia can be treated with tepid water baths.

8. Methods to hasten the elimination of salicylates

   a. Forced diuresis is of little benefit, and the patient should not be subjected to a larger fluid load than necessary to achieve a reasonable urine output (see sec **C.2.b**).

   b. Alkalinization of the urine is discussed in sec **C.2.b.(5)**. Despite its theoretical advantages, it has no practical use in salicylate poisoning.

   c. Peritoneal dialysis is about as efficient as the normal kidneys in eliminating salicylate from the blood. Its primary use is in the setting of renal failure, especially in young children, where hemodialysis is technically difficult and risky. The addition of albumin to the dialysis solution hastens the elimination of salicylate, but there is no evidence that its benefit outweighs the expense and added complexity of the dialysis.

   d. Hemodialysis is the most efficient means available for the elimination of salicylate. The generally accepted indications for hemodialysis are:

   (1) Salicylate level higher than 70 mg/100 ml or known absorption greater than 5 gm/kg.

   (2) Profound coma with respiratory failure.

   (3) Severe metabolic acidosis.

   (4) Renal failure.

   (5) Failure to respond to conservative therapy.

SELECTED READINGS

Hepatic Encephalopathy
Breen, J. J., and Schenker, S.   Hepatic Coma: Present Concepts of Pathogenesis and Therapy, in *Progress in Liver Disease,* Vol. 4. New York: Grune Stratton, 1972. Pp. 301–332.
Lunger, M., et al.   Treatment of chronic hepatic encephalopathy with levodopa. *Gut* 15:555, 1974.
Sherlock, S.   Hepatic Pre-coma and Coma, in *Diseases of the Liver and Biliary System.* London: Blackwell, 1975.

Victor, M., et al.   The acquired (non-wilsonian) type of chronic hepatocerebral degeneration. *Medicine* 44:345, 1965.

Renal and Electrolyte

Arieff, A. I., et al.   Neurological manifestations and morbidity of hyponatremia: Correlation with brain water and electrolytes. *Medicine* 55:121, 1976.

Bartler, F. C., and Schwartz, W. B.   The syndrome of inappropriate secretion of antidiuretic hormone. *Am. J. Med.* 42:790, 1967.

Cherrill, D. A., et al.   Demeclocylcine treatment in the syndrome of inappropriate antidiuretic hormone secretion. *Ann. Intern. Med.* 83:654, 1975.

Hantman, D., et al.   Rapid correction of hyponatremia in the syndrome of inappropriate secretion of antidiuretic hormone. *Ann. Intern. Med.* 78:870, 1973.

Tyler, H. R.   Neurologic disorders in renal failure. *Am. J. Med.* 44:734, 1968.

White, M. G., and Fetner, C. D.   Treatment of the syndrome of inappropriate secretion of antidiuretic hormone with lithium carbonate. *N. Engl. J. Med.* 292:390, 1975.

Acute Intermittent Porphyria

Perboth, M. G., et al.   Oral contraceptive agents and the management of acute intermittent porphyria. *J.A.M.A.* 194:135, 1965.

Tschudy, D. P., et al.   Acute intermittent prophyria: Clinical and selected research aspects. *Ann. Intern. Med.* 83:851, 1975.

Heavy Metals

Center for Disease Control.   Increased lead absorption and lead poisoning in young children. *J. Pediatr.* 87:824, 1975.

Chisholm, J., Jr.,   The use of chelating agents in the treatment of acute and chronic lead intoxication in childhood. *J. Pediatr.* 73:1, 1968.

Chisholm, J., Jr.   Lead Poisoning, in Henry L. Barnett (ed.), *Pediatrics.* New York: Appleton-Century-Crofts, 1972. Pp. 540–548.

Poskanzer, D. C., and Bennett, I. L., Jr.   Heavy Metals, in George Thorn, et al. (eds.), *Harrison's Principles of Internal Medicine* (8th ed.) New York: McGraw-Hill, 1977.

Vitale, L., et al.   Oral penicillamine therapy for chronic lead poisoning in children. *J. Pediatr.* 83:1042, 1973.

Alcohol

Mendelson, J. H.   Biologic concomitants of alcoholism. *N. Engl. J. Med.* 283:24, 71, 1970.

Seixas, F. A.   Alcohol and its drug interactions. *Ann. Intern. Med.* 83:86, 1975.

Sellers, F. M., and Kalant, H.   Alcohol intoxication and withdrawal. *N. Engl. J. Med.* 294:757, 1976.

Thompson, W., Leigh, D., et al.   Diazepam and paraldehyde for treatment of severe delirium tremens. *Ann. Intern. Med.* 82:175, 1975.

Drug Intoxication

Anderson, R. J., et al.   Unrecognized adult salicylate intoxication. *Ann. Intern. Med.* 85:745, 1976.

Done, A. K., and Temple, A. B.   Treatment of salicylate poisoning. *Mod. Treatment* 8:528, 1971.

Gardner, A. J.   Withdrawal fits in barbiturate addicts. *Lancet* 2:337, 1967.

Goodman, L. S., and Gilman, A. (eds.)   *The Pharmacological Basis of Therapeutics* (5th ed.). New York: Macmillan, 1975.

Granacher, R. P., et al.   Physostigmine treatment of delirium induced by anticholinergics. *Ann. Family Practice,* May, 1976.

Henderson, L. W., and Merrill, J. P.   Treatment of barbiturate intoxication. *Ann. Intern. Med.* 64:876, 1966.

Hill, J. B.   Salicylate intoxication. *N. Engl. J. Med.* 288:110, 1973.

Robinson, R. R., et al.   Treatment of acute barbiturate intoxication. *Mod. Treatment* 8:561, 1971.

Setter, J. G., et al.   Barbiturate intoxication. *Arch. Intern. Med.* 117:224, 1966.

15

Robert D. Helme

Movement Disorders

I. A SIMPLIFIED OVERVIEW OF MOTOR CONTROL SYSTEMS

The rational management of movement disorders requires some understanding of the anatomic and physiologic substrate necessary for normal movement. Beneficial therapeutic maneuvers are limited by our lack of knowledge of human anatomy and physiology.

The traditional concept of motor control is that of an upper motor neuron arising in the precentral gyrus; descending in the posterior limb of the internal capsule, cerebral peduncle, and pyramidal tract; and then descending in the medulla before entering the contralateral corticospinal tract to influence the lower motor neuron directly (Fig. 15-1). To this pyramidal system are added local feedback systems in the spinal cord whereby the α-motor neuron is influenced through the γ-loop and sensory input from the same or nearby segmental levels.

This pyramidal system arises from much of the posterior frontal lobe, the sensory strip of the parietal lobe, and other areas of sensorimotor cortex. A parapyramidal system also arises in part from these motor areas and acts on the lower motor neuron through multisynaptic pathways through the red nucleus (rubrospinal system) and reticular formation of the pons and medulla (reticulospinal system). The third major parapyramidal system is the vestibulospinal system, which has its major input from vestibular, reticular, and cerebellar sources. The neurotransmitters in these systems are not known (Fig. 15-2).

The basal ganglia influence motor control through these pathways, generally by means of input into the motor areas of the cerebral hemispheres (see sec **IV**). The cerebellum acts through the same pathways, especially via the vestibulospinal systems and through relays in the thalamus to the same motor areas of the cerebral hemispheres (see sec **III**).

II. PARALYSIS AND HYPERTONIA (SPASTICITY)

A. Paralysis. Most symptoms and signs of motor dysfunction may be explained in the context of lesions of the pyramidal and parapyramidal systems. That is, paralysis and variations in tone seen in different body regions in such patients have been consistently correlated with pathologic lesions in these systems. Although paralysis in such patients cannot be altered, physical therapy is of benefit in retraining the remaining neuromuscular apparatus.

B. Hypertonia. Hypertonia may occur in some **metabolic diseases,** such as pernicious anemia, and respond to specific treatment if recognized early. However, our **ability to influence tone is usually restricted** to generalized pharmacologic manipulation of the whole neuromuscular apparatus, thereby causing generalized, and usually unacceptable, side effects such as weakness. Indeed, spasticity may be necessary for gait training in the rehabilitation of the stroke patient. Without rigid legs, splinting may be useless.

C. Useful therapeutic modalities include the following (Table 15-1).

1. **Dantrolene sodium** (Dantrium) can be used to **reduce spasticity,** especially in the wheelchair-bound patient with paraplegia, by its action to uncouple the muscle excitation-contraction phenomenon. The dose is increased gradually from 25 mg BID to 100 mg QID over at least one month. The transient nausea, diarrhea, and generalized muscle weakness often observed may be better tolerated by this course of administration. Hepatotoxicity has been reported.

2. **Baclofen** (Lioresal), a gamma-aminobutyric acid (GABA) derivative, may also be useful (as a substance P antagonist rather than as a GABA agonist) in the spasticity resulting from a lesion of the spinal cord. The drug is particu-

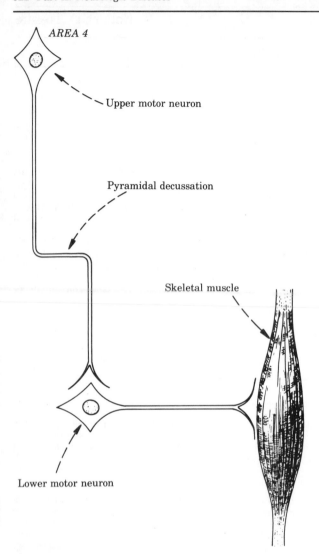

Fig. 15-1. Traditional concept of motor control. Upper motor neuron lesions produce paralysis, hypertonia, and hyperreflexia. Lower motor neuron lesions produce paralysis, hypotonia, areflexia, and muscle-wasting.

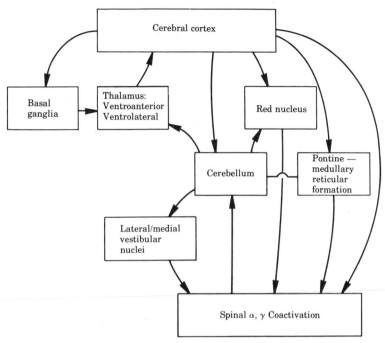

Fig. 15-2. Simplified outline of current concepts in motor control. The corticospinal and rubrospinal systems are excitatory for flexors. The vestibulospinal system is excitatory for extensors, and the reticulospinal system is variable at different levels.

larly useful **to relieve flexor spasms** and where there is **increased resistance to passive movements of the legs.** Probably baclofen is not useful for clonus, hyperreflexia, or other manifestations of spasticity. It is used in a dose of 30–100 mg daily following buildup from an initial dose of 10 mg daily, given in divided doses. Nausea, drowsiness, dizziness, and depression are common side effects.

3. **Diazepam** (Valium) may also be of some benefit when administered in high doses (10 mg QID). This drug is especially beneficial in the **"stiff man syndrome,"** in which spasticity is a principal motor sign, but no lesion of the descending motor systems has been demonstrated. The increased tone may be a result of abnormal function in the descending reticulospinal noradrenergic system.

4. **Phenytoin** (Dilantin) 300 mg every day, together with chlorpromazine (Thorazine) up to 100 mg TID, has recently been advocated as useful in the **treatment of spasticity.**

5. **Intrathecal phenol injection** may be useful for alleviation of **painful spasms in the lower extremities** (if drug treatment is ineffective), especially in the incontinent patient. (See also Chap. 13).

6. Individual **peripheral nerve blockade** (e.g., obturator, sciatic, femoral) with local anesthetic and then, if successful, with alcohol may be necessary to relieve severe spasticity in some patients.

III. **CEREBELLAR DYSFUNCTION.** Astride the pyramidal and parapyramidal motor control systems are two suprasegmental modulating systems, the **cerebellum and basal ganglia** (extrapyramidal system) (see Fig. 15-2).

Table 15-1. Drugs Useful for Spasticity

Drug	Dose (mg)	Major Use	Major Side Effects	Comments
Dantrolene sodium (Dantrium)	25 BID, slowly increased to 100 QID over 1 month	Wheelchair-bound paraplegic	Generalized weakness, nausea, diarrhea, hepatotoxicity	Uncouples muscle excitation contraction phenomenon
Baclofen (Lioresal)	10 QD, slowly increased to 30–100 QD in divided doses	Spinal cord lesions; flexor spasms; increased tone to passive movement (not clonus or hyperreflexia)	Nausea, drowsiness, dizziness, depression	? Substance P antagonist; ? GABA agonist
Diazepam (Valium)	10 QD, slowly increased to 40–60 QD in divided doses	Stiff man syndrome	Sedation	? Acts on norepinephrine; spinal cord pathways
Phenytoin (Dilantin)	300 QD	Uncertain	Rash, gingival hypertrophy, ataxia, pseudolymphoma, macrocytic anemia	Effectiveness not fully documented
Chlorpromazine (Thorazine)	50 QD, slowly increased to 300 QD in divided doses	Uncertain	Sedation, parkinsonism	Effectiveness not fully documented

A. The **anatomy** and **cellular physiology** of the cerebellum are well known, largely because of its relatively simple design. Input comes from all levels of the central nervous system. Vestibular and spinal cord sensory input is especially important, as are descending frontal motor relays. Output is directed to the pyramidal system via the ventrolateral and ventroanterior nuclei of the thalamus, and to the brainstem parapyramidal systems, especially the lateral vestibulospinal tract.

B. However, the method by which the cerebellum exerts control over the motor system is unknown, and **therapy is generally ineffective** when function of the cerebellum is abnormal. The following may be of some use.

1. **Limb weights** up to a few hundred grams may reduce the intention tremor (3–8 cycles per second) of cerebellar disease.

2. **Destructive lesions of the ventrolateral thalamus** (i.e., in the area of the thalamus that relays to cortical motor control systems) may alleviate congenital rubral tremor and cerebellar intention tremor.

IV. THE BASAL GANGLIA

A. **Overview.** The anatomic arrangement of the basal ganglia suggests that it functions primarily through a closed loop (Fig. 15-3). Afferents come to the small neurons of the neostriatum (caudate and putamen) from the cerebral cortex either directly or through connections with the nucleus centromedianum of the thalamus. Efferents from the large neurons of the neostriatum pass to the cerebral cortex by way of sequential connections in the globus pallidus and ventroanterior and ventrolateral nuclei of the thalamus, influencing ipsilateral cortical motor control centers and thus contralateral motor function. The neurotransmitters of this pathway are not all known, but it seems clear that acetylcholine is of major importance.

A number of other circuits influence the activity of the cholinergic system. Of primary importance is the nigroneostriatal system, which utilizes dopamine as an inhibitory neurotransmitter at terminals situated on dendrites of small, presumably cholinergic, neurons in the neostriatum. The afferent systems that influence the dopaminergic neurons in the pars compacta of the substantia nigra are not well documented, except for a descending pathway from the globus pallidus (pallidonigral pathway) containing gamma aminobutyric acid as neurotransmitter. There also may be a striatonigral cholinergic pathway. Other reciprocal connections exist between the striatum and the subthalamus and between the prerubral nucleus and the mesencephalon (part of which contains 5-hydroxytryptamine as neurotransmitter).

From this simplified outline it is clear that drugs that influence cholinergic and dopaminergic systems would be expected to have an influence on motor control as effected by the basal ganglia, and it is not surprising that such effects are antagonistic.

B. **Drug-induced extrapyramidal syndrome.** With the introduction of the phenothiazines, drug-induced extrapyramidal symptoms (EPS) became common. Phenothiazines and other more recently developed antipsychotic drugs act primarily as dopamine-receptor blockers in the treatment of psychotic disorders and produce many of the drug-induced EPS. The **abnormal movements** produced include:

1. **Acute idiosyncratic dyskinesias and dystonia** occurring within the first few days of treatment may be reversed by stopping treatment. **Acute dystonia** can be treated with a parenteral anticholinergic agent, such as benztropine (Cogentin) 1 mg IM or IV or with diphenhydramine (Benadryl) 50 mg IV.

2. **Dose-related akinesia, rigidity,** and **tremor** (3–5 cycles per second) typical of parkinsonism can occur after a few days of treatment, and usually occur within the first month. This activity may be **reversed** by:

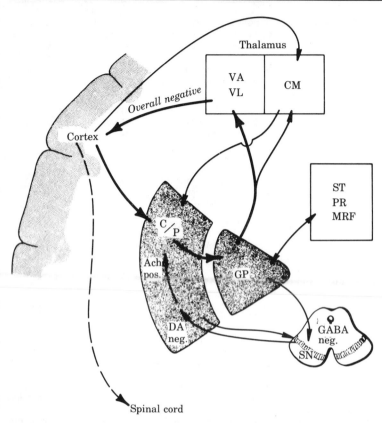

Fig. 15-3. Simplified outline of connections within the basal ganglia. C/P, caudate, putamen; CM, nucleus centromedianum of thalamus; GP, globus pallidus; MRF, mesencephalic reticular formation; PR, prerubral nucleus; SN, substantia nigra; ST, subthalamus; VA, ventroanterior nucleus of thalamus; VL, ventrolateral nucleus of thalamus. Presumptive neurotransmitters; DA, dopamine; Ach, acetylcholine; GABA, gamma-aminobutyric acid.

    a. **Decreasing the antipsychotic drug dosage.**

    b. **Adding anticholinergics:**

        (1) Benztropine (Cogentin) 0.5–4.0 mg BID.

        (2) Biperiden (Akineton) 1.0–2.0 mg TID.

        (3) Trihexyphenidyl HCl (Artane) 1–5 mg TID.

        The half-life of these drugs is benztropine > biperiden > trihexyphenidyl HCl.

        (4) These anticholinergics may partially **reverse the antipsychotic effects** of the primary drug. They are not necessary for all patients and are rarely required for more than 2 or 3 months. There is **no indication for prophylactic use** of anticholinergic agents when using antipsychotic drugs.

Table 15-2. Severity of Induced Parkinsonism with Commonly Used Antipsychotic Drugs

Types of Phenothiazines	Drugs	Relative Severity
Aliphatic	Chlorpromazine (Thorazine)	+ +
Piperidines	Thioridazine (Mellaril)	+
Piperazines	Perphenazine (Trilafon)	+ + +
	Trifluoperazine (Stelazine)	+ + +
	Fluphenazine (Prolixin)	+ + +
Thioxanthenes	Chlorprothixene (Taractan)	+ +
	Thiothixene (Navane)	+ +
Butyrophenones	Haloperidol (Haldol)	+ + +

3. **Akathisia** is another side effect of antipsychotic drugs that occurs during the first few weeks of treatment. The term refers to the restlessness seen in these patients: they are literally unable to sit still. The etiology is obscure, and the treatment is that for the parkinsonism state (see sec **IV.D.3**).

4. **The so-called tardive (late) dyskinesias** include facial and limb chorea, athetosis, and dystonia.

   a. **Mechanism.** L-dopa–induced dyskinesias are probably secondary to increased dopamine receptor activity induced by L-dopa or an L-dopa metabolite. For the tardive dyskinesias, a similar mechanism of **dopamine receptor overactivity** is presumed. It may be dopamine receptor hypersensitivity or breakthrough of hyperactive nigrostriatal feedback mechanisms, or it may be related to false transmitter production.

   b. **Treatment** of tardive dyskinesias depends on either stimulating the cholinergic mechanism or decreasing dopamine transmitter content, since often the involuntary movements of the tardive dyskinesias are restricted to movements involving the head and neck, such as head-turning and bobbing, and buccolingual movements, such as chewing and tongue-thrusting. (Further dopamine receptor blockade achieved by increasing the dose of antipsychotic drug may help this disorder in the short term, but often the symptoms cannot be controlled adequately in this way, and eventual dose reduction becomes necessary.)

     The **symptoms may fluctuate** and take months or years to resolve. It is said that 40% are reversible within 15 months, but some may never resolve. Treatment is difficult, and many medicines have been advocated.

    (1) **Reserpine** (Serpasil), starting with 0.5 mg daily, or tetrabenazine (a reserpinelike synthetic drug not currently available in the United States.)

    (2) **Choline** or **lecithin,** given in increasing oral dosage to a maximum of several grams per day.

    (3) **Deanol** (Deaner), 100 mg TID, increasing to 1000 mg daily. There is some evidence that if a single dose of parenteral physostigmine (1 mg IV) improves the condition, an even better response to deanol may be anticipated.

    (4) Other drugs said to be useful include cyproheptadine HCl (Periactin) and methyldopa (Aldomet).

C. **Idiopathic dyskinesias.** There is a group of idiopathic dyskinesias that appear to mimic the movements induced by drugs (e.g., spasmodic torticollis and retrocollis, and blepharospasm). Also grouped with these disorders, for diagnostic convenience, are other local muscle spasms, tics, and writer's cramp. It is fortunate that many of these problems may not require treatment, as therapy is limited in scope and success.

The most dramatic tic is that of **Gilles de la Tourette syndrome.** A tic may be defined as a quick, coordinated, repetitive movement, in contrast to the irregular and nonrepetitive quasi-purposeful jerky movements of chorea. In the Gilles de la Tourette syndrome tics are first noted between the ages of 2 and 13 years and intermittently worsen during the life of the individual. These patients may develop echolalia and—in about half the cases—uncontrolled use of offensive language (coprolalia).

Haloperidol (Haldol) is the **treatment** of choice; however, success is limited by the frequent side effects of drug treatment. The starting dose is 0.5 mg TID; the maximum dose, determined by observation of the onset of side effects (e.g., sedation, hypotension, and parkinsonism), is usually between 8 and 16 mg QID. There have been rare reports of leukopenia.

In disease presenting with **intermittent spasm,** diazepam, anticholinergics, and alcohol may be tried. Tetrabenazine, haloperidol, and lithium carbonate have been reported to be useful. Behavior modification techniques have been used. Thalamotomy is probably of little benefit. Often the **final treatment** is production of a lesion of the lower motor neuron outflow tract, for example, in spasmodic torticollis, section of the spinal accessory fibers and intradural section of C1-3 anterior roots.

D. Parkinson's disease. The classic diseases that illustrate disordered function of the basal ganglia are Parkinson's disease and Huntington's chorea (see sec **IV.E**). It is useful to consider these diseases in the context of the drug-induced effects described previously.

    1. Clinical description. Parkinson's disease is a movement disorder characterized by the slow development of **decreased voluntary movements** (akinesia), **abnormal tone,** and **involuntary movements.** Poverty of voluntary movements is noted particularly in the initiation of movements such as walking and rolling over in bed. Patients have decreased facial expression, monotonous speech, and decreased blinking. The gait is shuffling, with poor arm swing and reduced postural balance. The abnormal tone is referred to as *cogwheel rigidity.* Most characteristic and easily recognized early, however, is the asymmetric, coarse (3–7 cycles per second) resting tremor known as "pill-rolling." A later development is a symmetric action tremor at 7–12 cycles per second.

    Other features of Parkinson's disease include increased sweating and salivation. The presence of oculogyric crises is associated with postencephalitic Parkinson's disease and antipsychotic drug ingestion. It is often difficult to decide whether there is a concurrent dementia (more common in long-term patients), because of the difficulty with communication (see Chap. 3). Major long-term disabilities may include increasing postural instability and unusual breathing patterns.

    2. Differential diagnosis (Table 15-3)

        a. Common features. The differential diagnosis is usually not a problem in the 50 to 60-year-old person with slow onset of the typical features. A history of encephalitis lethargica between 1919 and 1926 is always difficult to document and rarely a cause of new disease. Neurofibrillary tangles are the characteristic neuropathologic finding of this postencephalitic disease. The more **usual pathology** is idiopathic degeneration of the substantia nigra and other pigmented brainstem nuclei, with the formation of Lewy bodies in affected areas. Whether the disease is a generalized body defect is currently being investigated.

        b. Other lesions and diseases. Atherosclerosis and syphilis are difficult to

Table 15-3. Differential Diagnosis of the Major Movement Disorders

Parkinsonism	Parkinsonism or Choreoathetosis	Choreoathetosis
Primary degenerative diseases Parkinson's disease Progressive supranuclear palsy Parkinson-dementia syndrome of Guam Shy-Drager syndrome Striato-nigral degeneration	Primary degenerative disease Childhood Huntington's chorea	Primary degenerative diseases Adult Huntington's chorea Pelizaeus-Merzbacher disease
Secondary to drugs or poisons Phenothiazine treatment (initial) Poisons (e.g., CO, cyanide, manganese)	Secondary to other processes Infection (e.g., encephalitis, syphilis) Metabolic (e.g., Wilson's disease, Fahr's disease, hypoparathyroidism, pseudohypoparathyroidism, Hallervorden-Spatz disease)	Secondary to drugs, poisons, or other processes Phenothiazine treatment (late) Anticonvulsant toxicity, L-dopa toxicity, poisons (e.g., mercury), thyrotoxicosis, vascular disease, kernicterus, Sydenham's chorea, Lesch-Nyhan syndrome

substantiate as the cause, and tumor must be extremely rare. Some cases of late-onset Huntington's chorea may be confused with Parkinson's disease, but these rarely present with rigidity, whereas the childhood form of Huntington's chorea may present with akinesia and rigidity. Other causes of parkinsonism, such as drug ingestion, carbon monoxide, cyanide, and manganese poisoning, are usually obvious. Striatonigral degeneration is rare and can be diagnosed only at autopsy. Other diseases in the differential diagnosis, those that may present with either parkinsonism or choreoathetosis (Wilson's disease, Fahr's disease, and Hallervorden-Spatz disease), usually present at a younger age and are discussed in sec **IV.F.**

    c. Associated syndromes. Association of a parkinsonlike state with the failure of conjugate upward gaze and dementia is known as **progressive supranuclear palsy** or **Steele-Richardson-Olszewski syndrome.** An association with dementia is also observed in the parkinsonism-dementia syndrome of Guam. Postural hypotension and other autonomic dysfunction may be also associated with a parkinsonism-type presentation in the Shy-Drager syndrome; the postural hypotension associated with this condition may be helped with 9-fluoro-cortisone (Florinef), 0.2–1.0 mg QID, as well as more standard measures used to treat the condition in other disease states.

3. Treatment. Treatment of Parkinson's disease is based on considerations of the dopaminergic-cholinergic balance discussed in **IV.B.** The object is either (1) to increase available dopamine or dopamine agonist at the cholinergic site in the neostriatum or (2) to reduce cholinergic activity with anticholinergic agents.

    a. Anticholinergics. Anticholinergics are thought by some to be useful early in the disease, when tremor is the most prominent problem. Commonly used agents include:

    (1) Ethopropazine (Parsidol), 10–20 mg TID.

    (2) Benztropine (Cogentin), 0.5–4.0 mg BID.

    (3) Biperiden (Akineton), 1.0–2.0 mg TID.

    (4) Trihexyphenidyl HCl (Artane), 1–5 mg TID.

    The **maximum dose** of these agents is determined by observation of the onset of side effects. The dosage is gradually increased to the tolerated maximum listed; for example, it may be possible to give up to 400 mg of ethopropazine daily. Common, well-tolerated **side effects** of anticholinergic drugs include dry mouth, blurred vision, and dizziness. Other, often serious, side effects are a toxic psychosis, constipation, urinary retention, and precipitation of glaucoma.

    b. L-dopa 2–8 gm daily administered in divided doses after meals, is best used for **akinesia.** The patient can usually start with 1 gm daily, and the dose is increased every few days until optimal control is attained. The most common side effects are nausea and vomiting; trimethobenzamide HCl (Tigan), 250 mg TID, may be useful in this situation.

    (1) Concurrent therapy. The concurrent use of a **peripheral decarboxylase inhibitor,** Carbidopa, has allowed reduction of the L-dopa dose to avoid peripheral side effects. In combination, begin the use of L-dopa 100 mg together with Carbidopa 10 mg (Sinemet 100/10) TID. Using Sinemet 250/25 tablets, increase dosage to a maximum of 2 gm of L-dopa over a period of approximately 1 month.

(2) Response to therapy. Approximately **80% of patients are improved** more than 25% by L-dopa therapy, but there appears to be no way to predict the response to therapy. Long-term studies suggest that there is a falloff in benefit from L-dopa after the first two or three years of treatment, such that after five years, about 60% of patients are more than 25% above their initial baseline. Nevertheless, **long-term treatment reduces mortality,** although the concomitant **effects on mentation** are not established. There are data suggesting that the patients who show the best initial improvement are those most likely to develop late side effects, such as the dose-related dyskinesias.

(3) Dose-related effects. Overdose of L-dopa results in dyskinesias as discussed in sec **B.4. Other side effects** include dysphonia, dry mouth, blurred vision, postural hypotension, agitation and confusion, gout, and, in rare cases, myocardial ischemia and psychosis. Most dose-related effects (including therapeutic effects) are **readily reversed** within days by stopping the drug, decreasing its dose, or giving vitamin B_6, 20 mg PO, which has an even more rapid effect. (Obviously, vitamin supplementation in patients receiving L-dopa therapy *should not* contain vitamin B_6, e.g., Larobec (2 tablets daily). This caution does not apply to patients taking Sinemet, however.

L-dopa–induced **dyskinesias** also may be controlled with deanol (Deaner) 100 mg TID, increasing to a maximum of 900 mg QID over 1 week.

(4) The **"on-off" phenomenon** is another complication of L-dopa therapy; it does not appear to be dose-related, but rather becomes more likely to occur with extended duration of therapy. This disability occurs in about 50% of patients treated for 5 or more years, who are generally those with relatively severe disease who tend to have late-onset dyskinesias. It consists of **periods of severe akinesia, hypotonia,** and **apprehension,** of rapid onset and termination, which last from 30 minutes to a few hours and are **unrelieved by further doses of L-dopa.** The **cause is unknown,** although "off" episodes have been correlated with low plasma concentrations of L-dopa. There is some evidence that fluctuation in L-dopa effectiveness may be related to direct absorption of the drug. Therapy is difficult, but increasing the frequency of L-dopa administration, using Sinemet rather than L-dopa alone, and restricting dietary intake of protein to 0.5 g/kg/day may help.

(5) Contraindications. The contraindications to L-dopa therapy are relatively few. They include **narrow-angle glaucoma** (most glaucoma cases are of the chronic, wide-angle type) and concurrent **use of monoamine oxidase inhibitors. Caution** should be used in patients who have arrhythmias or evidence of endocrine disease, or if surgery is planned.

c. Amantadine hydrochloride (Symmetrel) 100 mg daily, increasing to 100 mg BID, has also been found to be helpful in the treatment of Parkinson's disease. The benefit obtained is occasionally short-lived. **Intermittent use** has been advocated. The drug may act by increasing dopamine release at the synapse in the neostriatum. Prominent **side effects** include depression, congestive cardiac failure, pedal edema, and urinary retention. The drug is excreted unmetabolized in the urine.

d. Other drugs that cause release of endogenous dopamine at the receptor site include **amphetamines**—these have been said to have some beneficial effect in disabled patients and, in decades past, the treatment of oculogyric crises. For action tremor, a common accompaniment of Parkinson's disease, the treatment is **propranolol** (Inderal). Other new dopamine receptor agonists are currently under investigation: *bromocriptine* (an ergot alkaloid) may help by reducing the need for high-dose L-dopa, and **piribedil** (a piperazine derivative) also may reduce high-dose L-dopa requirements but has been considered too toxic for clinical use.

e. **Surgery.** **Ventrolateral thalamotomy** may be useful in patients with severe unilateral tremor, not controlled with drugs, who have the intellectual capacity for gainful employment. Bilateral thalamotomy has led to severe speech defects.

E. Huntington's chorea

1. **Clinical description. Huntington's chorea** is an inherited, autosomal dominant, dementing disease in which, in adult-onset cases, the associated movement disorder typifies relative overactivity of the dopaminergic system. Hypotonia is a frequent concomitant of chorea.

   Chorea and athetosis may be considered together, as the two commonly coexist in this and in other extrapyramidal syndromes. Severe chorea is virtually indistinguishable from athetosis, and there does not appear to be a distinct anatomic substrate for each involuntary movement. **Chorea** refers to rapid, jerky, semi-purposive movement, usually of the extremities; **athetosis** is used to describe slower, less purposeful, and continuous sinuous movements.

   L-dopa 1 mg/day, given PO or IV, has been suggested as a **provocative test** for producing chorea in persons at risk for developing the disease. However, the widespread pathology in the disorder does not clearly indicate the anatomic site where this induced effect might occur. Indeed, loss of the substrate of the caudate nucleus as a major manifestation might suggest loss of aminergic and cholinergic influences. However, dysfunction of other affected sites in the thalamus and brainstem are probably integral to the production of the movement disorder. Recent biochemical and anatomic data suggest that, while dopamine content of the striatum is normal, acetylcholine manufacture and the GABA inhibitory system are deficient and probably contribute to the chorea. Thus, the **site of action** for producing relative overactivity in the dopaminergic system may be loss of a descending inhibitory GABA influence on dendrites of the pigmented neurons of the substantia nigra.

2. **Differential diagnosis** (see Table 15-3). Other affections of the basal ganglia that may result in similar movements are **mercury poisoning, Sydenham's chorea of acute rheumatic fever, thyrotoxicosis, posthemiplegic athetosis, Lesch-Nyhan syndrome** in childhood, senile chorea, and diseases that may present as parkinsonism or choreoathetosis (see sec IV.F.). **Management** of these movement disorders is the same, in principle, as for Huntington's chorea.

3. **Treatment. Pharmacologic treatment** with dopamine receptor blockade is helpful in the early stages of Huntington's chorea.

   a. **Haloperidol** (Haldol), 1–4 mg QID.

   b. **Chlorpromazine** (Thorazine), 50 mg TID.

   c. **Tetrabenazine** (Nitoman), which depletes central aminergic stores much as reserpine does, also may be effective. The **maximum dose** is about 200 mg daily, increased slowly over several weeks from 25 mg BID. Drowsiness, depression, and extrapyramidal symptoms are common **side effects.** This drug is not yet commercially available in the U.S.

   d. **Propranolol** (Inderal), in high dosage, may be useful for action tremor, which may be a component of the disorder.

F. **Diseases presenting with parkinsonism or choreoathetosis.** There is **a group of**

uncommon diseases that may present with either choreoathetosis or parkinsonism as the primary movement disorder. At post mortem these diseases demonstrate widespread pathology in the basal ganglia, usually in a distribution that does not clearly implicate any of the specific connections previously discussed. These diseases should be considered in the differential diagnosis of any patient presenting with either parkinsonism or choreoathetosis (the onset is generally at a younger age than for Parkinson's disease).

Management is treatment of the underlying disease as well as of the movement disorder. However, it is intuitively apparent that parkinsonism secondary to a lesion of the neostriatum is unlikely to respond to L-dopa therapy if the postsynaptic elements for neurotransmission in that system have been destroyed by the disease process.

1. Wilson's disease

a. **Clinical description.** Wilson's disease is a rare, inherited, autosomal recessive disorder with onset between the ages of 10 and 40. It is characterized by progressive liver and neurologic disease, Kayser-Fleischer rings of the cornea, and occasional renal dysfunction.

(1) The **neurologic presentation** has been subdivided into two major categories. The **younger patients** have a rapid progression of either athetosis or of rigidity and dystonia. Myoclonus can also occur, and this form of the disease is more difficult to treat. **Adults** are more likely to have a more benign course, with tremor (action and intention); dysarthria, which may have spastic, cerebellar, and hypokinetic components; and dysphagia as prominent symptoms. This form of the disease is more amenable to treatment. **Asterixis** (see sec **VI**) may occur concomitant with progressive hepatic dysfunction.

b. The **diagnosis** is established by documenting the Kayser-Fleischer ring by slit-lamp examination, establishing disordered liver function, and evaluation of copper metabolism. Useful screening tests include decreased levels of serum copper and ceruloplasmin as well as increased urinary excretion of copper. Liver biopsy may help to establish cirrhosis and an increased liver copper concentration. Heterozygotes are best defined by measurement over several days of fecal excretion of intravenously administered radioactively labeled copper.

c. **Treatment**

(1) D-penicillamine (Cuprimine), 0.5 gm TID, retards the progression of the disease in most patients with the late-onset form. Medication is continued for life, but dosage may be reduced during pregnancy. Toxic reactions are more common with doses exceeding 2 gm/day. Acute sensitivity reactions occur in one-third of patients. Reported **side effects** are nausea and vomiting, rashes, adenopathy, arthralgia and leukopenia, and thrombocytopenia. The nephrotic syndrome and optic neuropathy have been reported following treatment with the *dl*-isomer; optic neuropathy may improve with pyridoxine 100 mg daily. Acute sensitivity responses can be treated with corticosteroids. A recently documented side effect is Goodpasture's syndrome.

(2) A **diet low in copper** (less than 1.5 mg/day) may decrease the requirement for penicillamine.

(3) **Triethylenetetramine dihydrochloride** has been suggested for use in patients with serious toxic reactions to penicillamine.

(4) **Treatment of metabolic acidosis** may help the neurologic disease in those patients with renal tubular acidosis.

(5) **Symptomatic treatment of the movement disorder** is outlined in sec **IV. D.** and **E.**

2. **Calcification of the basal ganglia and dentate nucleus** commonly occurs in the elderly and may account in part for the frequency of mild abnormal movements in that population. **When calcium deposition is severe,** a major progressive movement disorder may result that presents as either parkinsonism or choreoathetosis.

   a. The **differential diagnosis** depends on the history and examination, as well as on evaluation of the chemical data outlined in Table 15-4. In the presence of hypocalcemia, such as in postsurgical hypoparathyroidism, idiopathic hypoparathyroidism, or pseudohypoparathyroidism, the progress of the movement disorder appears to be arrested by restoring serum levels to the normal range by use of vitamin D, 50,000 to 100,000 units per day, and calcium supplements.

   b. **Management. Serum chemistries** should be monitored regularly to avoid vitamin D intoxication. Regression of the movement disorder is rare except, perhaps, in idiopathic hypoparathyroidism. In striopallidodentate pseudocalcification **(Fahr's disease),** the serum chemistries are normal, and no treatment is available. Calcification also occurs rarely in hyperparathyroidism and pseudopseudohypoparathyroidism (normocalcemic pseudohypoparathyroidism).

3. **Hallervorden-Spatz disease.** In Hallervorden-Spatz disease iron-containing pigments are deposited in the globus pallidus and pars reticularis of the substantia nigra. **The disease presents in childhood** as progressive parkinsonism or choreoathetosis and occasionally with other motor control system abnormalities. Iron-chelating agents are not useful in reversing the pigmentary deposits. The **movement disorder is treated** as outlined in sec **IV.D** and **E,** above.

G. **Dystonia,** as applied to a fixed postural rigidity, may be considered the end point of most of the diseases that affect the basal ganglia. The prototypical disease that produces the picture of truncal dystonia, which is more like axial athetosis, is **dystonia musculorum deformans.** The best **treatment** appears to be ventrolateral thalamotomy. L-dopa has been used to good effect in some familial cases with an autosomal dominant inheritance pattern, and in cases due to manganese poisoning.

H. **Hemiballismus.** The **flinging rotatory movements** of hemiballismus arise following lesions of the subthalamus—usually hemorrhage. Even without therapy the symptoms often resolve considerably over a few weeks. **Initial pharmacologic approaches** include reserpine or tetrabenazine for the acute disability; phenothiazines; and haloperidol (Haldol). However, the most effective treatment for chronic hemiballismus is probably ventrolateral thalamotomy.

V. TREMOR

A. **Description.** Tremor may be defined as *involuntary regular and repetitive shaking of a body part around a fixed point.* The anatomic substrate of most tremors is not known, although progress has been made in physiologic classification.

B. **Classification.** Tremors may be classified according to the following criteria:

   1. Distribution.

   2. Rate.

   3. Amplitude.

   4. Relationship to voluntary movement, i.e., tremor at rest, tremor with sustained posture (action tremor), or intention tremor.

C. **Action tremor**

   1. **Description.** The most common group of tremors to be managed are **action tremors,** which are usually of high frequency (7–12 cycles/sec) and low am-

Table 15-4. Differential Diagnosis of Calcification in the Basal Ganglia

Disease	Frequency of Disease of Basal Ganglia	Chemical Data			Urine Cyclic AMP to PTH Infusion	General
		Ca	Phosphorus	PTH		
Hypoparathyroidism	Uncommon	↓	↑	↓	↑	Postsurgical effects take 15 yr
Pseudohypoparathyroidism	Half of cases	↓	↑	N or ↑	0	Characteristic facies, extremities, and stature
Pseudopseudo-hypoparathyroidism	Rare	N	N	N	↑	Characteristic facies, extremities, and stature
Hyperparathyroidism	Very rare	↑	↓ or N	↑	—	Chemistries vary with renal impairment
Fahr's disease	Always (required for diagnosis)	N	N	N	—	

↑ = Increased   ↓ = Decreased   N = Normal   PTH = parathormone.

Table 15-5. Drugs Commonly Used for Movement Disorders

Drug	Availability	Frequency of Administration	Comments
Amantadine HCl (Symmetrel)	100 mg capsules	BID	Excreted unchanged in urine; initial effect reached 48 hr after administration; half-life, 2–4 hr; adjunct to main therapy; initial dose 100 mg daily
Baclofen (Lioresal)	10 mg tablets	TID	Begin with 10 mg daily and gradually increase to 30–100 mg daily
Benztropine mesylate (Cogentin)	0.5, 1.0 and 2.0 mg tablets; injectable, 1 mg/ml	BID	Initial effect of PO dose requires 24 hr; if given parenterally, effect takes only minutes; cumulative action; initial dose 0.5 mg BID; half-life, 12–24 hr
Biperiden (Akinetin)	2.0 mg tablets; injectable, 5 mg/ml	TID	Initial effect of PO dose requires 24 hr; if given parenterally, effect takes 1 hr; cumulative action
Clonazepam (Clonopin)	0.5, 1.0, and 2.0 mg tablets	TID	Begin with 0.5 mg TID, increase gradually to maintenance dose of about 6 mg daily
Dantrolene Na⁺ (Dantrium)	25, 50, 75, and 100 mg capsules	BID to QID	Watch for hepatotoxicity; half-life, 9 hr; start with 25 mg BID, slowly increase dosage
Deanol Acetamidobenzoate (Deaner)	25 and 100 mg tablets	TID	Slowly increase dosage over 3 weeks, to maximum of 1 gm

336

Drug	Preparations	Frequency	Comments
Diazepam (Valium)	2, 5, and 10 mg tablets; injectable, 5 mg/ml	BID to QID	High dose needed for muscle relaxation
L-Dopa (Dopar, Larodopa)	100, 250, and 500 mg capsules and tablets	QID or more often	Half-life less than 2 hr; cumulative action; start with 250 mg TID after meals
L-Dopa with carbidopa (Sinemet)	100/10-mg tablets 250/25-mg tablets	TID	Supplements of carbidopa or L-dopa may be needed
Ethopropazine (Parsidol)	10, 50, and 100 mg tablets	TID or QID	Initial effect requires 24 hr; cumulative action; start with 10 mg TID
Haloperidol (Haldol)	0.5, 1, 2, 5, and 10 mg tablets Injectable 5 mg/ml	TID or QID	5-day half-life; hepatic toxicity; start with lowest dose
D-Penicillamine (Cuprimine)	500 mg tablets	TID	Dose kept under 2 gm to avoid toxicity
Propranolol HCl (Inderal)	10, 40, and 80 mg tablets	TID to QID	Onset of effect within 30 min; half-life 3 hr; hepatic toxicity; start with 20 mg TID
Reserpine (Serpasil)	0.1, 0.25, and 1.0 mg tablets; 0.05 mg/ml elixir	QD	Several days for initial effect; start with 0.5 mg daily
Trihexyphenidyl HCl (Artane)	2.0 and 5.0 mg tablets; 0.4 mg/ml elixir; 5 mg sustained-release capsules	TID for tablets and elixir; QD or BID for sustained-release capsules	Initial effect requires 24 hr; half-life 6–12 hr; cumulative action; start with 1 mg TID

plitude. They may be asymmetric. Such a tremor may be induced in normal individuals under appropriate postural conditions, such as movements requiring extremes of precision or power. The tremor is increased in states of fatigue, anxiety, weakness, hypercapnia, drug withdrawal, and some metabolic and endocrine conditions (hypoglycemia, uremia, severe hepatic disease, and thyrotoxicosis). It may be familial. When it first appears in the elderly it is known as *senile tremor*. Otherwise, if there is no demonstrable cause, it is known as *essential tremor*.

2. **Mechanism.** The anatomic substrate of action tremor is not clear. It appears that peripheral mechanisms are involved in the genesis of both physiologic action tremor and that associated with thyrotoxicosis. In addition, central mechanisms are also involved in essential, familial, and senile tremor. Tricyclic antidepressants, lithium carbonate, and phenothiazines may produce or increase essential tremor.

3. **Management,** as with all tremors, involves distinguishing of factors that may underlie the tremor and their treatment with appropriate drugs.

D. **Treatment**

1. **Tranquilizers** may be used for anxiety-induced tremors: diazepam (Valium), 6–15 mg daily, in divided doses.

2. A single dose of **alcohol** will reduce an action tremor for 3–4 hours; its therapeutic effect begins within 10 minutes of ingestion.

3. **Propranolol** (Inderal), 60–240 mg daily in divided doses, usually will reduce action tremors within 48 hours of initiation of treatment. A useful starting dose is 20 mg TID. However, propranolol is **contraindicated** in asthma and insulin-dependent diabetes, and **side effects** include congestive cardiac failure, intensification of AV heart block, and bradycardia. Other side effects include hypotension, nausea, diarrhea, insomnia, and hallucinations.

4. **Ventrolateral thalamotomy** has been of benefit in severe action tremor and in congenital rubral and cerebellar intention tremor of the limbs, but not in head tremors.

VI. **ASTERIXIS.** Asterixis may be considered a **variant of tremor** in which the rate of limb flexion and extension is irregular and usually slow. The EMG data indicate that this disorder arises from temporary loss of tone in the outstretched limb. The anatomic substrate is unknown. The disorder arises in metabolic diseases (renal and hepatic), in pulmonary disease, and in Wilson's disease. **Treatment** is that of the underlying disorder.

VII. **MYOCLONUS**

A. **Definition and description.** The term *myoclonus* refers to the rapid, irregular, jerking movements familiar to everyone as "night start," which interrupts the steady drift into sleep. The anatomic substrate for myoclonus is not known, but aminergic mechanisms have been implicated. Physiologically it often appears to be temporally related to an epileptiform slow wave on the EEG. The myoclonic jerk is followed by a transient inhibition of normal postural mechanisms. Myoclonus has many causes and is characterized (1) by **brief shocklike contractions,** resembling the EMG of the tendon jerk and the EMG of a normal muscle contraction, and (2) by **stimuli** that induce the myoclonus. For example, intention myoclonus is found in patients with hypoxic brain damage. This type has brief shocklike contractions.

B. **Treatment. Treatable causes** of myoclonus include toxoplasmosis, neuroblastoma, thallium poisoning, uremia, hepatic encephalopathy, and drug intoxications (imipramine, penicillin, L-dopa, and piperazines). Unfortunately, **specific treatment** of myoclonus is generally unsatisfactory. Occasionally effective drugs include:

1. **Clonazepam** (Clonopin), 7–12 mg daily in divided doses, starting with 1.5 mg daily and increasing over four weeks, may be useful.

2. **5-hydroxytryptophan,** 150–400 mg PO daily divided into 2–4 doses with and without carbidopa, has been used in the treatment of myoclonus with some success. Gastrointestinal upset is a common problem but can frequently be managed with antiemetics.

SUGGESTED READING

Anatomy and Physiology of Normal Movement
Brodal, A. *Neurological Anatomy in Relation to Clinical Medicine,* 2nd ed. New York: Oxford University Press, 1969.
Lance, J. W., and McLeod, J. G. *A Physiological Approach to Clinical Neurology,* 2nd ed. London: Butterworth, 1975.

Spasticity
Cohan, S. L., Anderson, R. J., and Raines, A. Diphenylhydantoin and chlorpromazine in the treatment of spasticity. (Abstr.) *Neurology* (Minneap.) 26:367, 1976.
Duncan, G. W., Shahani, B. T., and Young, R. R. An evaluation of baclofen treatment for certain symptoms in patients with spinal cord lesions: a double-blind cross-over study. *Neurology* (Minneap.) 26:441, 1976.
Gelenberg, A. J., and Poskanzer, D. C. The effect of dantrolene sodium on spasticity in multiple sclerosis. *Neurology* (Minneap.) 23:1313, 1973.
Nathan, P. W. Chemical rhizotomy for relief of spasticity in ambulant patients. *Br. Med. J.* 1:1096, 1965.
Schmidt, R. T., Stahl, S. M., and Spehlmann, R. A pharmacologic study of the stiff-man syndrome. Correlation of clinical symptoms with urinary 3-methoxy-4-hydroxy phenyl glycol excretion. *Neurology* (Minneap.) 25:622, 1975.

Cerebellar Dysfunction
Meyers, R. *Handbook of Clinical Neurology,* Vol. 6, *Diseases of the Basal Ganglia.* Amsterdam: North Holland Publishing Co., 1968. Pp. 844–878.

Basal Ganglia Anatomy and Physiology
Hattori, T., Singh, V. K., McGeer, E. G., and McGeer, P. L. Immunohistochemical localization of choline acetyltransferase containing neostriatal neurons and their relationship with dopaminergic synapses. *Brain Res.* 102:164, 1976.
Kanazawa, I., and Toyokura, Y. Topographical study of the distribution of gamma-amino butyric acid (GABA) in the human substantia nigra. A case study. *Brain Res.* 100:371, 1975.

Drug-induced Extra-pyramidal Syndromes
Coleman, J. H., and Hayes, P. E. Drug induced extrapyramidal effects. A review. *Dis. Nerv. Syst.* 36:591, 1975.
Davis, K. L., Berger, P. A., and Hollister, L. E. Choline for tardive dyskinesia. *N. Engl. J. Med.* 293:152, 1975.
DeSilva, L., and Huang, C. Y. Deanol in tardive dyskinesia. *Br. Med. J.* 3:466, 1975.
Kobayashi, R. M. Drug therapy of tardive dyskinesia. *N. Engl. J. Med.* 296:257, 1977.
Neurologic syndromes associated with antipsychotic drug use. *N. Engl. J. Med.* 289:20, 1973.

Idiopathic Dyskinesias
Cleeland, C. S. Behavioural technics in the modifications of spasmodic torticollis. *Neurology* (Minneap.) 23:1241, 1973.
Couper-Smart, J. Lithium in spasmodic torticollis. *Lancet* 2:741, 1973.
Hankinson, J. Surgery of dyskinesias. *Proc. R. Soc. Med.* 66:876, 1973.
Shapiro, A. K., Shapiro, E., and Wayne, H. Treatment of Tourette's syndrome with haloperidol, review of 34 cases. *Arch. Gen. Psychiatry* 28:92, 1973.

Parkinson's Disease

Barbeau, A.   Potentiation of levodopa effect by intravenous 1-prolyl-1-leucyl-glycine amide in man. *Lancet* 2:683, 1975.

Barbeau, A., Campanella, G., Butterworth, R. F., and Yamada, K.   Uptake and efflux of ^{14}C-dopamine in platelets: evidence for a generalized defect in Parkinson's disease. *Neurology* (Minneap.) 25:1, 1975.

Bauer, R. B., and McHenry, J. T.   Comparison of amantadine, placebo, and levodopa in Parkinson's disease. *Neurology* (Minneap.) 24:715, 1974.

Callaghan, N., Fitzpatrick, E., and O'Mahony, J. B.   Piribedil (ET-495) in the treatment of Parkinson's disease combined with amantadine or levodopa. *Acta Neurol. Scand.* 52:179, 1975.

Hohol, R. D., Frame, B., and Schatz, I. J.   The Shy-Drager variant of idiopathic orthostatic hypotension. *Am. J. Med.* 39:134, 1965.

Hornykiewicz, O.   Parkinson's disease: from brain homogenate to treatment. *Fed. Proc.* 32:183, 1973.

Lieberman, A., Miyamoto, T., Battista, A. F., and Goldstein, M.   Studies on the antiparkinsonian efficacy of lergotrile. *Neurology* (Minneap.) 25:459, 1975.

Mawdsley, C.   Parkinson's Disease, in *Recent Advances in Clinical Neurology*, W. B. Matthews (Ed.). Edinburgh: Livingstone, 1975. Pp. 118–162.

Mena, I., and Cotzias, G. C.   Protein intake and treatment of Parkinson's disease with levodopa. *N. Engl. J. Med.* 292:181, 1975.

Parkes, J. D., Tarsy, D., Marsden, C. D., Boyill, K. T., Phipps, J. A., and Rose, P.   Amphetamines in the treatment of Parkinson's disease. *J. Neurol. Neurosurg. Psychiatry* 38:232, 1975.

Shy, G. M., and Drager, G. A.   A neurologic syndrome associated with orthostatic hypotension: a clinico-pathological study. *Arch. Neurol.* 2:511, 1961.

Sweet, R. D., and McDowell, F. H.   Plasma dopa levels and the "on-off effect" in Parkinson's disease. *Neurology* (Minneap.) 24:953, 1974.

Sweet, R. D., and McDowell, F. H.   Five years' treatment of Parkinson's disease with levodopa. Therapeutic results and survival of 100 patients. *Ann. Intern. Med.* 83:456, 1975.

Teychenne, P. F., Leigh, P. N., Reid, J. L., Calne, D. B., Greenacre, J. K., Petrie, A., and Bamji, A. N.   Idiopathic Parkinsonism treated with bromocriptine. *Lancet* 2:473, 1975.

Yahr, M. D.   Levodopa. *Ann. Intern. Med.* 83:677, 1975.

Huntington's Chorea

Barbeau, A.   Progress in understanding Huntington's chorea. *Can. J. Neurol. Sci.* 2:81, 1975.

Hiley, C. R., and Bird, E. D.   Decreased muscarinic receptor concentration in postmortem brain in Huntington's chorea. *Brain Res.* 80:355, 1974.

Klawans, H. L., Paulson, G. W., Ringel, S. P., and Barbeau, A.   Use of L-dopa in the detection of presymptomatic Huntington's chorea. *N. Engl. J. Med.* 286:1332, 1972.

McLellan, D. L., Chalmers, R. J., and Johnson, R. H.   A double blind trial of tetrabenazine, thiopropazate and placebo in patients with chorea. *Lancet* 1:104, 1974.

Urquhart, N., Perry, T. L., Hansen, S., and Kennedy, J.   GABA content and glutamic acid decarboxylase activity in brain of Huntington's chorea patients and control subjects. *J. Neurochem.* 24:1071, 1975.

Wilson's Disease

Denny-Brown, D.   Hepatolenticular degeneration (Wilson's disease). *N. Engl. J. Med.* 270:1149, 1964.

Marecek, Z. and Graf, M.   Pregnancy in penicillamine-treated patients with Wilson's disease. *N. Engl. J. Med.* 295:841, 1976.

Strickland, G. T., and Leu, M.-L.   Wilson's disease: clinical and laboratory manifestations in 40 patients. *Medicine* (Baltimore) 54:113, 1975.

Walshe, J. M.   Copper chelation in patients with Wilson's disease. A comparison of pencillamine and triethylene tetramine dihydrochloride. *Q. J. Med.* 42:441, 1973.

Walshe, J. M.   Drugs for rare diseases. *Br. Med. J.* 3:701, 1975.

Calcification of the Basal Ganglia

Chase, L. R., Melson, G. L., and Aurbach, G. D.   Pseudo hypoparathyroidism: defective excretion of 3′5′-AMP in response to parathyroid hormone. *J. Clin. Invest.* 48:1832, 1969.

Frame, B.   Parkinsonism in postoperative hypoparathyroidism. *Arch. Intern. Med.* 166: 424, 1965.

Knuth, W. P., and Kisner, P.   Symmetrical cerebral calcification associated with parathyroid adenoma. *J.A.M.A.* 162:462, 1956.

Lowenthal, A., and Bruyn, G. W.   Calcification of the Striopallidodentate System, in *Handbook of Clinical Neurology,* Vol. 6, *Diseases of the Basal Ganglia.* P. J. Vinken and G. W. Bruyn (Eds.). Amsterdam: North Holland Publishing Co., 1968. Pp. 703–729.

McKinney, A. S.   Idiopathic hypoparathyroidism presenting as chorea. *Neurology* (Minneap.) 12:485, 1962.

Muenter, M. D., and Whisnant, J. P.   Basal ganglia calcification, hypoparathyroidism, and extrapyramidal motor manifestations. *Neurology* (Minneap.) 18:1075, 1968.

Hallervorden-Spatz Disease

Dooling, E. C., Schoene, W. C., and Richardson, E. P.   Hallervorden-Spatz syndrome. *Arch. Neurol.* 30:70, 1974.

Dystonia

de Yebenes, J. G., and Logan, W. J.   Familial dystonia musculorum deformans: response to levodopa therapy. *Neurology* (Minneap.) 25:353, 1975.

Hemiballismus

Gilbert, G. J.   Response of hemiballismus to haloperidol. *J.A.M.A.* 233:535, 1975.

Tremor

Young, R. R., Growdon, J. H., and Shahani, B. T.   Beta-adrenergic mechanisms in action tremor. *N. Engl. J. Med.* 293:950, 1975.

Myoclonus

Chadwick, D., et al.   Clinical, biochemical, and physiological features distinguishing myoclonus responsive to 5-hydroxytryptophan, tryptophan with a monamine oxidase inhibitor and clonazepam. *Brain* 100:455, 1977.

Goldberg, M. A., and Dorman, J. D.   Intention myoclonus: successful treatment with clonazepam. *Neurology* (Minneap.) 26:24, 1976.

Van Woert, M. H., and Sethy, V. H.   Therapy of intention myoclonus with L-5-hydroxytryptophan and a peripheral decarboxylase inhibitor, MK486. *Neurology* (Minneap.) 25:135, 1975.

16

Thomas M. Walshe

Diseases of Nerve and Muscle

Disorders of muscle, of the myoneural junction, of the peripheral nerve, or of the motor neuron often have specific therapy. However, when there is not a specific therapy, the treatment is aimed at controlling symptoms, retarding progression, increasing the time of remission, and improving the quality of the patient's life. Treatment plans are complex and depend on the severity and progression of the disorder.

I. **ELECTROPHYSIOLOGIC TESTS** may be useful in the diagnosis and assessment of therapy of neuromuscular disorders and, in general, are used to support the clinical data. There are four parts in the neurophysiologic evaluation of a patient with a neuromuscular disorder.

A. **Motor conduction velocity** in large myelinated fibers can be calculated by recording the time a standard current takes to produce a twitch when the distance between the stimulus and the reacting muscle is known. Thus nerves in the upper and lower extremities as well as the facial nerve can be tested.

Nerve conduction velocity may remain normal for up to 7 days following section of a nerve, and denervation changes may not appear for 10–21 days following section. Most patients with chronic polyneuropathy may have slightly reduced conduction velocity, but the reduction may be so slight that it is only in the low normal range. Neuropathies that affect myelin early (and show segmental demyelination pathologically) reduce nerve conduction velocities. Landry-Guillain-Barré syndrome, diphtheria, Charcot-Marie-Tooth disease, metachromatic leukodystrophy, and entrapments show definite slowing regularly. When the nerve is completely degenerated, there is no way to measure nerve conduction velocity.

B. **Sensory conduction time** reflects the time it takes for an evoked potential to be recorded at a site that is distal along a nerve. In the upper extremity the median and ulnar nerves are tested; in the lower extremity the sural nerve is tested. Sensory conduction time is prolonged in the segmental demyelination-type neuropathy and is slightly reduced in the other polyneuropathies.

C. **Late responses**

1. The **Hoffman reflex** (H reflex) is an electric equivalent to a deep tendon reflex. It can only be elicited in the leg in adults. A submaximal stimulus is applied to the tibial nerve, which follows the afferent nerves to the cord, where it synapses with the motor neurons and causes a direct motor response and a delayed or H-reflex response. The latency of the H reflex may be absent or prolonged in neuropathy when other conduction studies are normal. All patients with Landry-Guillain-Barré disease have an abnormal H reflex.

2. The **flexor response** (F response) can be measured in both upper and lower extremities. It is elicited by supramaximal stimulation to a nerve, so the impulses travel antidromically in the efferent parts of the nerve. There is no synapse. In normal patients the F response and the H response vary with the size of the patient. Abnormal F-response latency may occur in neuropathy even when the other studies are in the normal range.

D. **The electromyogram** (EMG) assesses the electric characteristics of muscle. Signs of denervation include fibrillations, positive sharp waves, reduced interference pattern, and polyphasic units and may support the suspicion of neurogenic disease. Primary muscle disorders have nonspecific and variable EMG patterns, usually with reduced amplitude. Myotonia and myasthenia gravis show a distinct EMG pattern, which is described in secs **VI** and **XII**.

II. MUSCLE BIOPSY is safe and may resolve a diagnostic problem, allowing correct diagnosis and treatment.

A. Indications for muscle biopsy

1. Progressive muscular atrophy.

2. Localized or diffuse inflammatory disease of muscle.

3. Systemic disease that is suspected to be vasculitis or collagen-vascular in nature.

4. Occasionally to determine the state of a muscle after injury to nerves and vessels of a limb.

5. To diagnose congenital and metabolic myopathies; histochemical stains may be useful.

B. Ideally, the neurologist responsible for making the diagnosis should be present when the biopsy is done to ensure that the correct muscle is sampled and that the sample is handled correctly. The studies to be performed are set up in advance; and the specimen is fixed in the operating room. The specimen must be suitable for light and electron microscopy as well as for histochemical stains. Muscle biopsies taken from an area tested with an EMG needle are often uninterpretable due to trauma.

III. NERVE BIOPSY is done when a specific etiology is suspected. However, the diagnosis can often be made by other means to avoid the painful dysesthesia that may occur after sural nerve biopsy.

A. Nerve biopsy may be pathognomonic in:

1. Sarcoidosis

2. Metachromatic leukodystrophy

3. Amyloidosis

4. Polyarteritis nodosa

5. Leprosy

6. Toxic and hereditary neuropathy

B. In the majority of cases of neuromuscular disease, nerve biopsy yields nonspecific information and is of limited value. Electron microscopy is essential to separate axonal degeneration from segmental demyelination.

IV. GENERAL PRINCIPLES ON THE CHRONIC USE OF CORTICOSTEROIDS. Corticosteroid therapy requires careful thought about its indications, and when it is started, it requires careful observation of the patient. The complications and adverse responses to corticosteroids are time and dose-related. Therefore long-term corticosteroid therapy is avoided unless it produces a definite advantage.

As a general rule, other therapeutic agents are tried before corticosteroids are begun. However, in neuromuscular diseases there are few choices, and a corticosteroid is often needed. Thus less hazardous agents should be used in addition to corticosteroids to allow the lowest possible dose to be given.

A. Complications of corticosteroid use. Iatrogenic Cushing's syndrome, diabetes mellitus, osteoporosis, activation of tuberculosis, hypertension, psychosis, and increased susceptibility to infection are seen in some patients treated with corticosteroids. Also, some patients treated with high doses of corticosteroid for long periods have a tendency for gastric ulceration and bleeding.

B. Considerations in stopping corticosteroid. Three problems may arise when corticosteroids are stopped.

1. **Suppression** of the adrenal gland (hypothalamic-pituitary-adrenal axis) occurs regularly when the duration of therapy is longer than 1 week, with doses equivalent to prednisone 20–30 mg/day in divided doses. Complete recovery may take up to 1 year. With doses closer to the physiologic level, suppression may not occur for a month.

   Patients who have been treated with pharmacologic doses of corticosteroids usually need no replacement therapy, but they may require steroid coverage during acute illness or other stress.

2. Steroid **withdrawal symptoms** (anorexia, nausea, vomiting, lethargy, headache, fever, arthralgia, myalgia, or weight loss) may occur following the discontinuation of chronic steroid use. Symptomatic treatment and small doses (10 mg) of cortisol for several weeks may help.

3. Acute **exacerbation** of the underlying disease is a major concern when steroids are stopped. Very gradual reduction of the dosage helps to avoid acute flare-ups.

C. Choice of drugs

1. **Prednisone** is the standard short-duration oral corticosteroid used in the treatment of neuromuscular disorders. Prednisone (and cortisone) are activated in the liver, and in severe liver failure the active parenteral form (prednisolone or cortisol) are given.

2. **Corticosteroids** are preferred to ACTH because they can be given PO and the dose is more precise. With corticosteroids, adrenal gland function does not determine the blood level of hormone, and there are fewer side effects. Although ACTH does not suppress the adrenal gland, neither does corticosteroid therapy used on alternate days or once early in the morning.

D. Treatment course

1. Corresponding doses of various corticosteroids are given in Table 16-1. Corticosteroids can be given in divided daily doses, a single morning dose, or a morning dose every other day. In short treatment courses of less than 1 month, the dose schedule does not matter. In chronic treatment, divided daily doses produce iatrogenic Cushing's syndrome, adrenal suppression, and increased susceptibility to infection.

   The short-acting corticosteroids used chronically as a single morning dose produce less suppression of the adrenal gland, but they do not prevent iatrogenic Cushing's syndrome. The therapeutic effect of a single morning dose is the same as divided doses in most illnesses. Thus when chronic daily therapy is required, the single-dose schedule is preferred.

2. Alternate-day corticosteroid therapy (twice the daily dose given on alternate days) helps to prevent suppression of adrenal function and iatrogenic Cushing's syndrome. There is some evidence that it also prevents increased susceptibility to infection.

   Most neuromuscular diseases respond favorably to alternate-day therapy. In early morning single-day therapy and alternate-day therapy, long-acting

Table 16-1. Common Corticosteroid Drugs

Generic Name	Equivalent Doses	Duration	Mineralocorticoid Effect
Cortisol	20 mg	Short	Yes
Prednisone	5 mg	Short	Little
Dexamethasone	0.75 mg	Long	No

corticosteroids (e.g., dexamethasone) are not suitable, because they do not allow a sufficient period of low steroid level in the blood to prevent side effects.

3. To change from a daily dose to the alternate-day plan, merely increase the dose gradually on one day, while reducing the dose by the same amount on the alternate day. At the same time, in the case of divided daily doses, the frequency of the dose is reduced until the whole dose is given in the morning.

V. MUSCULAR DYSTROPHY

A. Description

1. A dystrophy is a chronic inherited myopathy characterized by progressive muscular weakness and loss of muscle bulk. Pathologically, the number of muscle fibers is reduced, and the remaining fibers are variable in size. Loss of muscle bulk from defects in the nerve or motor neuron, usually called *atrophy*, shows a different pathologic change. There are several types of dystrophy (Table 16-2).

2. The rate of progression and severity varies with both the type and the individual case. The Duchenne dystrophies are usually the most severe, and the majority of these patients die by the age of 20 years. Patients with other dystrophies survive into adulthood. Those with mild, restricted dystrophies may live a nearly normal life.

3. The pathophysiology of the muscular dystrophies is unknown. However, recent investigations suggest that a defect in the muscle cell membrane is the underlying abnormality. Further studies are in progress to isolate an enzymatic or metabolic defect, but none has been found. Until the underlying problem is recognized, it is impossible to develop specific therapy.

B. Diagnosis

1. The history and signs of muscle weakness and wasting in a child or young adult suggest the diagnosis. However, there are no absolute clinical criteria for separating neurogenic atrophy from dystrophy.
   Separation of the various dystrophies is made by the distribution of muscle involvement, speed of progression, and other clinical characteristics (Table 16-2). Table 16-3 lists some differences that may be useful in distinguishing atrophy and dystrophy.

2. Muscle biopsy is helpful in diagnosing dystrophy and in identifying certain benign myopathies (e.g., central core, nemaline) that may resemble dystrophy.

3. The muscle biopsy is taken from an involved muscle, but not one that is severely weak. The deltoid or gastrocnemius is often used in dystrophy, but the rectus abdominus may be a better choice, because there is less problem with postoperative immobilization, which causes disuse weakness.

C. Treatment

1. Mild cases need no therapy early in the course. Careful motor assessment at 6–12-month intervals is usually enough.

2. In severe cases, especially in patients with Duchenne dystrophy, the family must be made aware of the natural history of the disease.

   a. Knowledge that faithful compliance with therapeutic directions helps to prolong the patient's independence should encourage the family to help. However, when the disease is obviously progressing, there is often disappointment. Thus it is important to maintain a guarded hope for stabilization so the physical program will be maintained.

   b. Since many dystrophy patients are children, a treatment plan should

Table 16-2. Types of Muscular Dystrophy

Characteristic	Duchenne	Facioscapulohumeral	Limb-girdle	Myotonic Dystrophy
Sex	Male	Both	Both	Both
Age at onset	Before 5 years	Adolescence	Adolescence	Childhood or later
Initial symptoms	Pelvic	Shoulder girdle	Either	
Facial involvement	No	Always	No	Always
Pseudohypertrophy	Common	No	Rare	Never
Progression	Rapid	Slow	Slow	Slow
Inheritance	X-linked recessive	Autosomal dominant	Autosomal recessive	Autosomal dominant
Muscle enzymes	Very high	Normal	Normal or little increased	Normal
Abnormal ECG	Common	Rare	Occasional	Occasional
Myotonia	No	No	No	Yes

Other forms of dystrophy are less common and include oculopharyngeal dystrophy, progressive dystrophic ophthalmoplegia, and late distal dystrophy of Wielander.

Table 16-3. Separation of Neurogenic from Myopathic Disorders

Sign	Neurogenic	Myopathic
Weakness, wasting, decreased reflexes	Yes	Yes
Distribution	Distal	Proximal
Twitching	Yes	No
Hyperreflexia	Yes, in amyotrophic lateral sclerosis	No
Sensory loss	Yes	No
Nerve conduction	Slow	Normal
EMG	Fibrillation, decreased number of potentials	Decreased amplitude and duration of potentials
Elevated CSF protein	Yes	No
Elevated muscle enzymes	No	Yes
Muscle biopsy	Group atrophy	Degeneration

include education and social needs. For example, children can usually remain in normal schools until they cannot climb stairs easily. However, in Duchenne dystrophy the IQ is often reduced (most are below 90), and earlier transfer to special schools may be indicated.

  c. The goal of therapy **is more than keeping the patient ambulatory.** The patient who must spend most of his time concerned with his disease misses the purpose of therapy. The family and the patient should be encouraged to maintain as normal a life as possible for as long as possible.

3. **Physical treatment**

  a. Intensive physical therapy is begun early, and the family and patient are instructed in home exercises. Physical therapy is accepted better before contracture and deformity occur.

  b. Goals are to maintain good alignment in the weight-bearing joints and to prevent contractures. Flexion contractures are common around hips, ankles, and knees, since the flexors are often slightly less involved than the extensors.

  c. Range-of-motion exercises, instruction in proper positioning in bed and in a chair, frequent change of position, and early use of splints, when necessary, help prevent contractures that make nursing care difficult and impede ambulation.

  d. There is no evidence that physical therapy retards the progression of muscular dystrophy. Independent ambulation can be maintained, however, for several years longer in patients who have it. The cost-effectiveness of physical therapy has not been studied.

4. **Respiratory care**

  a. Swallowing and respiratory difficulty occur in severe, generalized dystrophy and in pharyngeal dystrophy. Respiratory decompensation is usually a gradual process and occurs late in the course.

  b. Pulmonary function tests are often abnormal, even in patients with superficially normal respiratory reserve. Patients are encouraged to develop diaphragmatic breathing by using blow bottles or playing wind instruments (e.g., harmonica). Breathing exercises taught by a therapist are also useful.

    c. Later in the course of the disease intermittent positive-pressure breathing (IPPB) and postural drainage may become necessary.

    d. A rising Pco_2 in patients without pulmonary infection is usually a bad prognostic sign in dystrophy, because about 80% of severe muscular dystrophy patients die from respiratory causes. Muscular dystrophy patients are rarely intubated late in the course of illness.

5. Gait maintenance

    a. Obesity is treated vigorously to improve the patient's ability to walk and to prevent hypoventilation.

    b. Patients are asked to walk for at least 3 hours each day, and if they are not ambulatory, they are instructed to stand for 3 hours in divided periods (30 minutes every 4 hours).

    c. As the disease progresses, independent ambulation can be maintained with crutches, braces, and surgical procedures. The wheelchair is avoided as the primary means of mobility until ambulation is impractical.

    d. Patients may become weaker during acute illnesses, but bedrest is usually contraindicated, since weakness invariably follows prolonged bedrest, and it may become permanent.

6. Preventive therapy—Genetic counseling. When the inheritance of a disease is known, it is often possible to predict the probability of the disease occurring in offspring of affected parents. An important aspect in the care of muscular dystrophy is advising the family about recurrence rates in future generations.

    a. Sex-linked recessive disorders (Duchenne dystrophy)

        (1) Inheritance. A known carrier can be told that there is one chance in two of producing a dystrophic male or a carrier female.

        (2) Carrier detection. Carriers of Duchenne dystrophy often have elevated creatinine phosphokinase (CPK). CPK is measured before, during, and after exercise to increase the chance of showing an abnormally high value. The CPK and the family history are enough in most cases to identify a carrier.

        Muscle biopsy and EMG are usually not necessary to identify a carrier. However, there is an abnormality of the red cell membrane in carriers and patients with Duchenne dystrophy. These data are incomplete, but they may provide a future means of detecting dystrophic males in utero.

        (3) Prevention. Several choices are open to families who carry the abnormal gene:

            (a) Voluntary sterilization or contraception.

            (b) In utero determination of sex may allow abortion of all male offspring, thus eliminating the possibility of a dystrophic child.

        (4) Spontaneous mutation occurs in one-third of Duchenne dystrophy patients: Either the affected offspring or the mother may be a mutant. The more normal children a woman has before a dystrophic child is born, the smaller the probability that she is a carrier. If the mother of a dystrophic child is not a carrier, the chances of her having another dystrophic child are small.

    b. Autosomal dominant disorders (facioscapulohumeral [FSH] dystrophy, myotonic dystrophy, and late distal dystrophy)

        (1) Inheritance. Although the typical halting FSH dystrophy is usually an autosomal dominant trait, there are others that are similar clinically, which may be autosomal recessive or sex-linked traits. The severity of the disease may vary. The affected person has one chance in two of having an affected offspring when there is autosomal dominant inheritance.

(2) There are no carriers.

(3) Prevention is by contraception. If the male partner is affected, artificial insemination may be used to produce normal offspring.

c. **Autosomal recessive disorders (limb-girdle)**

(1) Inheritance. Both parents must have the trait before the offspring are affected. If both parents are carriers, then one in four children will have the disease, two out of four will be carriers, and one will not be affected at all.

(2) Prevention. Avoidance of consanguineous marriage and contraception can help to prevent these diseases.

VI. MYOTONIA AND MYOTONIC DYSTROPHY

A. Description

1. Thinning of the muscles of the face and neck cause an expressionless countenance, with poor movement of the mouth and ptosis. The muscles of the hands and forearms are also thinned.

2. Stiffness of the muscles on contraction and relaxation may be detected. Percussion myotonia may be elicited in thenar muscles or the tongue. The myotonia is not usually severe.

3. The myotonia of myotonic dystrophy and congenital myotonia (Thomsen's disease) are treated with the same drugs. In congenital myotonia without dystrophy the myotonia is usually much more severe. Myotonia is also seen in hyperkalemic periodic paralysis.

4. The EMG shows a decremental pattern without a plateau on repetitive stimulation as well as the characteristic myotonic irregular pattern after-potentials.

5. Hypogonadism, cataracts, mental retardation, and esophageal dysfunction are often associated problems.

6. The disease is usually an autosomal dominant trait, and it may appear in childhood or early adult life.

B. Treatment of myotonia

1. Drugs that act on the muscle cell membrane are used for myotonia.

a. Dilantin 5 mg/kg/day PO is effective and has fewer cardiac side effects than the other agents. It is the usual first choice.

b. Procainamide 50 mg/kg/day PO divided into two to three doses.

c. Quinine 5–10 mg/kg/day PO per day divided into six doses.

d. Corticosteroids have been used in severe cases. (See sec **IV.**)

e. Valium has no effect.

2. **Respiratory care.** Intercostal myotonia may interfere with regular breathing and present respiratory complications, even when there is little myotonia in the limbs. Patients with myotonic dystrophy often have oropharyngeal dysfunction and may develop aspiration pneumonia.

3. Treatment of the dystrophy depends on the severity. Usually the weakness is much more of a problem than the myotonia, and often the myotonia needs no therapy.

VII. POLYMYOSITIS

A. Description

1. Polymyositis is an inflammatory disease of unknown etiology that causes weakness and fatigue. The natural history of the disease remains somewhat unclear, but most authorities report that untreated polymyositis occasionally improves but relapses occur.

2. The clinical features of polymyositis are variable, but proximal muscle weakness is the rule. The disease is occasionally acute and may progress in weeks to complete disability. Some patients have a subacute course that evolves over several months; those with acute cases may have associated myoglobinuria. The face is often spared, and muscle atrophy is a late sign. Pharyngeal muscle involvement may produce dysphagia, but speech usually remains normal. Also, the posterior neck muscles are often weak. Some patients develop an erythematous skin eruption on the dorsum of the hands, proximal digits, knees, or elbows or a purple discoloration and edema of the eyelids. Patients with skin involvement are said to have **dermatomyositis,** but the therapeutic approach is the same as for polymyositis.

B. Diagnosis

1. **Muscle enzymes** (creatinine phosphokinase, transaminase, and aldolase) are usually elevated, but they may be normal in some cases.

2. The **erythrocyte sedimentation rate** (ESR) does not correlate reliably with the activity of the disease.

3. The **EMG** is nonspecific, but it usually suggests a primary myopathic process with brief, small-amplitude polyphasic motor units. However, positive sharp waves, fibrillations, and high-frequency repetitive discharges are also frequently seen.

4. **Muscle biopsy** shows an inflammatory infiltrate and necrosis of muscle fibers in about 85–90% of patients. Often several biopsies must be taken to get a diagnostic specimen.

5. **Differential diagnosis.** Other diseases that may be confused with polymyositis initially are:

   a. Paroxysmal myoglobinuria

   b. Parasitic myositis

   c. Polymyalgia rheumatica

   d. Muscular dystrophy

   e. Thyrotoxic and other endocrine myopathies

   f. Diabetic amyotrophy

   Appropriate study and muscle biopsy usually separates these diseases from polymyositis.

6. **Relation to cancer.** Polymyositis has been linked to occult cancer, but recent reports have refuted the high incidence of occult cancer in patients with polymyositis. However, patients with true polymyositis, rather than muscle wasting from cachexia, have a 20% incidence of cancer. Patients with a rash and those who have evidence of denervation on EMG may have a higher incidence of cancer.

C. Treatment

1. **Use of corticosteroids in polymyositis**

   a. Corticosteroids have been found to benefit patients with polymyositis, although there are no controlled trials available. Mortality is not affected by corticosteroids, but remission is more rapid, and there is less morbidity when corticosteroids are used.

   b. Patients with an acute onset who have had the disease for a short time are most likely to benefit from corticosteroid therapy. However, those with chronic polymyositis and atrophy may not improve with steroid therapy. In chronic cases, when there is no improvement in 2 months, there will usually be no success with corticosteroids. (See sec **2.b.**)

   c. Dose

      (1) The usual beginning dose of prednisone is 60 mg PO every morning until improvement occurs; then the dose may be reduced to 40 mg and maintained for several months.

      (2) The prednisone dosage is reduced slowly, by 5–10 mg every 3–7 days, to prevent flare-up of the disease. At low total dosage, each change represents a larger decrement. Thus, as the dosage is decreased, longer intervals are used, and a period of 2–3 weeks at a given dosage (20–30 mg range) is allowed for signs of relapse to appear. If there is no sign of flare-up, the dosage is dropped to the maintenance level (15–20 mg every morning) and kept there for about 1 year.

        Alternate-day therapy (30–40 mg every other day) is recommended for most patients. If exacerbation occurs, high dosages are resumed and maintained until signs of improvement occur. Response to therapy and relapse can be monitored in most cases by muscle enzyme determination.

      (3) Attempts at steroid withdrawal should be made after the first 24 months of therapy, since activity of the disease often subsides after 2 years. Most cases are quiescent after 8 years.

      (4) Low doses of corticosteroids are not useful in bringing active polymyositis into remission.

   d. Steroid myopathy. The occurrence of steroid-induced myopathy in patients with chronic polymyositis may complicate therapy. It should be suspected if the patient's weakness seems to increase while muscle enzymes and EMG remain unchanged. Management requires reduction of steroids to a maintenance level and observation for a rise in muscle enzymes. If the enzymes rise and further deterioration occurs, high-dose corticosteroid therapy is restarted.

   e. Follow-up. The muscle enzymes (SGOT, CPK, and aldolase) are useful indicators of disease activity, although in some cases all the enzymes or all but one may remain normal. The enzyme levels may fall several weeks before clinical improvement is seen, and they may rise before weakness occurs in a relapse.

2. Immunotherapy

   a. Immunosuppressive drugs may be of benefit in chronic progressive polymyositis, in cases that are not improved by corticosteroid therapy, and in cases that have intolerable complications of steroid therapy.

   b. Immunosuppressive drugs may allow a smaller dosage of corticosteroid, or they may be effective if used alone.

      (1) Methotrexate. Up to 75% of steroid-resistant patients respond when methotrexate is added to corticosteroid therapy. The drug must be given IV over 20–60 minutes. In patients with normal liver and kidney function, the starting dose is 0.4 mg/kg per treatment, and it is increased to a maximum of 0.8 mg/kg per treatment in 2–3 weeks. Methotrexate is given weekly at the onset and, as improvement occurs, the frequency is reduced to biweekly and then triweekly. When improvement is maximal, monthly doses are given for 10–24 months. Corticosteroids may be reduced as improvement occurs.

Toxicity of methotrexate includes stomatitis and gastrointestinal complaints, which usually subside with reduction of the dosage. Leukopenia and hepatotoxicity may occur and, when severe, require that the drug be stopped.

  (2) Azathioprine (Imuran). 1.5–2.0 mg/kg PO is the usual starting dose. Then the dose is increased until the white cell count becomes depressed, and therapy is continued until remission occurs. Major side effects include bone marrow depression, anorexia, nausea, vomiting, and jaundice. Corticosteroids are used concomitantly as with methotrexate.

3. Other therapeutic measures

  a. Bedrest is essential in acute cases.

  b. As the patient improves, physical therapy is indicated for range-of-motion exercises.

  c. Patients with chronic weakness may benefit from braces and other physical measures.

VIII. TRICHINOSIS

A. Description

  1. In the United States there are about 300 cases per year of infestation with *Trichinella spiralis*, a nematode that affects skeletal muscle.

  2. The clinical syndrome varies as the parasite moves from the gastrointestinal tract, through the lymphatics, to the bloodstream, and, finally, it ends as an encapsulated embryo in the skeletal muscle. Nausea, vomiting, and diarrhea may occur acutely, with a low-grade fever. Fatigue and edema of the eyelids and face are common. Myalgia and muscle tenderness occur later. Occasionally isolated muscle weakness may produce a focal sign (e.g., diplopia), but weakness is generalized and mild. Eosinophilia is present early and muscle biopsy often demonstrates the parasite.

  3. Onset of the syndrome is usually within 2–3 days of ingestion of the parasite, and improvement begins at 4 weeks. By 2 months symptoms are usually gone. The disease is seldom fatal, and its severity depends on the size of the inoculum.

  Undercooked pork is the most common source of infection (pigs are rarely fed uncooked garbage, so there is less trichinosis in the pig population). Bear and walrus have also been implicated as sources of trichinosis.

B. Treatment

  1. Corticosteroids can be used to improve the symptoms. Prednisone 60 mg in the first 24–48 hours may be given with subsequent reduction to 20 mg/day for 7–10 days, or until the patient improves.

  2. Thiabendazole 25 mg/kg BID PO for 10 days may relieve the acute symptoms. Also, it acts to destroy the capsule of the *Trichinella* embryo. Side effects occur in about half the patients treated with thiabendazole and include anorexia, nausea, vomiting, dizziness, lethargy, headache, and elevation of liver enzymes.

IX. RHABDOMYOLYSIS

A. Description. Any process that disrupts the muscle cell may lead to the release of myoglobin and other muscle protein into the plasma. Major associated conditions

include trauma, strenuous exercise, heat stroke, polymyositis, alcohol ingestion, licorice ingestion, McArdle's disease, diabetic acidosis, and hyperkalemia. There are also familial cases (Myer-Betz disease) in which myoglobinuria may follow exercise or infection.

Three major complications of rhabdomyolysis may occur that require treatment:

1. **Respiratory distress** from weakness of respiratory muscles is a rare problem.

2. **Hyperkalemia** may occur because of the necrosis of muscles and may lead to lethal cardiac arrhythmia.

3. **Acute renal failure** occurs when plasma myoglobin concentration is high.

B. **Treatment.** Treatment is strict bedrest, osmotic diuresis for preventing renal failure, and maintenance of electrolyte balance.

X. GLYCOGEN STORAGE DISEASES

A. **McArdle's disease** (deficient muscle phosphorylase)

1. **Description.** Pain and stiffness on physical exertion in young adults is the mark of deficient muscle phosphorylase. Blood lactate does not rise following exercise, and weakness and wasting are rare. When the stiffness is severe, shortening of the muscles may occur. EMG of the shortened muscles shows physiologic contracture with electric silence; muscle glycogen is elevated on biopsy.

2. **Treatment**

   a. The amount of exercise is reduced automatically by the patient, and that alone may provide relief in the early stages.

   b. Ingestion of glucose or fructose (20–45 gm TID) may increase exercise tolerance, but the treatment may lead to obesity.

   c. Drugs that raise the concentration of free fatty acids may be used, including:

      (1) Fenfluramine 20 mg BID.

      (2) Isoprenaline 10–20 mg daily.

   d. Glucagon has been used to produce hyperglycemia, and it may increase tolerance in some patients.

B. **Pompe's disease** (acid maltase deficiency)

1. **Description.** Pompe's disease usually occurs in the first few months of life; it is associated with an enlarged heart from cardiomyopathy and hypotonia. Death usually occurs before 12 months, and diagnosis is made on muscle biopsy.

2. **Treatment.** No specific treatment is available.

XI. EPISODIC MUSCLE WEAKNESS

A. **Familial hypokalemic periodic paralysis**

1. **Description**

   a. Familial hypokalemic periodic paralysis is transmitted as an **autosomal dominant** trait. The disease is three times more common in males, and it usually appears in the late teens or early twenties.

   b. The **onset** is usually sudden with weakness of all four limbs. However, the muscles of respiration and swallowing are usually spared. The distribution of weakness may be asymmetric.

The attacks often occur in the morning and, untreated, last from 1–36 hours. The muscles are weak and flaccid, and the deep tendon reflexes may be absent. Large amounts of carbohydrate ingestion or exercise followed by rest may precipitate attacks. Cold weather may also precipitate attacks.

c. The **serum potassium** level is usually between 2–3 mEq/L. Other laboratory tests are normal.

d. EMG shows decreased muscle excitability. Muscle biopsy during attacks may reveal large vacuoles in the affected muscle fibers.

e. **Hyperaldosteronism** and **thyrotoxicosis** may be associated with episodic weakness and hypokalemia. Hyperthyroidism occurs with episodic weakness in Oriental persons.

2. Treatment

a. **Acute attack.** High doses of potassium are given either PO (10–15 gm KCl mixed in fluid) or IV in a potassium chloride solution (40–60 mEq in 500 ml 5% D/W infused over several hours) to reverse the acute attack.

b. **Prophylaxis**

(1) High-potassium, low-carbohydrate, and low-sodium diet.

(2) Spironolactone (Aldactone) 100 mg PO daily or BID.

(3) Thiamine HCl 50–100 mg daily.

(4) Treatment of hyperthyroidism when present.

(5) Acetazolamide (Diamox) 250–500 mg PO every 4–6 hours to cause a mild metabolic acidosis.

B. Familial hyperkalemic periodic paralysis

1. Description

a. Hyperkalemic periodic paralysis affects females and males equally, and it is transmitted as an autosomal dominant trait. Onset is usually during childhood.

b. The attacks are similar and shorter (30–90 minutes) than in hypokalemic paralysis. Respiratory muscles are spared, but trunk and proximal limb muscles are involved. Mild myotonia may be present clinically in the tongue, hands, and eyelids.

c. EMG shows hyperirritability between attacks and myotoniclike discharges during attacks. Serum potassium is either high or high normal.

2. Treatment

a. **Acute attack**

(1) Most attacks are of short duration and require no specific therapy.

(2) Attacks can be stopped with IV infusion of 10% calcium gluconate 10–20 ml.

b. **Prophylaxis**

(1) Acetazolamide 250 mg PO QID.

(2) Chlorothiazide 50–100 mg PO daily.

XII. MYASTHENIA GRAVIS

A. Description. Weakness and progressive fatigue with exercise are the hallmarks of generalized myasthenia gravis. However, diplopia may be the only symptom of ocular myasthenia, and the pupil is never involved. Muscle wasting may occur late, but it is not prominent. The course is variable, but it is marked with remissions and exacerbations, making evaluation of the therapy difficult. Classification into several general groups helps to predict the course and to determine the type of therapy.

1. **Group I.** Ocular myasthenia only.

2. **Group IIA.** Mild generalized myasthenia with ocular signs.

3. **Group IIB.** Moderately severe generalized myasthenia, with mild bulbar and ocular involvement.

4. **Group III.** Acute, severe myasthenia, with bulbar and respiratory complications. Tracheostomy is required.

5. **Group IV.** Late, severe myasthenia, usually developing from other groups within 2 years.

B. Diagnostic tests

1. Edrophonium (Tensilon) test

a. **Initial diagnosis.** When there is a defect that is easily observed, such as grip strength, neck power, extraocular muscle function, ptosis, diplopia, swallowing, vital capacity, and occasionally electromyogram, edrophonium chloride (Tensilon) may cause transient improvement and support the diagnosis of myasthenia gravis. The Tensilon test is not used in apneic patients.

   (1) For best results a placebo control is used, and the trial is done by a double-blind method. The placebo can be nicotinic acid (100 mg/10 ml saline), which gives a systemic response, or saline alone. Atropine (0.4 mg) is often used both as a control and to protect against excessive muscarinic side effects, such as:

   (a) Excessive sweating

   (b) Excessive salivation

   (c) Lacrimation

   (d) Diarrhea

   (e) Abdominal cramps and nausea

   (f) Incontinence of stool and urine

   (g) Bradycardia

   (h) Hypotension

   (i) Small pupils (less than 2 mm)

   (2) Tensilon 10 mg is used in the adult (0.2 mg/kg in children). To begin, 2 mg is infused into a secure IV line, and the patient is observed for excessive muscarinic side effects. If there are no severe effects, the remaining drug is infused in about 30 seconds.

   (3) The patient is observed for improvement. The duration of action is 2–20 minutes, but, occasionally, in patients treated with prednisone, it may be longer (up to 2 hours). The clinical improvement should coincide with the drug's expected duration of action.

b. Smaller doses of Tensilon (1 mg) are used to diagnose cholinergic crisis. If there is no improvement, more drug is infused 1 mg at a time, up to 5 mg. Improvement is judged clinically, as in the diagnostic test. Respiratory function must be assessed carefully before the test, and if Tensilon causes apnea, facilities for tracheal intubation must be at hand.

    c. Evaluation of oral anticholinesterase therapy can be done in some patients by infusing Tensilon 2 mg 1 hour after the last oral dose and watching for improvement and side effects. If there is improvement and there are no increased side effects, the oral dose is increased by 25–50%. If there is no change in the patient's power but there are mild side effects, the dose is kept the same. When the side effects are prominent and the patient's power is worse following the Tensilon, the oral dose is reduced by 25–50 percent.

2. Neostigmine test

    a. If the duration of the action of edrophonium is too short to evaluate the patient's response, the anticholinesterase neostigmine (Prostigmine) may be used. Prostigmine 0.04 mg/kg is injected IM and reaches its maximum activity in 1–2 hours. The effect is gone at 3–4 hours. Pretreatment with atropine may prevent muscarinic side effects.

3. EMG. If a nerve is stimulated at 3–10/sec repeatedly and an EMG is recorded, the amplitude of contraction is temporarily diminished in myasthenia gravis. When myasthenia patients are relaxed so that several muscles (at least one of which is proximal) are rested, 95% will show a pathognomic EMG pattern. In myasthenia, a decrement in response is followed by a plateau or an increment, whereas in other disorders that may show a decrement (myotonia, poliomyelitis, amyotrophic lateral sclerosis, neuropathies, and McArdle's disease), the decrement is continuous.

4. Curare test

    a. The use of curare in systemic low doses to uncover latent myasthenia is dangerous. This test should only be done in an intensive care unit, if at all.

    b. A regional curare test can be done safely in patients with ocular myasthenia. A blood pressure cuff is applied to the arm and the artery is occluded. A dose of D-turbo-curarine (curare) 0.2 mg is injected by rapid IV infusion into the ischemic arm.

    c. In the myasthenic patient the initial evoked potential is decreased in amplitude if there is repetitive supramaximal percutaneous stimulation of the medial or ulnar nerve. Succeeding potentials show 10% decrements at rates of 3, 5, or 15 stimuli per minute.

C. Treatment

1. General measures

    a. Patients with generalized myasthenia should be hospitalized and kept at rest while anticholinesterase medication is begun.

    b. Drugs that have mild neuromuscular blocking effects and sedatives, which may cause respiratory depression, are contraindicated. Common drugs of this type include:

        (1) Quinine

        (2) Quinidine

        (3) Procainamide

        (4) Propranolol

        (5) Lidocaine

        (6) Aminoglycoside antibiotics

        (7) Polymixin

        (8) Viomycin

        (9) Colistin

(10) Morphine

(11) Barbiturates

(12) Other tranquilizers

c. The goals of therapy in myasthenia vary with the severity of the illness. Improvement in strength or increased time spent out of the hospital are goals in more severe cases. However, complete remission may occur in patients in groups I and II.

d. Thyroid abnormalities occur in association with myasthenia gravis; and antithyroid antibodies and antimuscle antibodies have been detected in some myasthenics. However, no clinical correlation between the abnormalities and these antibodies has been made yet.

In thyrotoxic patients, thyrotoxic myopathy is more common than myasthenia gravis. However, in patients with myasthenia, thyrotoxicosis must be treated before the myasthenia gravis will improve.

e. Ephedrine 25 mg TID or other stimulant drugs are occasionally beneficial to patients in conjunction with other therapy.

2. Respiratory care

a. Acute generalized myasthenia is a medical emergency and, even when the patient appears to have normal respiratory function, decompensation can occur rapidly. Thus myasthenics with generalized disease are kept under close observation in an intensive care unit until treatment is seen to be effective.

b. Measurement of maximum voluntary ventilation (patient breathes as rapidly and as deeply as possible for 15 seconds, while expired gases are collected and analyzed) gives the best indication of effects of myasthenia on respiratory muscles. Measurement of vital capacity with a hand spirometer is also a satisfactory way of following respiratory function.

c. Ocular myasthenia (group I) is a benign illness. It is not associated with respiratory failure.

3. Anticholinesterase therapy remains the first choice in all cases of myasthenia. It is often used in conjunction with corticosteroid therapy.

a. **Pharmacology**

(1) Anticholinesterase drugs inhibit the destruction of acetylcholine and allow its accumulation at the synapse. Therefore the effects are limited to the cholinergic nerves. The motor nerves are the primary therapeutic target, but autonomic cholinergic fibers are also affected and produce side effects. The drugs used do not cross the blood-brain barrier, so there are insignificant central effects. The parasympathetic postganglionic effects predominate, since the ganglionic sites are less sensitive to inhibition. Both the dose of drug given and the level of activity in the nerve determine the degree of parasympathetic activity.

(2) Side effects may be reduced by avoiding factors that increase parasympathetic activity (e.g., motion). Atropine 0.4–0.8 mg PO may be useful in reducing side effects in certain circumstances, but chronic use is usually not helpful because of atropine toxicity. However, patients should have atropine on hand for occasional use.

(3) Smaller doses of anticholinesterase, taken more frequently, or doses taken with food to delay absorption may help to reduce side effects. The patient often becomes tolerant of the side effects with prolonged therapy.

(4) The common anticholinesterase drugs are listed in Table 16-4.

Table 16-4. Anticholinesterase Drugs Commonly Used for Myasthenia Gravis

Drug	Route	Adult Dose	Child's Dose[b]	Neonatal and Infant Dose	Frequency
Neostigmine bromide (Prostigmin)	PO	15 mg	10 mg	1–2 mg	Every 3–4 hours
Neostigmine methyl sulfate (Prostigmin injectable)	IM, IV	0.5 mg[a]	0.1 mg[b]	0.05 mg	Every 2–3 hours
Pyridostigmine bromide[c] (Mestinon)	PO IM, IV	60 mg 2 mg[a]	30 mg 0.5–1.5 mg/kg	4–10 mg 0.1–0.5 mg	Every 2–3 hours Every 2–3 hours
Mestinon/Timespan	PO	180 mg	—	—	Every 8–10 hours
Ambenonium chloride (Mytelase)	PO	30 mg	5 mg	—	Every 3–6 hours

[a] The parenteral dose is usually one-thirtieth of the oral dose.
[b] The dose in children varies so much that it must be determined for each case. Small amounts of the drug are given and increased as indicated by the clinical improvement.
[c] Also available as a liquid and as the chloride.

b. Administration

(1) The oral dosage and frequency of administration depend on the severity of the disease and the patient's sensitivity to the drug. Therapy is by trial and error initially, but a usual starting dose is pyridostigmine (Mestinon) 60 mg every 4 hours or its equivalent (Table 16-4).

(a) If one anticholinesterase drug is ineffective, usually the others will be also. Side effects may be less bothersome with one preparation, but there is no way of determining which will be tolerated best.

(b) The patient should be instructed to observe and record his response to the drug so adjustments can be made.

(2) Parenteral therapy may be required during an acute attack, after surgery, or if dysphagia is a problem. Supplementary subcutaneous injection of anticholinesterase 1 hour before meals may improve dysphagia. The parenteral dose is one-thirtieth the oral dose for neostigmine and pyridostigmine.

4. Crisis (acute weakening in a myasthenic)

a. Myasthenic crisis. Changes in the absorption of medication or the natural worsening of the disease may cause increased weakness, requiring an increase of anticholinesterase drugs.

b. Cholinergic crisis. Anticholinesterase drugs may occupy the same receptors as acetylcholine, and an excess of anticholinesterase will reduce neuromuscular transmission. The curarelike effect of anticholinesterase drugs gives them a bell-shaped dose-response curve and creates a serious hazard in therapy.

A slight decrease in neuromuscular transmission can produce severe weakness in the myasthenic patient. The clinical syndrome is much like that of a myasthenic crisis. Many patients may give a history of recent cholinergic side effects, suggesting excessive anticholinesterase therapy. If the patient is treated with atropine, the warning side effects may not occur, and increased weakness is the only sign of toxicity.

Chronic use of anticholinergic medication damages the synapse, and some patients become refractory to the medication. Usually after a time off the medication (often with respiratory support), the patient again responds to anticholinergic medication.

c. Treatment of crisis

(1) Crisis is an emergency and requires intensive care. The patient's respiratory function must be maintained, and if respiratory (or swallowing) dysfunction is present, elective endotracheal intubation is done before emergency intubation is necessary. When the airway is secure, diagnosis of the type of crisis can continue.

(2) The Tensilon (edrophonium) test can be used in the nonapneic patient, and if unequivocal improvement occurs, the anticholinesterase dosage can be increased while the patient remains under close observation. In severe cases the patient is unable to cooperate, so improvement with Tensilon is seldom consistent.

(3) When there is doubt about the result of the Tensilon test, all anticholinesterase medications are stopped for 72 hours. The patient may be followed with serial Tensilon tests until a definite improvement is seen. At that time longer-acting drugs may be started.

(4) Often less medication is required following crisis, because the patient is more sensitive to the drugs.

d. Patient education. The patient is taught not to increase the dosage of anticholinesterase in response to increased weakness. He or she should be aware that the smallest possible amount of drug is best and that full strength dosage may be too much.

5. Immunotherapy

a. Exciting advances in the understanding of the pathophysiology in myasthenia gravis have occurred following the development of an acceptable animal model. For example, animals immunized with a purified acetylcholine receptor develop a myasthenic syndrome. This syndrome can be transmitted by means of injection of lymphocytes but not serum, and it does not occur in thymectomized animals.

b. There are two groups of myasthenia patients. The peak incidence in one group is about the age of 30 years, and women are more commonly affected. The second group consists of elderly patients (peak incidence at the age of 70 years), with men and women equally affected. Most of the younger patients have thymic germinal centers, while the older patients have atrophied thymuses or thymomas. There is overrepresentation of the histocompatibility group HL-A8 in the younger patients and HL-A2 in the older patients.

(1) The younger group often responds to treatment with anticholinesterase and thymectomy but varies in response to corticosteroids.

(2) The older group is often benefited by corticosteroid therapy and responds less frequently to anticholinesterase or thymectomy. The patients in the older age group and those with thymoma have the highest cellular immunity to acetylcholine receptors. Young females do not differ from controls in their cellular immunity to acetylcholine receptors.

6. Corticosteroid therapy

a. Indications

(1) Failure of anticholinesterase medication to allow an acceptable level of function without excessive side effects.

    (2) To improve the patient's strength preoperatively in preparation for thymectomy.

    (3) Failure of remission following thymectomy.

    (4) Rarely in pure ocular myasthenia when diplopia is disabling.

  b. High-dose corticosteroid therapy

    (1) Prednisone 60–100 mg daily may produce increased weakness about 5 days after onset of therapy. Improvement begins at about 12 days. High-dose corticosteroids are as effective as ACTH, and with prolonged treatment longer remissions can be obtained.

    (2) High dosages are maintained until improvement is sustained (for about 2 weeks). There are seldom relapses after the first 2 weeks of therapy, and anticholinesterase drugs are gradually withdrawn over 1 month.

    (3) The corticosteroids are then gradually reduced to 5–15 mg daily (or the equivalent alternate-day dosage) over 1 or 2 months. Then the maintenance dosage is continued. Some patients may be able to stop the maintenance dosage without relapse.

    (4) Care must be taken early in the treatment to protect the patient from respiratory complications or aspiration. The incidence of such problems is smaller in corticosteroid treatment than in treatment with ACTH.

    (5) Dexamethasone 20 mg daily for 10 days and then repeated for a second course has been highly successful. Improvement or remission occurs in most cases and continues for 3 months or longer after the drug is stopped. Generally the higher the dosage of steroid used, the greater the remission rate. Dexamethasone is not often used as the first treatment, but it may be needed if prednisone treatment at lower dosages fails.

  c. Low-dose corticosteroid therapy

    (1) By starting with a low-dose alternate-day program (25 mg prednisone on alternate days) and gradually increasing the dosage by 12.5 mg every third dose until the total dosage reaches 100 mg on alternate days, or until optimal results occur, the initial period of worsening is avoided.

    (2) Improvement may not occur for 6–7 weeks of therapy with low-dose treatment, and therapy should be continued for 3 months before being abandoned.

    (3) If relapse occurs after withdrawing or reducing the corticosteroids, the full dosage should be resumed.

7. Other therapy

  a. ACTH therapy. ACTH was first introduced in the 1950s as a treatment for myasthenia gravis. However, because of severe acute deterioration early in the course, it was not pursued. In the 1960s it was reported that after the initial deterioration with ACTH therapy, the myasthenic patient improved significantly.

  b. The effectiveness of other immunosuppressive drugs has not been established in the treatment of myasthenia gravis.

  c. In severe myasthenics, who are maximally treated with other means, the use of gamma globulin has increased the time they have spent out of the hospital. Gamma globulin 5 ml in each hip every 3 weeks is currently used in patients with severe cases.

8. Surgical therapy

a. In patients without thymoma

(1) The thymus has been implicated in the etiology of myasthenia gravis. In 1939 a thymic cyst was removed from a patient, with coincidental improvement in the patient's myasthenia gravis. Since that time it has been found that, in young patients with generalized myasthenia, removal of the thymus often leads to a lasting remission. Also, as many as 90% of selected patients that have a thymectomy experience a remission or sustain improvement for 5 years. Many of these patients need less anticholinesterase medication, and some can discontinue it entirely.

(2) With continued reduction of operative morbidity and mortality, many authorities advocate thymectomy in all young patients early in their course, especially when anticholinesterase medications do not produce optimum improvement with minimum side effects. Young patients who have the disease for a short time improve most rapidly, and, pathologically, the thymus shows absent or few germinal centers. Patients with pure ocular myasthenia do not undergo thymectomy.

b. In patients with thymoma.
Mortality in patients with thymoma is much higher than in those without it, and removal of the thymoma may not improve myasthenia. Radiation therapy is used when the thymoma cannot be removed completely. About 30% of patients with thymoma have myasthenia; and 10% of myasthenic patients have thymoma.

c. Surgical approach.
There is some debate about the best approach for removal of the thymus.

(1) **Median sternotomy.** The classic approach is through a median sternotomy, and the method is safe in experienced hands.

(2) **Transcervical approach**

(a) The transcervical approach sacrifices the excellent exposure of the sternotomy, but it reduces the postoperative morbidity when it is successful.

(b) Hemorrhage, pneumothorax, and fragmentation of the gland with incomplete removal may complicate the transcervical approach and necessitate an unplanned open procedure.

(3) The procedure with which the surgeon is most comfortable is the best choice but when uncomplicated, the transcervical approach results in the least morbidity.

9. Postoperative treatment of the myasthenia patient

a. Tracheostomy is performed by many surgeons if there is:

(1) Oropharyngeal weakness.

(2) Previous myasthenic crisis.

(3) Previous history of respiratory complications.

(4) Vital capacity less than 2000 cc.

b. In patients without tracheostomy the nasotracheal tube is left in place for 48 hours following surgery.

c. After thymectomy the patient may show marked improvement for 12–24 hours.

(1) In the immediate postoperative period no anticholinesterase drugs are

given, keeping the patient slightly underdosed to reduce excess secretions.

(2) The medication is changed from the parenteral to the oral form as soon as possible. It is increased to the optimal dose level gradually (36–48 hours).

(3) Care must be taken not to overdose the patient, since previous doses of anticholinesterase drug may be excessive after thymectomy.

d. Sedatives and weak neuromuscular blockers must be used with extreme caution when the patient is intubated.

10. Treatment of myasthenia in pregnancy

a. During pregnancy myasthenic symptoms may become worse, improve, or remain unchanged. When change occurs, it is usually in the first trimester or postpartum.

b. Therapeutic abortion is not indicated, because it may cause worsening. Spontaneous abortion is common during the first trimester in women with myasthenia gravis.

c. Labor in myasthenic mothers is usually shorter than in normal mothers. Thus intramuscular anticholinesterases are used during labor.

d. Local or regional anesthetics are preferred to general anesthesia, and caution is required with sedatives.

e. Cesarean section is done only for obstetric indications.

f. The neurologist and obstetrician must help the myasthenic woman formulate plans for long-range family planning. Voluntary sterilization or contraception should be suggested when the myasthenia is severe.

11. Neonatal myasthenia

a. Description. Congenital myasthenia gravis is very rare, but neonatal myasthenia occurs in about 20% of babies born to myasthenic mothers. The condition is transitory and is usually gone in 24–36 hours. However, it may persist for weeks. Signs include masklike face, poor sucking, difficulty swallowing, regurgitation, and respiratory distress. Symptoms usually begin within 3 days of birth, but they may not appear for 10 days.

b. Treatment. Symptomatic treatment to prevent aspiration, provide nutrition, and maintain respiration are most important. Anticholinesterase drugs may be needed for a short time. Neostigmine 1–2 mg PO (parenteral dose is one-thirtieth the oral dose) every 4 hours or pyridostigmine 4–10 mg PO are the approximate dosages for infants.

XIII. OTHER NEUROMUSCULAR JUNCTION DISORDERS— EATON-LAMBERT SYNDROME

A. Description. A myasthenialike syndrome (Eaton-Lambert) occurs with carcinoma (usually oat-cell carcinoma of the lung). The syndrome is associated with generalized muscle weakness but, unlike myasthenia gravis, the weakness improves when the muscle is exercised. EMG is helpful in differentiating the syndrome from true myasthenia gravis.

B. Treatment

1. Removal of the tumor, when possible, may resolve the syndrome.

2. When the tumor is not resected or there is no improvement after removal, guanidine HCl (35–40 mg/kg/day divided into three or four doses) has been beneficial in some cases. Gastrointestinal upset is a frequent side effect and may require that the drug be stopped or the dose reduced. Bone marrow suppression has resulted from guanidine therapy.

XIV. BOTULISM

A. Description. Botulism is an intoxication caused by the exotoxin of *Clostridium botulinum,* an anaerobic gram-positive spore-forming rod that may contaminate foods.

   1. As in tetanus, the toxin rather than the bacterial infection produces the illness. Botulinus toxin is a powerful presynaptic blocker of acetylcholine release. There are six antigenically distinct toxins (A, B, C, D, E, and F) but only A, B, and E are associated with human illness.

   2. The clinical syndrome is one of progressive muscle weakness, often beginning in the extraocular or pharyngeal muscles and becoming generalized. Also, gastrointestinal complaints may be prominent. There are no sensory signs; dilated unreactive pupils are regularly seen, but the patient remains alert. Dry, erythematous mucous membranes are also seen.

   3. The diagnosis is confirmed when the disorder appears in a mouse injected with either serum from the patient or an aliquot of the suspected food.

   4. The course is usually rapid, with symptoms appearing within 18 hours of ingestion of the toxin. A more rapid onset is associated with more severe courses.

   5. The prognosis in treated patients is about 80% survival. Patients whose cases are not generalized usually do very well. Those who are over 20 years old and those with type A toxin have a slightly higher mortality.

B. Treatment

   1. Therapy against the toxin is begun as soon as possible.

      a. Specific typing of the toxin can be done, but treatment is usually started with trivalent (A, B, E) antitoxin.

      b. The antitoxin is horse serum, so skin-testing and precautions for anaphylaxis are necessary. 10,000 units of antitoxin are administered IV in one dose.

      c. 15–20% of patients will have minor allergic reactions that may require treatment with antihistamines or corticosteroids. However, some patients have severe reactions, so provision for emergency endotracheal intubation should be made when the antitoxin is given.

   2. Emetics, cathartics, and enemas are used with caution to eliminate any toxin that remains in the gastrointestinal tract.

   3. **Guanidine HCl,** an acetylcholine agonist, is useful in some patients to counteract the presynaptic blockade caused by the toxin; 35–40 mg/kg/day is given PO every 4 hours. The major side effect of guanidine is gastrointestinal upset, but suppression of blood counts has been observed in chronic treatment.

   4. **Respiratory care.** Maintenance of respiratory function is the most important aspect in treating severe cases of botulism.

      a. Patients who appear to have mild symptoms (diplopia and mild weakness) may rapidly develop respiratory failure, so respiratory function must be monitored frequently in all patients until there are signs of improvement.

      b. If vital capacity falls to 1000 cc, elective intubation is considered. Severe dysphagia also requires nasogastric or endotracheal intubation to prevent aspiration.

XV. TETANUS

A. **Description.** Tetanus is an intoxication that results from infection with *Clostridium tetani,* a gram-positive coccus that enters through a wound.

1. An exotoxin causes the neuromuscular irritability and the syndrome of tetanus.

2. The major presenting feature of generalized tetanus is muscle rigidity and discomfort in the jaws, neck, and lower back. The symptoms that may be mild at the onset progress over hours or days to a state of muscular hyperirritability and spasm, which may involve the respiratory and pharyngeal muscles. Convulsive seizures are common.

3. Tetanus may be localized to the area surrounding the wound rather than generalized. Often the jaw is involved early in both localized and generalized tetanus (lockjaw).

4. The prognosis is good in localized tetanus, but mortality reaches 50% despite therapy in patients with generalized disease.

B. **Treatment**

1. **Treatment directed against the toxin.** The major emphasis is on the neutralization of the toxin. Some patients with tetanus may have no *Clostridium tetani* in their wound cultures, and others may have no wound (20%) visible at the time of onset.

   a. **Human hyperimmune globulin** is the antitoxin of choice. 3000–10,000 units are given IM or IV, although lower doses may be effective. A single dose is adequate. Toxin already fixed in the neural tissues will not be eliminated by antitoxin, but circulating antitoxin will be neutralized by it.

   b. **Horse serum antitoxin** can be used, but prior skin tests for sensitivity are required. The usual dose is 50,000 units IM followed by 50,000 units in a slow IV infusion.

   If surgical excision of the wound is impossible, a small amount of antitoxin may be injected locally.

2. **Therapy directed against the bacteria**

   a. The area of the wound is surgically excised and drained.

   b. Cultures of the wound are taken, but they do not always grow the organisms.

   c. Penicillin is the antibiotic of choice: procaine penicillin, 1.2 million units IM or IV every 6 hours for 10 days.

   d. For patients unable to take penicillin, tetracycline 500 mg PO or IV every 6 hours for 10 days may be substituted.

3. **General measures**

   a. The treatment of tetanus, as with any paralyzed patient, includes care of skin, bladder, bowel, fluid management, nutrition, and respiration. Prevention of aspiration pneumonia and pain are particularly important.

   b. Spasms of generalized tetanus are painful and interfere with respiration. A dark, quiet room will help reduce the spasms. Sedation is important in controlling the spasms, and the patient should be kept asleep. Diazepam, in dosages determined by the patient's response (2–10 mg IV every 4–12 hours), is safe and effective. Meprobamate, barbiturates, and chlorpromazine have also been used with success. Diazepam may cause respiratory and cardiac arrest in a few patients if it is used with barbiturates, so the combination should be avoided.

c. Neuromuscular blockers are helpful when other methods fail to reduce the muscle spasm that interferes with swallowing or respiration. Thus the patient must be artificially ventilated when neuromuscular blockers are used. It is not safe to try to give a dose of neuromuscular blocker to stop spasm in the extremities while preserving respiratory function.

Pancuronium (Pavulon), succinylcholine, and other blocking agents may be useful when the patient is intubated. Sedation should be maintained or increased when blockers are used, because it is extremely unpleasant for the patient to be awake and paralyzed.

d. Autonomic dysfunction (hypertension, hypotension, hyperpyrexia, and cardiac arrythmia) is common. Treatment is directed at the symptoms.

4. Prophylaxis

a. All persons, beginning at 2 months of age, should be immunized against tetanus toxin. Initial immunization is tetanus toxoid 0.5 ml in three injections 4 weeks apart. Booster injections are required every 10 years.

b. In acute injuries thorough washing and debriding are necessary.

(1) In fresh, clean wounds the toxoid course should be completed if it has not been completed already. If the initial immunization is complete, a booster dose of toxoid is given if the patient has not had one in the past 10 years.

(2) In wounds that are dirty or infected, toxoid booster is given if none has been received for 5 years. Human antitoxin (250 units IM), in addition to the toxoid, is given to patients who have not received earlier immunization. Contracting tetanus does not confer immunity, and the series of toxoid injections is required in these persons.

XVI. NEUROPATHY

A. Description

1. Peripheral neuropathy of various types (polyneuropathy [PN], entrapment neuropathy [EN], mononeuritis multiplex [MNM]) is a symptom that may be associated with many systemic disorders, such as:

a. Multiple myeloma, PN

b. Carcinoma, PN

c. Myxedema, PN

d. Systemic lupus erythematosus, PN

e. Cryoglobulinemia, PN

f. Rheumatoid arthritis, PN, EN

g. Scleroderma, PN

h. Diphtheria, PN (Nerve conduction velocities greatly reduced)

i. Hepatic failure, PN

j. Renal failure, PN

k. Diabetes mellitus, PN, MNM, EN

l. Porphyria, PN

m. Refsum's disease, PN

n. Tangier disease, PN

o. Metachromatic leukodystrophy, PN (Nerve conduction velocities greatly reduced)

p. Polyarteritis nodosa, MNM
q. Sarcoidosis, MNM
r. Tuberculosis, MNM
s. Waldenstrom's disease, MNM, PN
t. Acromegaly, EN
u. Amyloidosis, EN, PN

2. Certain vitamin deficiencies are associated with polyneuropathy, such as:
   a. Thiamine
   b. Pyridoxine
   c. Pantothenic acid
   d. Riboflavin
   e. Vitamin B_{12}
   f. Folic acid

3. Intoxication from the following substances may cause polyneuropathy:
   a. Arsenic
   b. Lead
   c. Mercury
   d. Thallium
   e. Acrylamide
   f. Carbon tetrachloride
   g. Chlorinated hydrocarbons
   h. Methyl-n-butyl ketone
   i. Triorthocresyl phosphate
   j. Hexachlorophene
   k. Glue

4. Some commonly used drugs that may cause polyneuropathy are:
   a. Chloroquine
   b. Clioquinol (antidiarrheal patent medicines)
   c. Dapsone
   d. Phenytoin
   e. Disulfiram
   f. Glutethimide
   g. Gold
   h. Hydralazine
   i. Isoniazid
   j. Nitrofurantoin
   k. Stilbamidine (facial numbness)
   l. Vincristine
   m. Immunization (rabies, typhoid, smallpox, rubella, pertussis)

There are also several primary neurologic disorders that affect peripheral nerves or roots (e.g., Landry-Guillain-Barré disease and Charcot-Marie-Tooth disease). Thus the first step in management of polyneuropathy is to diagnose the underlying disease. The details of therapy depend on the underlying illness, the severity of the neuropathy, and the rate of progression. Patients with acute progressive motor neuropathy require observation in the hospital, whereas those with chronic neuropathy can be treated as outpatients.

5. **Polyneuropathy.** Symmetric loss of sensory function, motor function, or both, usually begins in the feet or finger tips in polyneuropathy. Deep tendon reflexes may be diminished early, especially in the ankles; later reflexes may be absent. Some neuropathies affect the proximal nerves early (diabetic amyotrophy), and these may be confused with myopathy.

6. **Mononeuropathy.** Mononeuropathy is the asymmetric dysfunction of one or more large nerves. There is usually pain, and the cranial nerves may be affected. The cranial nerves may also be involved in mononeuropathies.

7. The pathology of mononeuropathy and mononeuropathy multiplex is usually disruption of the vasa nervorum, whereas in the polyneuropathies the mechanism is often unknown. However, axonal degeneration occurs in some, and in others the myelin sheaths undergo segmental demyelination.

B. Diagnosis

1. The separation of chronic polyneuropathy from primary disease of muscle and other conditions that cause weakness is seldom a problem. However, identifying the cause of the neuropathy is difficult.

2. Muscle enzymes are normal in polyneuropathy.

3. Abnormal nerve conduction studies support the diagnosis of peripheral neuropathy, although normal studies do not exclude it. Mononeuropathy usually shows decreased conduction in the affected nerve, but other nerves are normal.

C. Acute idiopathic polyradiculoneuritis (Landry-Guillain-Barré-Strohl syndrome)

1. Clinical picture

a. Persons of all ages are affected in acute idiopathic polyradiculoneuritis. The syndrome may follow a mild viral illness by 10–12 days or appear without prodrome.

b. The earliest signs are motor weakness, paresthesias, and pain, progressing from lower extremities to upper extremities.

c. The cranial nerves are affected in 75% of cases. The facial nerve is involved in half of those with cranial neuropathy, and of those with facial palsies, it is bilateral in about 80%.

d. Autonomic disorders are not unusual (hypotension, hypertension, and hyperpyrexia).

e. CSF protein is often high, and occasionally a patient will have papilledema, which is thought to be the result of excess CSF protein blocking the arachnoid villi. Cell counts in CSF are always below 70 lymphocytes/cu mm; they are usually lower than 20/cu mm.

f. Nerve conduction velocities are reduced in 90% of patients.

2. Prognosis. Patients with normal nerve conduction studies have the best prognosis.

a. The disease progresses over 7–21 days. Patients with more rapid progression usually need respiratory support. Improvement follows the progressive period by 10–14 days, and recovery continues for 6–36 months.

b. Most patients recover enough to leave the hospital in 75 days or less. Atelectasis, aspiration, pneumonia, pulmonary abscess, venous thrombosis, and pulmonary embolus are serious complications of the paralysis. Despite these complications, overall mortality is only 5% with modern intensive care.

c. Recovery is complete in about one-half of patients and most of the remainder have only mild abnormalities. Severe disability occurs in about 10–15% of patients.

3. Treatment. There is no specific treatment for idiopathic polyradiculoneuropathy. The neuropathologic defect is an inflammatory perivascular mononuclear infiltrate that may involve the entire peripheral nervous system. Both axonal degeneration and segmental demyelination occur.

a. Corticosteroids have been used early in the course of the disease and during its progression to reduce edema and to decrease the inflammatory response. There is no evidence that they alter the severity or the duration of hospitalization, and the risks usually outweigh the advantages. It is not helpful to use corticosteroids at any time other than when the disease is progressing.

b. Respiratory care. The most important consideration is maintaining adequate respiration. Patients should be followed closely, with measurement of vital capacity, and endotracheal intubation is performed when the vital capacity drops to 25–30% of normal. (Normal vital capacity in males = 25 cc × height in centimeters; females = 20 cc × height in centimeters; children = 200 cc × age in years). When bulbar muscles are involved, feeding is done by IV administration, nasogastric tube, or gastrostomy.

c. Prophylactic anticoagulation is indicated in paralyzed patients. Subcutaneous heparin in low doses (5000 units every 12 hours) or coumadin helps to prevent thromboembolic complications of immobilization. Infants and small children need not be anticoagulated since they can be easily mobilized.

d. Fecal impaction is a painful problem that occurs in bedridden patients. Thus suppositories and enemas should be used from the outset, before problems arise.

e. Physical therapy. Bedrest is indicated in the acute phase of the illness until improvement begins.

(1) Positioning. Careful positioning of the patient in bed prevents bed sores and compression of nerves. A firm mattress or bedboard is necessary, and flexed positions are avoided for prolonged periods. Frequent (every 2 hours) change of the patient's position is necessary to prevent pressure sores.

(2) Prevention of contractures

(a) Range-of-motion exercises prevent the connective tissues from shortening, which is a natural tendency. A short, passive range-of-motion program twice daily is started early in the course of the illness. Stretching range-of-motion exercises are not needed early. However, as improvement occurs, most types of intensive physical therapy can be used.

(b) A footboard is necessary to prevent gastrocnemius and achilles tendon contractures. Pillows under the shoulders should be avoided, since they may promote kyphosis. Allowing the patient to lie face down periodically helps to prevent flexion contractures of the hips.

(c) If contractures begin to form, stretching range-of-motion exercises may relieve them. Once contractures are fully formed, however, surgical release is necessary.

f. Edema. Paralyzed extremities lack the normal muscle tone that keeps edema from occurring. Edema makes the skin less resistant to pressure necrosis, infection, or mild trauma. Edema may be painful when it forms rapidly.

(1) Intermittent elevation of the extremities (above the level of the heart) may help to prevent edema and reduce edema that is already present.

(2) Intermittent compression of edematous extremities for 60–90 minutes BID, followed by massage and elevation, is useful.

(3) Ace bandages applied tightly up to the trunk and unwrapped for 10–15 minutes TID or a pressure stocking can be used to prevent edema.

g. Pain. Myalgia and arthralgia are common in acute polyradiculoneuritis. Mild analgesics are usually effective (aspirin 600 mg every 3–4 hours), but occasionally codeine (30–60 mg every 4 hours) or morphine (5–10 mg IM) are needed. However, narcotics cause respiratory depression and constipation.

Heat applied before range-of-motion exercises and warm baths (Hubbard tank) may reduce pain.

h. Later phase of therapy. Maximum development of residual function is the goal of late therapy.

(1) Restorative surgical procedures may increase function.

(2) A brace can be used to maintain the limb (often the foot) in good position, but it cannot overcome a fixed deformity. A brace must be strong enough to function but light enough to allow easy ambulation. The weight of the brace is especially important in the patient with weakness of hip flexion. A brace that allows controlled motion is usually more comfortable than one that allows no motion.

(3) Management of physical therapy is done with the help of trained physical therapists and, if available, a competent physiatrist.

i. Autonomic syndrome. Occasionally paroxysmal hypertension, headache, sweating, anxiety, and fever occur in patients with acute polyradiculoneuritis. Phenoxybenzamine (20–60 mg in divided doses) has been used to relieve this syndrome. Also, diabetes insipidus and the syndrome of inappropriate antidiuretic hormone secretion have been reported to occur in patients with acute polyradiculopathy. In these patients observation of the urinary output, the state of hydration, and serum and urine electrolytes allows prompt therapy when needed.

D. Chronic neuropathies. The treatment of chronic neuropathy associated with a systemic disorder begins with treatment of the underlying disease or deficiency. Management of these patients is aimed at keeping them functional. For example, braces and splints are often used to maintain ambulation. The sensory neuropathies may not interfere with gait and do not require physical therapy as a rule. Also, care of the skin prevents ulcers from pressure and trauma. Respiratory failure does not occur in patients with chronic neuropathy.

1. Neuropathy associated with deficiency diseases (see sec XVI.A.2)

a. Alcoholic polyneuropathy probably results from multiple vitamin deficiencies or from thiamine deficiency. Alcohol, by itself, is probably not responsible for the neuropathy.

Adequate diet supplemented with multivitamins and thiamine (50–100 mg PO daily) is the usual method of treatment. Most patients improve in several months, but severe cases may take up to a year to improve.

b. **Other deficiencies**

(1) Pyridoxine deficiency occurs in patients treated with INH. It may cause a mild sensorimotor neuropathy and optic neuritis. A preparation of INH-B_6 combination prevents the neuropathy.

(2) **Folic acid deficiency** may occur with chronic phenytoin (Dilantin) administration or in persons with a low folate intake. 1 mg folic acid every morning prevents the neuropathy, but it may make the seizure disorder less responsive to phenytoin.

(3) **Niacin deficiency,** by itself, probably does not cause peripheral neuropathy, but pellegra patients with peripheral neuropathy have multiple vitamin deficiencies.

2. **Diabetes mellitis**

a. **Polyneuropathy.** Diabetes mellitis is the most common cause of neuropathy in developed parts of the world. The polyneuropathy associated with diabetes is usually mixed, but is often primarily sensory. Pain is common and both legs and feet are involved.

(1) Control of hyperglycemia may improve diabetic polyneuropathy. Treatment of the pain is difficult.
    Physical measures, such as warm compresses, massage, and whirlpool baths, may be temporarily helpful. Also, rest may help, and mild analgesics, such as aspirin, are often used.

(2) Narcotics are not generally used, because they are often ineffective and lead to addiction. Dilantin 300–400 mg daily may help, but if improvement does not occur in 10–14 days, therapy should be stopped.

b. **Autonomic neuropathy** is common in diabetes and causes decreased sweating, orthostatic hypotension, nocturnal diarrhea, fecal incontinence, constipation, urinary incontinence or retention, and impotency. Delayed gastric emptying may also occur, causing difficulty in controlling the blood sugar.

(1) **Orthostatic hypotension** may improve with pressure stockings or mineralocorticoid (Florinef 0.1 mg daily). **Ephedrine** (up to 25 mg TID) is also helpful in some patients. Diarrhea may be intermittent and may resolve spontaneously. Thus **denatured tincture of opium** 5–10 drops QID or other antidiarrheals are often helpful.

(2) When fecal incontinence is a problem, an enema each morning cleans the bowel and allows the patient relative safety, using only a pad.

(3) Treatment of urinary problems is discussed in Chapter 14.

c. **Mononeuritis.** The cranial nerves are frequently involved, particularly the oculomotor nerve. Diabetic oculomotor nerve palsy is usually painful. As a rule there is sparing of the pupil, a sign that helps to distinguish it from a posterior communicating artery aneurysm. Large peripheral nerves may also be involved, causing a pain syndrome.

(1) The pain is treated with analgesics, and often narcotics are required. This pain usually subsides spontaneously in a few days, and in the case of third-nerve palsy, the deficit improves in 1–4 months. An eye patch prevents diplopia until improvement is complete.

3. **Neuropathy associated with toxic diseases** (see sec **XVI.A.3**). Removal from exposure and, when possible, direct removal of the toxin is the treatment for all toxic conditions.

a. **Chronic arsenic toxicity** causes a painful mixed motor and sensory polyneuropathy.

(1) The treatment is dimercaprol (BAL) oil suspension. However, dimercaprol is contraindicated in hepatic insufficiency, and acute renal failure may occur during therapy. Alkalinization of the urine helps to prevent breakdown of dimercaprol-metal complexes and protects the kidney. Other side effects are hypertension, nausea, vomiting, and headache. Reduction of dosage reduces the side effects.

(2) For chronic arsenic poisoning dimercaprol 2.5 mg/kg is given QID for 2 days, BID on the third day, and then daily by deep intramuscular injections for 10 days. Dimercaprol therapy is thought to decrease the duration of the illness, but it has no effect on the recovery rate.

b. The sensorimotor neuropathy of **lead intoxication** is treated with EDTA.

(1) EDTA may cause renal failure, and daily urinalysis is indicated during therapy. If hematuria, proteinuria, or epithelial cell casts increase during treatment, the drug should be stopped.
EDTA is usually given IM 0.04 gm/kg BID. The prognosis depends on the amount of exposure and the degree of impairment. Early treatment results in the best prognosis.

c. **Mercury intoxication** neuropathy is predominantly a motor disorder. It can also be treated with dimercaprol, but it is usually treated with EDTA (Calcium Disodium Versenate). Mercury poisoning causes dementia, which may not be reversible.

(1) Penicillamine 25 mg/kg daily in divided doses also has been used to remove lead from the body in chronic intoxication.

4. Neuropathy associated with drugs (see sec XVI.A.4)

a. **Nitrofurantoin** (Furadantin) (400 mg daily for 2 weeks) has produced decreased conduction velocities in all patients tested. The polyneuropathy is primarily sensory at the onset, with pain and paresthesias. However, the polyneuropathy is reversible when the drug is stopped.

b. **Vincristine** is consistently associated with peripheral polyneuropathy, and the neurotoxicity is the dose-limiting factor. Absent achilles tendon reflex is the earliest sign that accompanies paresthesias in the fingers and toes. However, the cranial nerves may also be affected. The neuropathy usually improves within several months after the drug is stopped.

c. **Phenytoin** (Dilantin) is occasionally associated with a mild polyneuropathy, which is thought to be related to folate deficiency.

d. **Isoniazid** (INH) causes B_6 (pyridoxine) deficiency with polyneuropathy.

5. Entrapment neuropathy

a. **The carpal tunnel syndrome** is the most common entrapment. It is the result of compression of the median nerve by the volar ligament.

(1) Pain and tingling in the hand are the usual early signs, and retrograde distribution of the pain may cause arm and shoulder pain in some patients. There may be no objective neurologic signs and nerve conduction studies may be normal, but usually median nerve conduction is slowed across the wrist. Often the earliest objective sign is failure to appreciate textures. Later, clear deficits of sensation and muscle wasting occur in the distribution of the median nerve.

(2) There is a variety of diseases associated with carpal tunnel syndrome (see sec **XVI.A.1**). Thus before surgery is undertaken, underlying diseases that are treatable should be controlled.

(3) The treatment is usually surgical release at the site of entrapment. When the symptoms are mild and there are no objective signs of nerve damage, conservative measures may be enough. For example, splinting the wrist at night may relieve carpal tunnel symptoms, especially in the transient syndrome seen in pregnancy.

(4) Injection of corticosteroid into the volar ligament may relieve the symptoms temporarily. In some cases remission may last for several years. If nerve conduction is slow, however, surgery is usually required.

b. Pronator syndrome. The median nerve may also be entrapped as it passes into the forearm between the two heads of the pronator teres muscle.

(1) Pain is reported in front of the elbow and at the wrist. Also, weakness in apposition of the thumb and hypesthesia on the radial side of the index finger have been reported. However, this condition is rare. Treatment is surgical release.

c. The ulnar nerve may be entrapped at the wrist or in the palm, but most commonly entrapment occurs at the elbow. Paresthesia of the fourth and fifth fingers is a common symptom. Weakness of the hand with atrophy of the first interosseous muscle and the hypothenar eminence is less common; and weakness of abduction of the fifth finger may be the only sign. When entrapment is at the elbow, therapy is surgical transposition of the nerve anteriorly.

d. The radial nerve is entrapped very rarely, and most isolated radial palsies are caused by direct trauma.

(1) Weakness of finger extension without weakness of wrist extension has been attributed to entrapment of the radial nerve at the level of the supinator muscle. The extensor carpi ulnaris is weak, but the extensor carpi radialis is normal, so weakness of finger extension occurs with radial deviation of the hand. Sparing of the extensor carpi radialis occurs, because the branch of the radial nerve to the carpi radialis branches distal to the entrapment point.

(2) The onset of entrapment is slow as opposed to the sudden onset seen in the common traumatic palsies. Treatment is surgical release, but splints and physical therapy comprise the only therapy for traumatic lesions. Most patients with traumatic radial palsy recover in several months.

e. The lateral cutaneous nerve of the thigh may be entrapped between the two folds of the inguinal ligament. The syndrome produced is known as *meralgia parasthetica,* which is characterized by parasthesia, pain, or numbness in the lateral part of the thigh. There may be objective signs of decreased sensation in the region of numbness.

(1) The etiology varies, but trauma, use of a corset or truss, and other external mechanical compressions around the waist have been implicated. Intrapelvic tumor and acute abdominal enlargement from ascites or pregnancy have been implicated.

(2) Therapy is unnecessary if there is no pain. Evaluation for a definite etiology must be done, and if pain is severe, injection of local anesthetic into the nerve at the anterior iliac spine may help. Resection of the nerve is rarely necessary.

f. The **posterior tibial** nerve may be entrapped under the flexor retinaculum, behind and inferior to the medial malleolus at the "tarsal tunnel."

(1) The patient complains of pain or numbness in the sole of the foot; walking and standing increase the pain. A tender tibial nerve may be found behind the medial malleolus, and dorsal extension and pronation of the foot may provoke pain. The syndrome is rare, but it may occur following previous trauma. Treatment is surgical release.

6. Leprosy

a. **Description.** In underdeveloped parts of the world, leprosy is a common cause of neuropathy. ***Mycobacterium leprae,*** an acid-fast rod, causes a predominantly sensory neuropathy. **Lepromatous** leprosy is extensive, diffuse, and symmetric, involving skin and peripheral nerves. **Tuberculoid leprosy** is less extensive, with fewer skin lesions that are sharply demarcated, but the neurologic involvement is more severe. The nerves are often enlarged.

b. **Treatment.** Free treatment and hospitalization are available at the United States Public Health hospitals at San Francisco, California, Carville, Louisiana, or Staten Island, New York. Most cases require less than 2 months of hospitalization.

   (1) The drug of choice is dapsone 50–100 mg PO daily given to adults and 1 mg/kg to children. When there is no clinical evidence of activity and no acid-fast rods are seen on skin smears, treatment is continued for 18 months in tuberculoid leprosy and for 10 years in lepromatous leprosy. Patients who have features of both types are treated for lepromatous leprosy. Note that dapsone, by itself, may cause polyneuropathy.

   (2) Rifampin is a more effective agent, and it is used in many parts of the world. However, it has not been released for use in leprosy by the Federal Drug Administration. Patients who relapse on dapsone alone are often given rifampin in addition.

   (3) **Reactional states.** During therapy, tender inflamed subcutaneous nodules (erythema nodosum leprosum) may appear acutely. These nodules appear in groups and last 1 week or longer, and new groups occur as the older ones regress. Fever, myalgia, and other systemic symptoms also occur with these nodules. Treatment is with analgesics and antipyretics. Corticosteroids may be needed in some severe cases, and dapsone is continued.

   (4) **Treatment of household contacts.** Dapsone 50 mg twice weekly or 25 mg daily for 2–3 years is recommended for close contacts.

E. Idiopathic facial palsy (Bell's palsy)

1. Acute idiopathic facial palsy is a common disorder of the seventh cranial nerve.

   a. Isolated unilateral facial weakness is the most common feature, but pain, hyperacusis, and aguesia may occur in some cases. In about 90% of patients the deficits improve without therapy.

   b. Patients older than 60 years of age and those with hypertension and diabetes mellitus are at risk of not recovering completely. When the EMG shows signs of denervation, the prognosis for complete recovery is worse.

2. **Treatment.** Corticosteroid therapy is recommended, but since most patients recover, there is some controversy about the necessity for therapy. Prednisone 60 mg PO every morning for 5 days, then reduced gradually over 10–14 days, is standard and usually safe treatment.

   Evidence shows that the recovery time is shorter when steroids are used. If used, corticosteroids should be started as soon after the onset as possible, since the suspected effect of the drug is reduction of facial nerve edema.

3. **Complications.** Facial spasm is occasionally a late complication of Bell's palsy, and it is often refractory to medical treatment. Anxiety usually makes the twitches worse, and mild sedatives may help relieve them (Valium 5–10

mg QID or phenobarbital 30–60 mg TID). Phenytoin is occasionally helpful (300 mg PO every morning), but if no effect is seen in 10–14 days, the drug should be stopped.

F. Restless leg syndrome

1. **Description.** The restless leg syndrome is a rare condition, in which an unpleasant creeping sensation occurs deep in the legs (and occasionally in the arms). The problem occurs when the patient is at rest, so it interferes with sleep. The person is compelled to move the legs around to avoid the unpleasant feeling.

   The calf and pretibial areas are the usual sites of discomfort, and it is often bilateral. It may be intermittent, lasting several minutes or hours, and there is no pain. The cause of the syndrome is unknown, but it has been associated with iron deficiency anemia, cancer, and pregnancy. It is found in some families as an autosomal dominant trait.

2. **Treatment**

   a. The underlying condition is treated.

   b. Diazepam 20–40 mg/day helps occasionally.

XVII. MOTOR SYSTEM DISEASE

A. **Description.** Neuronal degeneration confined to the anterior horn cell motor neurons in the cerebral cortex and the corticospinal tract is called *motor system disease.* The course of motor system disease varies, depending on the age of the patient and the parts of the motor system that are involved. There are several distinct forms of motor system disease.

1. **Amyotrophic lateral sclerosis** (ALS) is the most common form of motor system disease. The disease is known as **progressive bulbar palsy,** and its etiology is unknown. It is easily recognized by atrophy, weakness, spasticity (from degeneration of upper motor neurons), and absolute lack of sensory signs. It occurs sporadically, but occasionally it may be found in families as a dominant trait. Males are affected more than females, and the onset is usually in middle age with rapid progression.

   Before making the diagnosis, treatable disease, such as spinal cord compression, must be sought. Myelography is necessary unless clear involvement of spinal and brainstem nuclei indicate a diffuse localization. Abdominal reflexes and bladder function are usually normal. The degenerative process may be localized only in the brainstem.

   In Guam and the Kii Peninsula of Japan, an exceptionally high incidence of amyotrophic lateral sclerosis has been reported.

2. **Progressive muscular atrophy** resembles amyotrophic lateral sclerosis, but without involvement of the upper motor neurons. Tendon reflexes are almost always absent, although spinal cord and brainstem neurons may be involved. This is a very rare form of motor system disease, with an earlier onset and slower progression than amyotrophic lateral sclerosis. Some forms of progressive muscular atrophy are hereditary, either as dominant or recessive traits. There is an infantile form, **Werdnig-Hoffmann disease,** which is manifested as a "floppy infant." A juvenile variety with proximal distribution is called **Kugelberg-Welander** syndrome.

3. **Primary lateral sclerosis** is an extremely rare form of motor neuron disease, in which the spinal motor neurons are spared but the upper motor neurons degenerate and cause spasticity. The pathology of this disease is not fully known. The progression is slow and it is usually not fatal. The disorder may be found in families, and the patient's kin may demonstrate other degenerative disorders.

B. Prognosis. Patients who have amyotrophic lateral sclerosis with only spinal involvement usually die within 3 to 5 years. Those who have bulbar involvement (alone or with spinal disease) usually die within 2½ years. Occasionally the progression of this form of the disorder seems to slow down; some patients are reported to have lived 10–15 years with the spinal form of the disease. Thus these cases may be cited when discussing the prognosis of the illness with the patient and his or her family.

Physical disability is usually complete earlier in bulbar cases (several months) than in spinal cases (up to 4 years). However, progressive spinal atrophy and primary lateral sclerosis, as they progress, often develop into the complete syndrome of amyotrophic lateral sclerosis. Patients with the juvenile form of progressive muscular atrophy (Kugelberg-Welander) may live for 20–40 years after diagnosis.

C. Management

1. Emotional

a. The psychological management of any terminal illness must be individualized. The general approach described for amyotrophic lateral sclerosis can be modified to be of use in other terminal illnesses as well. When the mind is spared and the patient can feel that he or she is becoming more disabled from one visit to another, there is a particularly severe sense of helplessness. Thus frequently the physician will tend to avoid the patient and appear only during catastrophe, when certain tangible action can help. However, the management of amyotrophic lateral sclerosis requires more availability and more support on the part of the physician than diseases that are directly treatable.

b. When the patient realizes the severity of the illness, a massive reorganization of his or her life must be undertaken. Also, once he or she realizes that death is inevitable, a variety of reactions will occur. For example, the patient may become depressed, with a sense of uselessness and hopelessness, and increased dependence on the family and physician may follow. Self-pity and low self-esteem may also contribute to the depression. The physician can help in these situations by being appropriately available and by serving as a listener for the patient to express his or her feelings. At times antidepressant medication (Elavil 100–300 mg at bedtime) is useful, but it should not be used as a substitute for the doctor-patient relationship.

Some patients react with denial of depression and present a front of pseudogaiety. In this case the physician can help by being receptive to the patient's underlying fears and anxieties and by not participating in the process of denial.

c. Initial denial gives way to feelings related to job, family, religion, finances, self-esteem, physical incapacity, and emotional vulnerability. The dying patient has fear of pain and abandonment, as well as anxiety about desertion of his or her family and concern over other responsibilities. These are subjects about which a patient may wish to talk with the physician. A psychiatric consultant or social worker may be needed if the neurologist is unable to provide enough time.

d. In general, the physician should avoid offhand reassurances and superficial denial of the illness. It does not help to commiserate with the patient, to grieve with him or her, or to provide false hopes. Instead, the physician should represent a warm, compassionate personal force, who is willing to help the patient.

The patient should be included in all major discussions and decisions regarding the illness, and he or she is encouraged to remain as active as possible. Also, the family need support and accurate information to allow them to adjust to the change in their lives with more ease.

   e. The patient with chronic progressive illness leaves many questions unasked. The physician should provide opportunities for the patient to acquire the knowledge he or she wants and at the rate at which it is needed.

   It is best to tell the truth, if not the whole truth, about the prognosis. Many answers need to be repeated and expanded as the illness progresses. Predicting the time of death is not possible and should be avoided, but the patient should be advised to arrange his or her affairs "just in case." When direct questions about death are asked, pleading ignorance is not sufficient. Turn the question back to the patient and allow him or her to express his or her feelings about the condition.

   f. There is often a point in a chronic illness at which the patient becomes angry. The anger may be directed at the family, physician, or hospital. The physician must allow the patient to express this hostility and refrain from counterattack, thus maintaining the therapeutic alliance. The family and hospital staff must also be aware of the process behind the patient's anger.

2. **Medical therapy.** There is no medication that alters the course of motor system disease. Guanidine is not used at present, because it has not been effective in past trials. However, most patients take vitamins and derive benefit from them. The use of harmless medicines that are not specifically therapeutic may act as a sign to the patient that an attempt is being made to help him or her. Early in treatment a tangible sign of help is useful to keep the patient in the supportive program.

3. **Treatment of weakness**

   a. The treatment of weakness in amyotrophic lateral sclerosis is purely mechanical. For example, a neck brace may help when neck muscles are too weak to hold the head up; and wrist splints occasionally improve grip in patients with weakness of wrist extension.

   b. Motorized and mechanical appliances (wheelchair, lifts, hospital beds) help to maintain maximal independence.

   c. Bracing is usually not done to preserve gait in amyotrophic lateral sclerosis. However, in cases of juvenile motor neuron disease (Kugelberg-Welander), bracing may be indicated, since the progression is very slow.

   d. Physical therapy helps to minimize disuse atrophy and prevent contractures. Fatigue should be avoided, and strength should be used for necessary activities of daily living rather than in useless attempts to "build up" the muscles.

   e. Muscle cramps are common and may be prevented with phenytoin 300 mg every morning or 300 mg daily, or diazepam 2–10 mg TID. Warmth and massage are helpful in releasing the cramps.

4. Most patients with motor system disease can be treated at home during most of their illness, with help from a visiting nurses association or other community agencies. It is expensive to keep these patients in acute care facilities. However, if the family is not able to manage the patient, placement in a chronic care facility for terminal care is necessary.

   In following patients with motor system disease, body weight, ability to cough, vital capacity, and swallowing ability are evaluated to measure change and to anticipate problems.

   Suicide is uncommon in these patients, perhaps because the weakness caused by the disorder renders them incapable of performing the act.

SUGGESTED READING

General
Adams, R. D. *Diseases of Muscle.* Hagerstown, Md: Harper and Row, 1975.
Howard, F. (ed.) Treatment of neuromuscular disorders. *Mod. Treatment* 3:224, 1966.

Murphy, E. G. *The Chemistry and Therapy of Disorders of Voluntary Muscles.* Springfield: Thomas, 1964.

O'Donohue, W. J., Baker, J. L., Bell, G. M., et al. Respiratory failure in neuromuscular disease: Management in a respiratory intensive care unit. *J.A.M.A.* 235:733, 1976.

Walton, J. (ed.) *Disorders of Voluntary Muscles.* Edinburgh: Churchill, Livingstone, 1974.

Muscular Dystrophies

Cohen, L., and Morgan, J. Diethylstilbestrol effects on serum enzymes and isoenzymes in muscular dystrophy. *Arch. Neurol.* 33:480, 1976.

Harris, S. E., and Cherry, D. B. Childhood progressive muscular dystrophy and the role of physical therapy. *Phys. Ther.* 54:4, 1974.

Hook, R., Anderson, E. F., and Noto, P. Anesthetic management of a parturient with myotonia atrophica. *Anesthesiology* 43:689, 1975.

Roses, A. D., Roses, M. J., Miller, S. E., Hull, K. L., and Appel, S. H. Carrier detection in Duchenne muscular dystrophy. *N. Engl. J. Med.* 294:193, 1976.

Sarnat, H. B., O'Connor, T., and Byrne, P. A. Clinical effects of myotonic dystrophy on pregnancy and the neonate. *Arch. Neurol.* 33:459, 1976.

Vignos, P. J., Spencer, G. E., and Archibald, K. C. Management of progressive muscular dystrophy of childhood. *J.A.M.A.* 184:89, 1963.

Zellweger, M. D., and Ionasescu, V. Myotonic dystrophy and its differential diagnosis. *Acta. Neurol. Scand.* Supplement 55, Vol. 49, 1973.

Polymyositis

Barwick, D. D., and Walton, J. N. Polymyositis, *Am. J. Med.* 35:646, 1963.

Benson, M. D., and Aldo, A. Azathioprine therapy in polymyositis. *Arch. Intern. Med.* 132:447, 1973.

Brown, M., Swift, T. R., and Spies, S. M. Radioisotope scanning in inflammatory muscle disease. *Neurology* 26:517, 1976.

Devere, R., and Bradley, W. G. Polymyositis: Its presentation, morbidity, and mortality. *Brain* 98:637, 1975.

Dubowitz, V. Treatment of dermatomyositis in children. *Arch. Dis. Child.* 51:494, 1976.

Metzger, A. L., Bohan, A., Goldberg, L. S., et al. Polymyositis and dermatomyositis: Combined methotrexate and corticosteroid therapy. *Ann. Intern. Med.* 81:182, 1974.

Winkleman, R. K., Mulder, D. W., and Lambert, E. H. Course of dermatomyositis-polymyositis: Comparison of untreated and cortisone-treated patients. *Mayo Clinic Proc.* 43:545, 1968.

Periodic Paralysis

Resnick, J. S. Episode muscle weakness. *Clin. Orthop.* 39:63, 1965.

Vroom, F. O., Jarrell, X. X., and Maren, T. H. Acetazolamide treatment of hypokalemic periodic paralysis. *Arch. Neurol.* 32:385, 1975.

Myasthenia Gravis

Flacke, W. Treatment of myasthenia gravis. *N. Engl. J. Med.* 288:27, 1973.

Genkins, G., Papatestas, A. E., and Horowitz, S. H. Studies in myasthenia gravis: Early thymectomy. *Am. J. Med.* 58:517, 1975.

Mann, J. D., Johns, T. R., and Campa, J. F. Long term administration of corticosteroids in myasthenia gravis. *Neurology* 26:729, 1976.

Millichap, J. G., and Dodge, P. R. Diagnosis and treatment of myasthenia gravis in infancy, childhood and adolescence. *Neurology* 10:1007, 1960.

Osserman, K. E., and Genkins, G. Critical reappraisal of the use of edrophonium chloride tests in myasthenia gravis and significance of clinical classification. *Ann. N.Y. Acad. Sci.* 135:312, 1966.

Ozdemir, C., and Young, R. R. Electrical testing in myasthenia gravis: An overview. *Ann. N.Y. Acad. Sci.* 183:287, 1971.

Perlo, V. P., Arnason, B. G., and Poskanzer, D. The role of thymectomy in treatment of myasthenia gravis. *Ann. N.Y. Acad. Sci.* 183:308, 1971.

Seybold, M. E., and Drachman, D. B. Gradually increasing dose of prednisone in myasthenia gravis. *N. Engl. J. Med.* 290:81, 1974.

Simpson, J. F., Westerberg, M. R., and Magee, K. R. Myasthenia gravis. *Acta. Neurol. Scand.* Supplement 23, 42:6, 1966.

Tetanus

Blake, P. A., Feldman, R. A., and Buchanan, T. M. Serologic therapy of tetanus in the United States, 1965–1971. *J.A.M.A.* 235:42, 1976.

Botulism

Donadio, J. A., Gangarosa, E. J., and Faich, G. A. Diagnosis and treatment of botulism. *J. Infect. Dis.* 124:108, 1971.

Neuropathy

Adour, K. K., and Wingerd, J. Idiopathic facial paralysis (Bell's palsy): Factors affecting severity and outcome in 446 patients. *Neurology* 44:1112, 1974.

Adour, K. K., Wingerd, M. A., Bell, D. N., Manning, M. D., and Hurley, J. P. Prednisone treatment for idiopathic facial paralysis (Bell's Palsy). *N. Engl. J. Med.* 287:1268, 1972.

Bradley, W. G. *Disorders of Peripheral Nerves.* Oxford: Blackwell Scientific, 1974.

Dyck, P. J., Lais, A. C., Ohta, M., Bastron, J. A., Okazaki, H., and Groover, R. V. Chronic inflammatory polyradiculoneuropathy. *Mayo Clin. Proc.* 50:621, 1975.

Freeman, F. R. Causes of polyneuropathy. *Acta. Neurol. Scand.* Supplement 59, Vol. 51:6, 1975.

McLeod, J. G., Walsh, J. C., Prineas, J. W., and Pollard, J. D. Acute idiopathic polyneuritis, *J. Neurol. Sci.* 27:145, 1976.

Pleasure, D. E., Lovelace, R. E., and Duvoisin, R. C. The prognosis of acute polyradiculoneuritis. *Neurology* 18:1143, 1968.

Ravn, H. The Landry-Guillain-Barré syndrome. *Acta. Neurol. Scand.* Supplement 30, 43:6, 1967.

Vinken, P. J., and Bruyn, G. W. *Handbook of Clinical Neurology,* Vols. 7 and 8. New York: *American Elsevier,* 1970.

Motor System Disease

Bonduelle, M. Amyotrophic Lateral Sclerosis, in P. J. Vinken and G. W. Bruyn (eds.), *Handbook of Clinical Neurology,* Vol. 22. New York: American Elsevier, 1975.

Mackay, R. P. Course and prognosis in amyotrophic lateral sclerosis. *Arch. Neurol.* 8:117, 1973.

Smith, R. A., and Norris, F. H. Symptomatic care of patients with amyotrophic lateral sclerosis. *J.A.M.A.* 234:715, 1975.

17   Thomas M. Walshe and Howard D. Weiss

Problems Associated with Chronic Neurologic Disease

Chronic neurologic disease may be stable or progressive. In mild cases almost normal existence is possible with proper bracing or other rehabilitation. However, in disorders that cause fixed deficits, management is aimed at maximizing the remaining function.

In progressive disorders the treatment is adjusted to the tempo and severity of the illness. For example, malignant brain tumor or amyotrophic lateral sclerosis (ALS) become fatal rapidly, but an understanding of the prognosis and care of the symptoms provide a real benefit to the patient and his or her family.

The following sections describe the management of the common problems seen in disabled neurologic patients. The guidelines discussed can be applied with slight modification regardless of the underlying neurologic process.

I. **TREATMENT OF DYSPHAGIA.** Weakness or spasticity or both of the pharynx and tongue causes dysphagia and a lethal tendency to aspirate secretions and foods.

   A. Early use of a feeding tube, either through a gastrostomy or cervical esophagostomy, is required. Nasogastric tubes can be used temporarily for feeding, but they are uncomfortable, cause pressure necrosis of the nares, and allow aspiration. If a nasogastric tube is used, the smallest possible diameter is best; the soft rubber pediatric tubes are large enough even for adults. The cervical esophagostomy may be useful in dysphagic patients who are ambulatory, since the tube can be inserted during feedings and the ostium can be covered with a dressing at other times. Patients with severe weakness are usually unable to feed themselves, so gastrostomy is the method of choice. However, multiple abdominal procedures, especially gastric operations, make gastrostomy more dangerous than cervical esophagostomy.

   B. Care of a gastrostomy is simple; 10–14 days after the tube is inserted, a well-defined fistula is established, and the tube can be changed easily. A 28Fr foley catheter or special gastrostomy tube may be used.

   C. Tube feedings with commercial products (e.g., Sustacal or Sustagen) are calculated to deliver the desired amount of calories each day. The caloric need is higher for active patients and ranges from 1200 to 2400 kcal every 24 hours. The liquid foods are usually concentrated to deliver 1 kcal/ml. If they cause diarrhea, they may need to be diluted. To avoid clogging of the tube, each feeding is followed with water.

   Tube feeding is best started with about one-half the total desired calories diluted in water. A gradual increase in concentration (and calories) avoids diarrhea and malabsorption. Before administering a feeding, the tube is aspirated to ensure that the previous feeding was absorbed. Small volumes are given at first at frequent intervals (every 1–2 hours). The maximum volume given is about 200 ml (150 ml of food followed by 50 ml of water).

   Large volumes may cause vomiting and aspiration, although larger individuals may require more volume. If the patient needs more water, small volumes may be given between feedings. Also, blended food mixed with milk or water may provide more bulk and prevent the feeling of hunger in patients with a gastrostomy.

   D. If aspiration of saliva and nasal secretions is a problem, a cuffed endotracheal tube is necessary. Anticholinergic drugs or tricyclic antidepressants may reduce salivation, prevent drooling, and in some cases the patient may be able to swallow the reduced volume of secretions safely. **Ligation** of the trachea above the tracheostomy may be necessary to prevent chronic aspiration of secretions and food.

E. The decision to undertake palliative surgery such as gastrostomy and tracheostomy depends on the **general level of function** of the patient. Patients with progressive illnesses are often not treated with tracheostomy late in the illness, when respiratory failure threatens. Patients with stable illnesses of brainstem or spinal cord often benefit from it.

II. BLADDER DYSFUNCTION. Spinal cord trauma is the most common cause of severe neurogenic bladder dysfunction, but other spinal cord conditions—such as multiple sclerosis, spinal cord tumor, ruptured disc, and tabes dorsalis—produce problems with micturition. In addition, disorders of **peripheral nerves,** such as diabetes mellitus and herpes zoster, may cause hyporeflexive bladder, and neurologic disease affecting higher centers, such as Parkinson's disease, frontal lobe tumors, and cerebrovascular disease, may cause abnormal micturition. In each incidence, a cystometrogram is necessary to define the type of bladder dysfunction so that appropriate therapy can be attempted. Early urologic consultation together with a cystometrogram are needed to define structural abnormalities.

A. Normal bladder function. The anatomy and physiology of the bladder are arranged to allow storage of urine until it can be conveniently excreted.

1. The majority of the detrusor muscle derives its **innervation** via parasympathetic fibers (S2-4). The area of the trigone, however, is innervated by sympathetic fibers (T11-L2). (Ascending fibers provide appropriate feedback control).

    a. Both somatic sensory fibers and parasympathetic ascending fibers leave the bladder to converge in the S2-4 levels. There are also some ascending sympathetic fibers that synapse at the T9-L2 levels. The lateral spinothalamic tracts and the fasciculus gracilis carry the ascending fibers to higher centers.

    b. The corticospinal tracts carry motor fibers to the external sphincter and pelvic floor muscles, which are under voluntary control. The primitive micturition reflex is at the S2-4 level via parasympathetic efferent fibers.

2. To maintain **continence of urine,** the urethral pressure must be higher than the vesical pressure. The muscles of the urogenital diaphragm and urethra may be flaccid or spastic. If they are flaccid there is little outflow obstruction, and incontinence is common even with low bladder pressure. If these muscles of the urogenital diaphragm and urethra are spastic, high bladder pressure is necessary to empty the bladder so that ureteral reflux and high volumes of residual urine do not occur. Optimal function requires a balance between the bladder and the urogenital musculature. In neurologic disease the balance among urethral pressure at the bladder neck, external sphincter and pelvic muscle tension, and detrusor pressure is disturbed, which can cause incomplete or unexpected voiding.

3. **Micturition** is the result of reflex and voluntary activity. In the normal bladder a pressure of 30–40 cm H_2O causes reflex reduction of urethral pressure and consequent micturition. As the bladder fills, wall tension increases but intravesicular pressure remains constant. At low volumes a normal person feels the bladder filling, and when it reaches 100–200 ml, the urge to void occurs. Voluntary control of the external sphincter and pelvic floor muscles helps to maintain continence, but there is also reflex inhibition of the detrusor, so pressure is kept constant. In normal persons the maximum bladder capacity is 400–450 ml, and at this point the detrusor contracts and all the urine is expelled. Initiation of micturition when the bladder is full is caused by reflex mostly. The latency between the decision to void and the initiation of flow is inversely related to the bladder volume.

B. **Goals for management of the neurogenic bladder**

1. Protect the kidneys from hydronephrosis and infection by reducing residual urine and reflux.

2. Relieve incontinence.

3. Maintain an acceptable functional capacity so voiding only occurs every 4–6 hours.

C. **Hyperreflexive bladder management** (lesions above S2–4). The hyperreflexive bladder is characterized by many subthreshold, uninhibited detrusor contractions, reduced capacity, and spontaneous voiding with a strong stream. Chronic spinal cord lesions above S2–4 cause a hyperreflexive bladder in which the patient has no sensation of bladder fullness. In these patients the bladder empties by reflex action when a critical volume is reached. If the urogenital diaphragm muscles are coordinated with the reflex detrusor contraction, complete spontaneous voiding occurs. However, if the urethral pressure is too high, there is reflux into the ureters; and if the urethral pressure is too low, there is incontinence.

In lesions that are higher (i.e., in the cortex, posterior hypothalamus, midbrain, or anterior pons), there may be a sensation of urgency and frequency without dysuria.

Dysynergy between the muscles of the urogenital diaphragm and the detrusor causes incontinence during small reflex contractions. In this case instillation of ice water into the bladder will produce reflex micturition.

Cystitis may cause bladder hyperreflexia because of irritation of nerves; and hyperactivity may occur in obstructive bladder disease, even without neurologic disease.

1. When a patient is incontinent with a hyperreflexic bladder or has an acute spinal cord injury with resolving spinal shock, **intermittent catheterization** is started. To avoid infection, an experienced person (or team) should perform the catheterization in the early stages.

   a. The patient is given large volumes of fluid either PO, through a nasogastric tube, or IV, and the bladder is drained every 2–4 hours. High-volume intake reduces the risk of infection and calculus formation.

   b. Bladder training is begun (see sec **II.C.2**), and as the patient begins to void on his own (usually by reflex) the frequency of catheterization is reduced until the patient voids by reflex and carries an acceptable residual volume (i.e., less than 100 ml).

   It usually takes less than 90 days for a patient with a complete spinal cord lesion to become catheter-free. Approximately 10–20% fail to improve because of either a very small bladder capacity or excessive bladder hyperreflexia. If intermittent catheterization fails, an indwelling catheter is placed or other methods are used to maintain continence.

   c. **Incomplete spinal cord lesions** have the most rapid and complete return of reflex micturition. Other patients may require chronic intermittent catheterization in addition to reflex voiding.

2. **Bladder training.** Intermittent catheterization prevents excess bladder distention. Bladder training helps to prevent bladder contracture, conditions a regulated reflex pattern, and causes the patient to take notice of bladder function.

   a. Regular attempts at initiating the reflex should be made. In patients with a complete sensory level below the waist, the best means of beginning the reflex varies. Squeezing the glans penis, scratching the scrotum, pulling the pubic hair, tapping over the bladder, and (most often successful) deep digital stimulation of the rectum, are useful methods.

384 Part II. Neurologic Diseases

b. High-volume intake keeps the urine dilute and helps prevent infection. However, once a patient is trained, fluid volume must be adjusted so voiding is not too frequent.

c. Observance of intake and output ensures fluid balance.

d. External compression of the bladder (Credé) helps reduce residual volume and, with triple voiding, increases the total amount voided.

e. Alternation of the patient's position increases the total volume voided.

3. Drug therapy. The use of drugs is limited because chronic use causes toxicity.

a. Bethanechol chloride (Urecholine), a cholinergic agonist, may increase detrusor function and facilitate reflex activity. The dose is 10–50 mg every 4–6 hours PO or 5–10 mg every 4–6 hours subcutaneously. A similar drug, **methacholine chloride** (Mecholyl), is used in doses of 200–400 mg every 4–6 hours PO or 10–20 mg every 4–6 hours subcutaneously. Methacholine chloride is used to lower threshold for reflex voiding when the reflex is not adequate to empty the bladder and early in spinal cord trauma to promote reflex activity.

b. When small bladder volumes cause excessive reflex activity, reduction in reflex may increase the time between voidings.

(1) Useful drugs are **methantheline bromide** (Banthine) and **propantheline bromide** (Pro-Banthine), which are anticholinergic agents that reduce detrusor reflex activity in doses of 50 mg QID (Banthine) or 15 mg PO QID (Pro-Banthine). Anticholinergic drugs such as these are most useful in partial spinal cord or higher lesions to reduce urgency and frequency.

The anticholinergic drugs may, however, increase residual volume and, paradoxically, cause more frequency because of reduced functional capacity. Increased residual volume also increases the risk of infection, which may lead to chronic cystitis or even pyelonephritis. Thus these drugs are discontinued if the residual volume is increased to more than 15% of the voided volume.

(2) Tricyclic antidepressants (150 mg at bedtime) may act to increase bladder capacity through their anticholinergic activity.

c. Phenoxybenzamine, an alpha-adrenergic blocking agent, acts on the proximal urethra and reduces urethra pressure. Residual volume may be reduced when phenoxybenzamine is given in doses of 20–40 mg TID. Also, bladder neck resection may be avoided when alpha blockers are effective.

d. Propranolol (Inderal), a beta-adrenergic blocker, increases urethral resistance and may be helpful when incontinence is caused by uninhibited contractions that overcome the urethral pressure. Usual doses are 20–40 mg QID or more.

e. Drugs to reduce spasticity of the pelvic floor may reduce residual volume and allow more complete voiding. **Dantrolene sodium** (Dantrium) has not been systematically tested, but **baclofen** (Lioresal), used for bladder training, has been reported to reduce residual urine volume.

4. Surgical therapy

a. When medical measures fail to allow reflex voiding or there is high bladder pressure with reflux of urine into the ureters, causing hydronephrosis, bladder neck resection or external sphincterotomy will reduce both resistance to flow and bladder pressure. However, removal of prostate or urethral valve obstruction may be necessary to allow adequate reflex voiding.

    b. Other procedures are available to increase the voiding pressure, reduce capacity, increase capacity, or divert the urinary stream. Urologic consultation is needed in all these cases.

    c. When a hyperreflexive bladder is severe and contracted so there is low functional capacity, alcohol block of the cauda equina or anterior and posterior rhizotomy of T12–S5 will cause it to become hypotonic. However, these procedures can only be done in paraplegics, and they often cause impotence. The major consideration is to spare the kidneys if there is hydronephrosis, in which case the patient is treated for hyporeflexive bladder.

D. Hyporeflexive bladder management. The hyporeflexive bladder is characterized by very low pressure, no contractions, high capacity, high residual volume, and poor stream. There is absent or decreased sensation of fullness. It is associated with lesions at either the S2–4 level or on the peripheral nerves and roots.

    Transient urinary retention may follow lumbar puncture or, more commonly, lumbar myelography. Men with prostate enlargement are particularly susceptible to retention. However, intermittent catheterization every 4–6 hours will keep the bladder trained. Occasionally urecholine (10–25 mg PO every 6–8 hours) is needed, but the retention usually resolves spontaneously in 24–48 hours.

    1. Chronic intermittent catheterization done by the patient on a timed schedule is effective in keeping the bladder empty. Also, it can be done, if necessary, using nonsterile technique without danger of serious infection. The patient can carry the catheter with him in a pocket or purse.

    Patients with ataxia, upper extremity weakness, excessive adduction spasticity in the legs, or dementia are often not able to catheterize themselves.

    2. The use of **external bladder compression** (Credé) and contraction of abdominal muscles may allow the patient to void sufficiently to reduce residual urine to an acceptable volume (usually less than 15% of voided volume). Since the patient may not perceive bladder fullness, regular attempts at voiding at specific times are important. In patients with weak abdominal muscles, a lumbosacral corset helps to increase intraabdominal pressure.

    3. Drug therapy

        a. Incomplete lesions in which there is diminished reflex activity may improve with Urecholine 10–25 mg PO every 8 hours. If the dose is ineffective PO, subcutaneous injection may be useful.

        b. Phenoxybenzamine may reduce urethral pressure so voiding is more complete (20–40 mg TID).

    4. Surgical therapy

        a. Bladder neck resection reduces physiologic obstruction and allows more complete emptying of the bladder.

        b. Relief of obstruction from prostate or urethral valves may also reduce residual volume.

E. Incontinence. Overflow incontinence occurs in hypotonic bladders and higher-volume reflex incontinence occurs in hyperreflexic bladders.

    1. Incontinence in the female is difficult to treat if the volume is great as in a hyperreflexic bladder, and an indwelling catheter may be necessary. If the volume is small and the patient can use intermittent catheterization, a pad may be sufficient between catheterizations.

    2. For the incontinent male, several **appliances** are available.

        a. The **condom collecting device** is useful for both temporary or chronic use. The device is attached around the shaft of the penis with cement or tape, and it can be left in place for up to 12 hours. A reservoir bag can be strapped to the leg and be hidden by clothing.

Most males with bladder dysfunction require a condom device when they are in public. Frequent changes of the condom (every 1–2 hours) and local care usually prevent local complications. However, if ulceration or maceration of the skin of the penis occurs, the device should be removed, the area kept dry, and a bland ointment used to help with healing. In hospitalized patients a diaper can be used instead of the device to allow the penis to heal.

    b. The **Cunningham clamp** is a device designed to occlude the urethra mechanically by external compression of the penis. However, the clamp should be released frequently. A major complication is pressure necrosis of the penis or urethra. Thus this device should not be used in patients who do not have tactile sensation on the penis.

3. Surgically implanted prosthetic devices to provide sphincteric effect are available. These devices are useful in patients with hyporeflexive and hyper-reflexive bladders.

4. Electrodes placed in the S2–4 area of the spinal cord have produced detrusor contraction in some cases of hyporeflexive bladder.

5. Chronic indwelling catheters should be avoided if possible.

    a. The catheter is inserted, using strict aseptic technique.

        (1) Teflon catheters have less chance of accumulating mineral deposits. Therefore they can be changed less frequently.

        (2) The standard rubber catheter is changed every 7–10 days.

        (3) A Foley balloon-type catheter is less desirable for chronic use, because the balloon may cause bladder irritation and pressure damage. In women the Foley catheter is usually necessary, since there is no effective way of securing a straight catheter. In males, a straight catheter taped to the penis can be substituted for the bag type.

    b. In all cases the drainage system should remain closed; and the reservoir should never be raised above the bladder to prevent reflux into the bladder. A disinfectant may be added to the reservoir.

    c. Irrigation of the bladder through a double-lumen catheter at 40–50 ml QID or TID with a volume that is equal to the bladder capacity. Any sterile solution is suitable. A citric acid solution (e.g., Renacidin) helps to prevent calcium salts from aggregating on the catheter, and solutions of acetic acid or neomycin are also available. When the patient is ambulatory, continuous irrigation may be stopped by clamping the inflow tube.

    d. A 16 French catheter or smaller is optimal. Large catheters are associated with urethral abcess in men, but in women the urethra will dilate if larger catheters are used. If a balloon catheter is used, 5 ml volume in the balloon is sufficient.

In males the catheter should be taped to the abdomen to prevent extreme angulation, causing pressure necrosis at the penoscrotal junction.

    e. Drainage of the upper urinary tracts is facilitated by:

        (1) Early ambulation or wheelchair activity.

        (2) Frequent changes of position.

        (3) Elevation of the head of the bed.

    f. High fluid intake helps to prevent infection and calculus formation. Intake of 3000–4000 ml of fluid each day is indicated for persons with indwelling catheters in place, unless there is a strong medical contraindication to this fluid load.

F. Stone prevention

1. Good nutrition and high fluid volume are important to the recovery of a patient with bladder dysfunction. If hypercalciuria is present, a reduction in the amount of dietary calcium may help to prevent stone formation.

2. Acidification of the urine helps to prevent infection as well as to keep mineral salts in solution. Thus most patients with bladder dysfunction, especially those with indwelling catheters, should have their urine acidified to prevent precipitation of mineral deposits and help to prevent infection.

   a. Cranberry juice lowers the pH irregularly and is not as useful as other agents; 250 ml TID has been used in selected cases.

   b. Ascorbic acid 250 mg PO QID will lower urine pH if there is no infection present. Methenamine mandelate (Mandelamine) 1 gm PO QID will lower urine pH if there is no infection present; 1 gm PO QID, used with ascorbic acid, is useful in keeping urine acidified when infection is present. It also has bactericidal action.

   c. Hippuric acid 12–14 gm daily acidifies the urine and has a weak bacteriostatic effect.

G. Urine infection

1. It is not necessary to treat asymptomatic, chronic urinary infection rigorously while a catheter is in place. Acidification of the urine and use of suppressive agents, such as Mandelamine 1 gm QID, Hiprex (methenamine hippurate 1 gm BID), or Gantrisin 1 gm QID are sufficient to keep the bacterial count as low as possible. Prevention of reflux is critical to protect the upper tracts from infection.

2. When acute infection occurs or the patient becomes febrile, specific therapy is necessary. If the patient is on intermittent catheterization, a Teflon catheter is inserted and kept in place until the infection is under control. If the patient is on continuous drainage, the old catheter is replaced and specific antibiotics are used. However, frequent aseptic change of the catheter may be necessary.

   Although the urine may never become sterile, the goal of therapy is to eradicate the bacteria in the tissue and upper tracts. Bladder urine may remain infected.

III. BOWEL DYSFUNCTION

A. Fecal impaction occurs in a variety of illnesses, but it is especially common in neurologic disease.

1. **Predisposition**

   a. Bedridden patients.

   b. Elderly patients, especially those with a history of fecal impaction or constipation.

   c. Patients with abdominal weakness from neuromuscular, neuropathic, spinal cord, or other disorders.

   d. Patients receiving narcotics or other drugs that reduce bowel motility (anticholinergics).

   e. Dehydrated patients, such as those on glycerol, mannitol, or alumina gels.

2. **Signs and symptoms**

   a. The urge to defecate but the inability to do so is a common complaint in fecal impaction.

  b. Frequent watery stools.

  c. Crampy abdominal pain.

  d. Bowel obstruction with air-fluid levels seen on abdominal x-rays.

  e. A hard mass in the rectum or an abdominal mass that moves easily with palpitation.

3. Treatment

  a. Adequate hydration softens the stool and prevents impaction.

  b. Natural laxatives (e.g., whole bran and prunes) in the diet are useful to keep the stool soft. Drugs, such as dioctyl sulfosuccinate (Colace), also increase stool water and soften stools.

  c. Digital removal of the impaction or removal through a sigmoidoscope is necessary once it forms.

  d. Enemas, using a large volume with soap or oil and repeated three or four times, may relieve the impaction.

  e. Oral mineral oil 30 ml PO daily or BID for several days also helps to move impactions.

B. Fecal retention and incontinence

 1. Paralyzed patients often have no problem with fecal incontinence or constipation, even when bladder dysfunction is severe.

 2. Diarrhea may precipitate fecal incontinence in an otherwise controlled patient. When diarrhea is controlled, the bowel is often continent.

 3. Bowel training is necessary in some patients.

  a. Regular enemas or a suppository each day until a bowel pattern is established.

  b. Regular attempts at defecation, using an abdominal corset if necessary.

  c. Maintenance of a soft stool, using prunes, bran cereals, and stool softeners (Colace 100 mg TID) helps to promote bowel function.

  d. An abdominal corset may help to increase intraabdominal pressure in patients with weak abdominal muscles.

  e. In severe idiopathic polyradiculitis (Landry-Guillain-Barré syndrome) regular enemas and suppositories are often necessary until the patient can contract the abdominal muscles. Vacuetts suppositories are very useful when the stool is soft. These suppositories release CO_2 gas, increase pressure in the lumen of the bowel, and help stimulate reflex defecation.

  f. Avoid constipating medications, such as narcotics.

 4. Patients with chronic fecal incontinence (e.g., diabetics) can be helped occasionally.

  a. Use of denatured tincture of opium (5–10 drops BID) may reduce motility of the bowel.

  b. A regular morning enema to cleanse the bowel may allow the patient to go through the day with only a pad, with little risk of an unexpected loss of stool.

  c. Biofeedback techniques have been used to train some patients to use the external sphincter and the other voluntary muscles to maintain fecal continence.

IV. MANAGEMENT OF TRACHEOSTOMY

A. Placement

1. Acute respiratory distress is managed by endotracheal intubation. Tracheostomy can be done as an elective procedure if improvement is not expected to occur within 7–10 days.

2. **Indications.** Patients with neuromuscular, motor system, or brainstem lesions often require tracheostomy to:

   a. Maintain airway.

   b. Prevent aspiration.

   c. Permit deep suctioning.

   d. Reduce dead space and reduce the work of breathing.

B. Complications

1. Mortality is 1.6% in adults and 1.4% in children. Hemorrhage and a displaced tube are the most common causes of death.

   Death rarely occurs as a late complication unless there is obstruction or detachment of the tube from the ventilator.

2. **Causes of obstruction**

   a. **Secretions.** Secretions harden and occlude the lumen of the tube, especially when inadequate humidity is administered or the tube is not changed frequently.

   b. **The cuff.** In metal tubes the cuff is separate from the tube, and it may slip down and occlude the lumen.

   c. **The cannula.** If the tracheostomy is low in the neck, the cannula may obstruct at the carina. If a tube is used that is too long, it may intubate only a single bronchus. Postintubation auscultation and chest x-ray are important to guard against this complication.

   d. **Trauma.** Injured mucosa causes collection of tissue debris and granulation at the lumen of the tube, which may obstruct it.

3. **Hemorrhage**

   a. Acute postoperative hemorrhage around the wound may be life-threatening.

   b. Later, hemorrhage caused by erosion of the mucosa or erosion into an artery or vein, causing massive hemorrhage, may be fatal because of aspiration or exsanguination.

4. Subcutaneous or mediastinal emphysema usually needs no treatment but, if excessive, change of tube position and repair of the rent may be indicated. At times pneumothorax may follow subcutaneous emphysema, and appropriate x-rays of the chest should be obtained in all patients with subcutaneous or mediastinal air.

5. **Infection**

   a. **Wound infections.**

   b. **Chronic tracheitis.** Culture of bacteria in the secretions of a tracheostomized patient is not enough to diagnose infection. Most patients with tracheotomies harbor a number of potential pathogens.

C. Choice of tube

1. Metal tubes usually have an outer cannula that remains in the trachea and an inner cannula that can be removed and cleaned. Metal tubes have no

built-in cuff, but one can be added. These tubes are used for permanent tracheotomies. Patients with chronic tracheotomies can be instructed in self-management of these tubes at home if they have arm function.

2. Valved tubes are also metal. They are used so the patient can speak. At night a nonvalved inner cannula can be inserted.

3. Plastic tubes are becoming more popular and are used for tracheostomy when a cuff is necessary. However, the whole tube must be changed when secretions accumulate. Most neurologic patients require a cuff, since protection against aspiration is an important consideration.

D. Management of the cuffed tube

1. Choice of a low-pressure, high-volume cuff helps to prevent pressure necrosis of the trachea.

2. The cuff is never inflated with an arbitrary volume. The volume is determined by leakage of air around the cuff. When positive-pressure ventilation is used, the cuff is inflated until no leakage is heard around the cuff and then several milliliters are withdrawn until there is a slight leak.

3. The cuff will cause pressure necrosis unless it is deflated for 5–10 minutes every 1–2 hours. Also, if a high-volume, low-pressure cuff is used, there is less chance of necrosis.
   When aspiration is a problem, the patient is placed in the Trendelenburg position, or at least supine, when the cuff is deflated. Note that suctioning above the cuff is necessary before it is deflated.

4. The patient requires adequate fluid intake, and when a plastic cuffed tube is used, hydration in the form of aerosol is necessary to keep the patient's secretions thin. Room humidity should be kept high and the room temperature, warm. A tracheostomy mask is useful to deliver warm humidified air to the patient.

5. Frequent suction of secretions keeps the accumulation on the tube to a minimum. Instillation of 5–10 ml of sterile saline may help when secretions are very thick.

6. Postural drainage helps to remove secretions from the bronchi.

7. Speech is possible with any tracheotomy if the tube is occluded and the cuff is deflated.

8. Tracheotomy wounds close spontaneously in several days when the tube is removed. If healing is slow, taping the edges of the wound together or using a bandage with petroleum jelly to make an airtight seal will speed healing. In a few cases the tracheotomy must be closed surgically.

9. Trials of tube occlusion with mouth breathing for several minutes, increasing to hours, test the need for a tracheotomy. Once artificial respiration is not necessary, the tracheotomy can be allowed to close unless aspiration or prophylactic use (as in severe myasthenia) requires continuation.

10. In chronic aspiration the trachea can be ligated and the tube is left in place. Then the patient can take fluid and food by mouth.

11. Otolaryngology consultation is helpful in management of a chronic tracheotomy.

E. Changing the tracheostomy tube

1. Plastic tubes must be changed every 5–10 days. Metal tubes can be cleaned daily and changed less frequently.

2. The orifice at the neck communicates with the trachea and is well formed

after about 3–5 days postoperatively. If the tube is changed earlier, a surgeon should do it.

3. Gentle, firm pressure slips the tube into place and usually causes a cough reflex.

4. It is best to use the same size tube with each change. There is a tendency for staff members to use a smaller tube at each change, because the larger tubes are not as easily inserted. However, if progressively smaller tubes are used there will be a point at which the orifice is not adequate and surgical dilatation is needed.

V. DECUBITUS ULCER

A. Prevention

1. Neurologic patients who are paralyzed and those with sensory deficits are highly susceptible to pressure necrosis of the skin. The most important preventive measure is frequent turning of the patient and frequent changing of the patient's posture.

   In quadraplegic patients the Stryker frame is useful, and the patient can be rotated easily every 1–2 hours. Careful turning and positioning alone will prevent decubitus ulcer in these patients. Thus prevention of decubitus ulcer depends on the quality of nursing care.

2. Protection of bony prominences (e.g., heels, ischial tuberosities, and sacral areas) from trauma is necessary. In infants with chronic compensated hydrocephalus, care must be taken to shift the enlarged head and keep it protected; otherwise decubitus ulcer will occur.

3. Sheep's skin, water mattress, and other soft material help to protect the skin. However, cushions in donut shape may cause ischemia of the central area and actually **promote** decubitus ulcer formation.

4. The patient's skin should be kept dry, and urinary incontinence must be controlled. A diaper can be used to keep the patient dry without using an indwelling catheter.

5. Use of bland ointment, such as petroleum jelly, in areas exposed to dampness may help to prevent maceration of the skin.

6. Good nutrition is important to maintain healthy skin.

7. If edema forms, the skin becomes thin and vascularity decreases. Aggressive treatment of dependent edema in a paralyzed limb and special protection of it will help to prevent skin breakdown.

B. Treatment of established pressure sores

1. Pressure must be removed from the area of the skin that is involved. As long as pressure is maintained, the ulcer will fail to heal and may progress.

   The area of the ulcer is gently scrubbed with saline or hydrogen peroxide and mechanically debrided if there is necrotic tissue present. Wet to dry dressings are useful for large necrotic ulcers until there is a fresh area of granulation tissue. Also, lytic enzyme ointment (e.g., Biozyme, Elase, Penafil, and Travase) can be applied to the ulcer or in solution with a wet to dry dressing, which may be enough to debride the lesion. The enzyme is applied BID or TID, and the ulcer is washed before application. Large ulcers usually require surgical débridement. After débridement the area is kept dry, using a light 4 × 4-inch dressing or other lightly applied bandage.

2. Petroleum jelly or zinc oxide can be used as an occlusive dressing. A paste of magnesium aluminum gel can be made by pouring off the supernatant liquid of a bottle of antacid. This paste can be applied to the ulcer and will dry, forming a crust that protects the area. Application TID is adequate.

3. Capillary circulation is thought to be defective in patients with pressure sores. Warmth from a lamp and gentle massage around the ulcer may improve circulation and promote healing.

4. Patients with poor nutrition or anemia have more difficulty healing.

5. In severe deep ulcers with undermined edges, surgical débridement and skin-grafting may be necessary.

6. Infection in decubitus ulcer is usually not a contributing cause of the ulcer, but in severe undermined ulcers septicemia and death can occur. Topical antibiotics are not useful in these cases.

VI. SEXUAL DYSFUNCTION

A. **Introduction.** Sexual performance and enjoyment depend on a complex interplay of psychological, neurologic, endocrine, vascular, and anatomic factors. The evaluation and treatment of patients with sexual dysfunction require expertise in several disciplines of medicine. This section will outline an approach to sexual function in healthy patients and those with chronic disabling diseases of the nervous system.

B. **Initial evaluation.** Initial evaluation of patients with sexual dysfunction should include:

1. **History.** The nature and duration of the patient's complaint are clarified, and the strength of the patient's sexual desire is evaluated. Severely reduced sexual drive is a common manifestation of depression, but it may also be related to chronic physical illness, endocrine disturbances, drug side effects, extreme sexual inhibition, or adaptation to the unavailability of a partner. The spouse's sexual functioning and expectations must also be assessed to gain accurate insight into the patient's problem.

2. **Examination.** General physical examination might reveal stigmata of systemic illness, endocrine disturbances, or peripheral vascular disease. A careful neurologic examination is performed, looking particularly for evidence of peripheral neuropathy, autonomic dysfunction, or spinal cord disease. Urologic or gynecologic examination should be done to search for local structural-anatomic abnormalities or signs of gonadal atrophy; and vascular examination may reveal evidence of arterial insufficiency.

C. **Classification.** The classification of sexual dysfunction may be based on impairment of specific aspects of sexual physiology.

1. **Impotence.** Impotence is defined as the inability to have a penile erection that is adequate for sexual intercourse.

a. **Physiology of penile erection.** Erection takes place on a segmental reflex basis, involving centers in the lower spinal cord. The afferent sensory inputs that initiate the reflex may be psychic stimuli, local stimulation of the genital region, or interoceptive stimuli arising from the bowel or bladder. The efferent impulses of the erection reflex travel mainly by means of sacral parasympathetic fibers from segments S2, 3, and 4. These impulses result in a greatly increased blood flow into the erectile tissues of the penis. Eventually a steady state is reached, where the rate of arterial inflow and venous outflow are equal, and the penis stops enlarging but remains rigid.

b. **Psychogenic impotence**

(1) **Clinical features.** Depression, anxiety, phobias, and partner problems are the most common causes of impotence. Although psychological factors can inhibit the erection reflex, it may still occur under specific

circumstances. Thus the patient may report that he occasionally awakens in the morning with a full erection, is potent with some sexual partners but not others, or is able to obtain a full erection by masturbation. The occurrence of these erections implies that the neurologic and circulatory pathways are intact and suggest a psychogenic etiology for his impotence.

Many patients with psychogenic impotence lose interest in sex, thereby leading to nonperformance. Impotence can also result from untreated premature ejaculation.

(2) Therapy. Therapeutic nihilism is no longer warranted, because many patients regain penile potency following appropriate treatment. The approach to therapy and its success depend largely on the patient's underlying problem. A word of reassurance is sometimes all that is needed, especially in the "anxious-inhibitory" impotence of young men. Also, psychotherapy, dual-team sex therapy (Masters and Johnson method), and behavior therapy have been claimed successful in certain cases of psychogenic impotence.

Skepticism about the personal integrity, background, and skills of sex therapists is justifiable, considering the newness of the field and its potentials for patient exploitation. The referring physician should, therefore, be personally familiar with the local resources available for dealing with sexual problems before sending the patient to a sex clinic.

(3) Drug therapy

  (a) Androgens. There is little rationale for the administration of androgens to men with psychogenic impotence. Testosterone is unlikely to be more effective than a placebo in this circumstance, and it carries the risk of many side effects (e.g., aggravation of prostatic cancer, sodium and water retention, and hypercalcemia).

  (b) Aphrodisiacs. Cantharides (Spanish fly) or herbal aphrodisiacs, such as yohimbine, can occasionally produce a joyless reflex erection by irritating the urethral mucosa. These drugs are potentially toxic and have no role in the treatment of impotence.

c. Neurologic impotence—Autonomic neuropathies

(1) Clinical features

  (a) Peripheral neuropathies that involve autonomic fibers may cause impotence. Diabetes mellitus is the most common cause of autonomic neuropathy, with impotence occurring in 10–25% of young diabetics and in over 50% of older diabetics. The incidence of impotence does not correlate well with the duration or severity of the diabetes. However, impotence is occasionally the **initial clinical manifestation** of diabetes, so diabetes should be strongly considered in the differential diagnosis of impotent men. There is a high correlation between neurogenic bladder abnormalities (as demonstrated on cystometrogram) and impotence, thereby verifying the presence of autonomic dysfunction in these patients. Patients with diabetes mellitus are certainly not immune from **psychogenic impotence,** and objective signs of autonomic dysfunction should be diligently sought in questionable cases.

  (b) Other disorders of the autonomic nervous system commonly associated with impotence include the Shy-Drager syndrome, pure pan-dysautonomia, familial dysautonomia (Riley-Day syndrome), and hereditary primary amyloidosis. Some cases of Guillain-Barré syndrome and alcoholic polyneuropathy may also be associated with autonomic dysfunction.

(2) Treatment. Unfortunately, there is no satisfactory treatment to reverse the underlying autonomic neuropathy. However, surgical implantation of a prosthesis into the penis has allowed some patients to resume coitus.

d. Neurologic impotence—Spinal cord disease

(1) Clinical features. Disorders of sexual function have been carefully studied in patients with spinal cord injuries. Sexual function in other spinal disorders, such as multiple sclerosis, has not been analyzed in great detail, but similar principles probably apply. The level and completeness of spinal transection are important in determining residual sexual function.

Most men with a clearcut transection in the cervical or thoracic region will retain the ability to have erections. These erections can occur spontaneously during a flexor spasm or by manipulating the penis during a spasm. Therefore they appear at inappropriate times and not in response to psychic stimuli unless the cord lesion is incomplete.

Patients with low lesions that involve the lumbosacral cord or cauda equina are less likely to have erections, and their erections may be more difficult to elicit.

(2) Treatment. The psychological reactions to spinal injury are devastating, and the patient must be reassured that sexual function may still be possible. However, there are many physical obstacles that must be overcome. For example, the erections in patients with spinal injury are often not well sustained; the patient may be incontinent of urine during erection; and flexor spasms in the legs may prevent satisfactory penetration. Also, patients with high cord transections can develop severe autonomic hyperreflexia, with marked hypertension and cardiac arrhythmias during intercourse.

Nevertheless, counseling by physicians familiar with the problems of sexual activity in paraplegics and tetraplegics often enables these patients to resume intercourse. Fertility is usually impaired in spinal-injured men, but there have been cases in which semen has been successfully obtained and used to impregnate the patient's wife.

e. Neurologic impotence—Drug induced. Dozens of drugs have been implicated as causes of impotence. The incidence of this effect is not known, and the evidence that impotence is drug-induced is usually circumstantial. It would seem appropriate, however, to discontinue medications if possible in evaluating patients with impotence.

(1) Anticholinergic agents may theoretically impair the autonomic impulses that initiate erection. Some drugs in this category include:

(a) Atropine

(b) Propantheline (Pro-Banthine)

(c) Methantheline (Banthine)

(d) Belladonna alkaloids

(e) Benztropine mesylate (Cogentin)

(f) Biperiden (Artane)

(2) Drugs that have significant **anticholinergic side-effects** have also been implicated in causing impotence. These include:

(a) The tricyclic antidepressants (e.g., amitriptyline, imipramine)

(b) The phenothiazines (e.g., chlorpromazine, thioridazine)

(c) The anti-vertigo drugs (e.g., meclizine, diminhydrinate)

(3) Men addicted to **narcotic stimulants** or **psychedelic** drugs are subject to reversible disturbances of potency.

(4) Drugs that induce **depression** as a side-effect, such as reserpine, methyl dopa, and propranolol, may disturb normal sexual appetite and potency. Other **antihypertensive medications,** including thiazide diuretics, chlorthalidone (Hygroton), spironolactone (Aldactone), prazosin (Minipres), and clonidine (Catapres), have been associated with impotence. The mechanism and incidence of impotence with these agents is uncertain.

(5) Shakespeare has commented on the relationship of **ethyl alcohol** to sexual activity (". . . provokes the desire, but it takes away the performance. . . ."—*Macbeth*). The malnourished chronic alcoholic with peripheral neuropathy is often impotent. The effect of alcohol in other circumstances is less predictable.

f. Neurologic impotence—Brain disorders. There have been reports of impotence associated with temporal lobe tumors or trauma. Some patients with temporal lobe epilepsy are described as "hyposexual," and the relation between psychogenic factors and impotence is not clear in these cases. However, effective treatment of temporal lobe seizures may reverse the hyposexuality.

Since the introduction of L-dopa, many previously impotent patients with Parkinson's disease have been able to resume sexual activity. This is not a result of any specific aphrodisiac effect of L-dopa, but rather it is related to the improved mobility of these patients following therapy.

g. Endocrine impotence. In general the endocrine disorders that affect male potency do so by impairing sexual drive rather than causing a direct dysfunction of the erection reflex. Addison's disease, hypothyroidism, hypopituitarism, Cushing's syndrome, acromegaly, hypogonadism, Klinefelter's syndrome, and myotonic dystrophy have all been associated with decreased libido and potency.

h. Vascular impotence. Adequate blood flow to the penis is necessary to maintain erection. Thus a progressive weakening of erection can be a prominent sign of impaired circulation due to atheromatous narrowing of the abdominal aorta or iliac arteries. Bruits, claudication of thighs or buttocks, leg weariness, and diminished pulses are other clinical features of this syndrome. Vascular surgery may restore potency in some of these patients.

2. Disorders of ejaculation

a. Physiologically, ejaculation is a spinal reflex mediated by pathways in the thoracolumbar segments. Sympathetic nerve stimuli provoke release of semen from the seminal vesicles; and the presence of semen in the posterior urethra causes reflex contraction of the periurethral muscles, resulting in ejaculation. Supraspinal connections can modify the ejaculation reflex, but they are not necessary for ejaculation to occur.

b. Premature ejaculation

(1) Definition. Premature ejaculation must be judged relative to the man's performance wishes and the woman's sexual desires. Thus a man with an average vaginal containment time of 5 to 10 minutes may label himself as premature or normal, depending on his partner's sexual response. These patients, who consider their vaginal containment time inadequate, can be classified as suffering from the sexual dysfunction "premature ejaculation."

(2) Differential diagnosis. Ejaculatory control is an acquired skill. It tends to be minimal during adolescence, at the onset of sexual activity, and improves considerably with intercourse experience. Also, a man might not be motivated to develop ejaculatory control because he views his partner's responsiveness as unimportant or impossible. Other psychological factors, such as performance anxiety, relationship deterioration, or hostility may also underlie premature ejaculation. Only rarely can premature ejaculation be attributed to organic causes, such as spinal cord diseases (e.g., multiple sclerosis, spinal tumors) or urologic disorders.

(3) Treatment. Premature ejaculation is frequently a curable sexual dysfunction, and the patient should be reassured about the possibilities for significant improvement.

Discussion of the underlying psychic problems may provide the patient with helpful insights, and emphasis should be placed on the importance of the man's relaxation while receiving sexual pleasure. Some commonly used remedies include masturbation before intercourse, attempts at more than one orgasm per sexual encounter, use of a condom, or use of a self- or partner-applied penile squeeze before ejaculation. Sexual therapies that utilize progressively more intense genital stimulation, stopping short of ejaculation, have also been helpful.

c. **Inability to ejaculate or achieve orgasm**

(1) Clinical features. The inability to ejaculate or achieve orgasm may be selective (e.g., inability to ejaculate under some circumstances but not others) or global (e.g., inability to ejaculate during either masturbation or intercourse).

(2) Differential diagnosis. A variety of organic disorders can cause a global inability to ejaculate.

(a) Conditions that **interfere with the sympathetic nerve supply** to the pelvis, such as sympathectomy or radical surgery, can prevent ejaculation. Many women with diabetes mellitus may be unable to achieve orgasm due to diabetic autonomic neuropathy.

(b) Spinal cord trauma can result in inability to ejaculate even when potency is not lost.

(c) Drugs that deplete sympathetic neurotransmitter stores, such as guanethidine, monoamine oxidase inhibitors, and alphamethyldopa, sometimes impair ejaculation.

(d) Aging may be associated with increasing ejaculatory control and, ultimately, with an intermittent inability to ejaculate. The pathophysiology of this change is uncertain.

Patients who are unable to ejaculate intravaginally or with a particular partner are likely suffering from a psychogenic disorder (e.g., fear of impregnating the partner, relationship deterioration).

d. **Retrograde ejaculation**

(1) Clinical picture. Retrograde ejaculation occurs when the internal vesical sphincter fails to close as the seminal secretions are discharged into the urethra. The patient may have an orgasm without producing an ejaculate, only later to find semen in the urine.

(2) Differential diagnosis. Retrograde ejaculation is caused by disorders that interfere with the sympathetic nerve supply or anatomic integrity of the bladder neck. For example, retrograde ejaculation may be an early sign of diabetic autonomic neuropathy. Some patients with impotence secondary to autonomic neuropathy give a prior history of retrograde ejaculation. Postganglionic sympathetic blocking agents, such as guanethidine, bilateral sympathectomies, and transurethral resections of the prostate or bladder neck may also cause retrograde ejaculation.

Professional and general literature as well as other services are available from the local chapters of the various neurologic disease charities. To locate the nearest office, just write or call the national office listed below. Most of the charitable organizations will help if the disease is similar to the one of their major interest, even if it is not exactly the same.

Muscular Dystrophy Associations of America
810 Seventh Avenue
New York, New York 10019
212-586-0808

Myasthenia Gravis Foundation
230 Park Avenue
New York, New York 10017
212-684-6387

National Multiple Sclerosis Society
257 Park Avenue South
New York, New York 10010
212-674-4100

ALS Foundation
915 East 17th Street
Suite 418
Brooklyn, New York 11230

SELECTED READING

Fecal Incontinence

Engel, B. T., Nikoomanesh, P., and Schuster, M. M. Operant conditioning of recto-sphincteric responses in the treatment of fecal incontinence. *N. Engl. J. Med.* 290:646, 1974.

Tracheostomy

Applebaum, E. L., and Bruce, D. L. *Tracheal Intubation.* Philadelphia: W. B. Saunders, 1976.
Egan, D. F. *Fundamentals of Respiratory Therapy.* St. Louis: C. V. Mosby, 1973.
Montgomery, W. *Surgery of the Upper Respiratory System.* Philadelphia: Lea & Febiger, 1973. Pp. 315–368.

Decubitus Ulcer

Guttmann, L. *Spinal Cord Injuries: Comprehensive Management and Research.* Oxford, Blackwell Scientific, 1973. P. 484.

Neurogenic Bladder Dysfunction

Bors, E., and Comarr, A. E. *Neurological Urology: Physiology of Micturition, Its Neurological Disorders and Sequelae.* Baltimore: University Park Press, 1971.
Boyarsky, S. (ed.) *Neurogenic Bladder: A Symposium.* Baltimore: Williams & Wilkins, 1967.
Bradley, W. E., Rockswold, G. L., Timm, G. W., and Scott, F. B. Neurology of micturition. *J. Urology* 115:481, 1976.
Firlit, C. F., Canning, J. R., Lloyd, F. A., Cross, R. R., and Brewer, R. Experience with

intermittent catheterization in chronic spinal cord injury patients. *J. Urology* 114:234, 1975.

Krane, R., and Olsson, C. Phenoxybenzamine in neurogenic bladder dysfunction. II. Clinical considerations. *J. Urology,* 110:653, 1973.

Orikasa, S., Koyanagi, T., Motomura, M., Kudo, T., Togashi, M., and Tsuji, I. Experience with non-sterile intermittent self-catheterization. *J. Urology* 115:141, 1976.

Perkash, I. Intermittent catheterization and bladder rehabilitation in spinal cord injury patients. *J. Urology,* 114:230, 1975.

Scott, F. B., Bradley, E., and Timm, G. W. Treatment of urinary incontinence by an implantable prosthetic urinary sphincter. *J. Urology* 112:75, 1974.

Sexual Dysfunction

Levine, S. B. Marital sexual dysfunction: Erectile dysfunction. *Ann. Intern. Med.* 85:342–350, 1976.

Levine, S. B. Marital sexual dysfunction: Introductory concepts. *Ann. Intern. Med.* 84:448–453, 1976.

Levine, S. B. Marital sexual dysfunction: Ejaculatory disturbances. *Ann. Intern. Med.* 84:575–579, 1976.

Masters, W. H., and Johnson, V. E. *Human Sexual Response.* Boston: Little, Brown, 1966.

Masters, W. H., and Johnson, V. E. *Human Sexual Inadequacy.* Boston: Little, Brown, 1970.

Mooney, T. O., Cole, T. M., Theodore, M., and Chilgren, R. A. *Sexual Options for Paraplegics and Quadriplegics.* Boston: Little, Brown, 1975.

Oliven, J. F. *Clinical Sexuality: A Manual for Physicians and the Professions* (3rd ed.). Philadelphia, Lippincott, 1974.

Silver, J. R. Sexual problems in disorders of the nervous system. *Br. Med. J.* 3:480–482 and 532–534, 1975.

Weiss, H. D. The physiology of human penile erection. *Ann. Intern. Med.* 76:793–799, 1972.

INDEX

Index

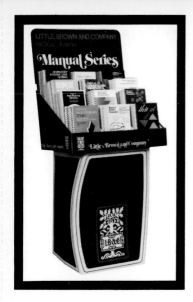

THE LITTLE, BROWN

MANUAL SERIES

Titles in Little, Brown's Manual Series are readily available at all medical bookstores throughout the United States and abroad. You may also order copies directly from Little, Brown and Company, 34 Beacon Street, Boston, Massachusetts 02106, by simply tearing out, filling in, and mailing this postage-free card.

☐ MANUAL OF CORONARY CARE—Alpert & Francis (#034991-88A1) $8.95

☐ MANUAL OF DERMATOLOGIC THERAPEUTICS: WITH ESSENTIALS OF DIAGNOSIS, 2nd Edition—Arndt (#052809) $10.95

☐ MANUAL OF PEDIATRIC THERAPEUTICS, 2nd Edition—Children's Hospital Medical Center, Boston; Graef & Cone, Editors (#139114) In press—Spring 1979 .... $10.95 T

☐ MANUAL OF SURGICAL THERAPEUTICS, 4th Edition—Condon & Nyhus, Editors (#152862) In press—Fall 1978 .... $9.95 T

☐ PROBLEM-ORIENTED MEDICAL DIAGNOSIS—Friedman & Papper, Editors (#293547-88AB1) $9.95

☐ MANUAL OF ACUTE BACTERIAL INFECTIONS: EARLY DIAGNOSIS AND TREATMENT—Gardner & Provine (#303275-88V1) $9.95

☐ MANUAL OF ACUTE ORTHOPAEDIC THERAPEUTICS—Iversen & Clawson (#434402-88Q1) $10.95

☐ MANUAL OF MEDICAL CARE OF THE SURGICAL PATIENT—Papper, Editor (#690473-91AD1) $9.95

☐ MANUAL OF NEUROLOGIC THERAPEUTICS: WITH ESSENTIALS OF DIAGNOSIS—Samuels, Editor (#769908) $12.50

☐ MANUAL OF PSYCHIATRIC THERAPEUTICS: PRACTICAL PSYCHOPHARMACOLOGY AND PSYCHIATRY—Shader, Editor (#782203-90AC1) .. $9.95

☐ MANUAL OF CLINICAL PROBLEMS IN INTERNAL MEDICINE: ANNOTATED WITH KEY REFERENCES, 2nd Edition—Spivak & Barnes (#807141) $10.95

☐ INTERPRETATION OF DIAGNOSTIC TESTS: A HANDBOOK SYNOPSIS OF LABORATORY MEDICINE, 3rd Edition—Wallach (#920444-88Z1) $9.95

☐ MANUAL OF MEDICAL THERAPEUTICS, 22nd Edition—Washington University Department of Medicine; Costrini & Thomson, Editors (#923966-88AD1) $9.95

☐ MANUAL ON TECHNIQUES OF EMERGENCY AND OUT-PATIENT SURGERY—Washington University Department of Surgery; Klippel & Anderson, Editors (#924032) In Press—Spring 1979 .... $9.95 T

NAME_____
(Please print)

STREET_____

CITY_____ STATE _____

ZIP CODE_____

PUBLISHER PAYS POSTAGE AND HANDLING CHARGES ON ALL ORDERS ACCOMPANIED BY A CHECK. (Please add sales tax if applicable.)

☐ Bill me.
☐ Check enclosed.

The symbol T following a price listing indicates that the price is tentative as of the printing of that particular book. All prices listed above are Little, Brown and Company prices as of printing and are subject to change at any time without notice. In no way do they reflect the prices at which books will be sold to you by suppliers other than Little, Brown and Company.